The
Breastfeeding
Book

Books by William Sears, M.D., and Martha Sears, R.N.

The Baby Book
The Healthy Pregnancy Book
The Attachment Parenting Book
The Family Nutrition Book
The Fussy Baby Book
The Discipline Book
The Birth Book
The Baby Sleep Book
The Portable Pediatrician
The Premature Baby Book
The Successful Child

The

Breastfeeding Book

Everything You Need to Know About Nursing
Your Child from Birth Through Weaning

MARTHA SEARS, R.N., AND WILLIAM SEARS, M.D.

Revised Edition

LITTLE, BROWN AND COMPANY

New York • Boston • London

LITTLE, BROWN AND COMPANY
HACHETTE BOOK GROUP
1290 AVENUE OF THE AMERICAS, NEW YORK, NY 10104
LITTLEBROWN.COM

FIRST EDITION: MARCH 2000
REVISED EDITION: AUGUST 2018

LITTLE, BROWN AND COMPANY IS A DIVISION OF HACHETTE BOOK GROUP, INC. THE LITTLE, BROWN NAME AND LOGO ARE TRADEMARKS OF HACHETTE BOOK GROUP, INC.

THE PUBLISHER IS NOT RESPONSIBLE FOR WEBSITES (OR THEIR CONTENT) THAT ARE NOT OWNED BY THE PUBLISHER.

THE HACHETTE SPEAKERS BUREAU PROVIDES A WIDE RANGE OF AUTHORS FOR SPEAKING EVENTS. TO FIND OUT MORE, GO TO HACHETTESPEAKERSBUREAU.COM OR CALL (866) 376-6591.

ISBN 978-0-316-41785-3
LIBRARY OF CONGRESS CONTROL NUMBER: 2018954122

10 9 8 7 6 5 4 3 2 1

LSC-C

PRINTED IN THE UNITED STATES OF AMERICA

To our breastfed children:

James
Robert
Peter
Hayden
Erin
Matthew
Stephen
Lauren

Contents

Gratitudes

WE WISH TO thank the many breastfeeding families who either directly or indirectly contributed to this book, with a special thanks to the wise founding mothers of La Leche League International. This organization has provided mothers around the world with support and information about breastfeeding, correcting the myths and bad advice that have made breastfeeding difficult for many women. Because of La Leche League's efforts, the world is now more sensitive to the needs of mothers and babies. Much appreciation goes to two of our special teachers, Kittie Frantz, formerly director of the breastfeeding clinic at the University of Southern California's Keck School of Medicine, in Los Angeles, and Chele Marmet, codirector of the Lactation Institute in Encino, California. Bill had the privilege of working with Kittie for four years in pediatrics practice. Chele was Martha's teacher. Hugs and thanks go to our research assistants, Lisa Marasco and Tracee Zeni, for their conscientious help in preparing this book. We also wish to thank our editor, Jennifer Josephy, our copyeditor, Pamela Marshall, who put the finishing touches on this book, as well as Barbara Clark, who copyedited the 2018 revised edition. Finally, this book would not have been possible without our eight children, who taught us so much about the art of breastfeeding and how it helps express and shape that most tender relationship between mother and child.

For this revised edition, our deep gratitude goes to Christine Betzold, R.N., M.S.N., a certified nurse practitioner who brought her expertise in the field of lactation to our efforts to give mothers the most up-to-date and intuitive help in breastfeeding their babies.

A Word from Dr. Bill and Martha

DURING OUR MANY YEARS as pediatrician and nurse, we've noticed that there is something wonderfully unique about breastfeeding babies and their mothers. Breastfed babies are healthier. When they do get sick, breastfeeding infants recover faster. But what's more, as we have observed these nursing pairs, we've learned that breastfeeding is not just a method of delivering nutrition, it's also a way of establishing a relationship. Breastfeeding requires a sensitive dialogue between mother and infant. Mother tunes in to baby, and baby tunes in to mother. They learn about each other's face and mannerisms. Most important, they learn to trust each other and to feel confident of each other's love. This is baby's first relationship in life and one that sets the tone for how baby learns to view the world.

Breastfeeding also gives mothers a biochemical boost to help them through the trying times of baby tending. The same hormones that make milk make mothers more intuitive about their babies. Breastfeeding empowers mothers. It helps them become experts on their babies. Lessons learned during breastfeeding are the first steps toward becoming wise parents. Breastfeeding will make it easier to guide and discipline your child in the years to come.

Much of this book was researched on the job.

In four decades of counseling breastfeeding parents, we have learned what works and what doesn't. As Bill has helped breastfeeding pairs get the right start after birth, or as Martha has counseled breastfeeding parents in our office's Breastfeeding Center, we have collected many practical tips for nursing mothers. We have also tried and tested many solutions to the problems that mothers experience with breastfeeding. What we have learned we have gathered into this book in the hope that it will help more mothers enjoy breastfeeding their babies.

The more we have learned about breastfeeding, the more passionate we have become about encouraging mothers to start breastfeeding and to continue breastfeeding for as long as possible. We know that when the mother of a newborn baby makes the commitment to give her baby her milk, she is offering her baby the best intellectual, physical, and emotional start in life.

Martha has happily logged eighteen years of breastfeeding our eight children through a variety of challenging circumstances. With our first three infants, she juggled breastfeeding and working. Jim and Bob (now pediatricians themselves) nursed for eight months each—considered a long time decades ago. And Peter (now practicing family medicine) was our first nursing toddler—a laid-back little guy who weaned fairly easily at seventeen months. Our fourth infant, Hayden—our high-need child—had the benefit of breastfeeding for four years. She (a mother of three now, all happily breastfed) taught us a lot and paved the way for her younger siblings Erin and Matthew to also enjoy extended breastfeeding. Stephen, our seventh child, was born with Down syndrome, yet for three and a half years Martha was able to give him the intellectual and developmental benefits that come with breastfeeding. For an encore, our eighth child, Lauren, came into our family as a newborn by adoption, and with a lot of support and a big dose of commitment Martha was able to breastfeed her for ten months, strengthening the bond between them. Martha cherishes the wonderful memories of babies at breast, knowing that she gave our children a gift that no one else in the whole world can give. Now we can sit back and enjoy the benefits, and Martha can pass on all she learned from her own breastfeeding years and from being both a La Leche League leader since 1980 and a student at the Lactation Institute in Encino, California, from 1984 to 1985. The work she has done in this field of health care has been the most rewarding of her career.

Based on our wealth of personal experience and the work we've done with thousands of breastfeeding families, we have written this book. We hope that what we have to share will cause our nation's greatest natural resource—mothers' milk—to flow more abundantly than ever, that new mothers will be inspired to give breastfeeding a try, and that with the tools in this book they will succeed. We hope that you will enjoy the time you spend giving your baby this wonderful gift and that you, too, will have memories to treasure for years to come.

Since the first edition of *The Breastfeeding Book* was published, in 2000, more discoveries have been made to make breastfeeding easier for mothers and babies. Nearly all top companies now provide lactation lounges to enable mothers to pump their "liquid gold" while at work. This makes economic sense: as these companies have discovered, a breastfeeding-friendly workplace means mothers miss less work because breastfed babies tend to be less sick. New laws protect a mother's right to breastfeed in public. More hospitals are becoming breastfeeding-friendly, and smart new mothers have access to professional lactation consultants for getting the best start in feeding their babies.

While we have always known that mothers' milk delivers many precious nutrients to babies, in recent years more magical nutrients have been discovered that help feed and fertilize babies' early "gut garden," programming the breastfed baby to enjoy better emotional, physical, and intellectual health for life. For example, on page 12 you will learn about the magical microbiome that breastfeeding babies enjoy. Get ready to read about these newly discovered nutrients in mothers' milk that have cute names: M.O.M. (milk-oriented microbiota) and H.M.O.s (human milk oligosaccharides).

After reading each page you will feel enriched with breastfeeding tools and empowered with breastfeeding knowledge to better enjoy what we believe is one of the greatest gifts a mother can give to her baby: the gift of health.

We wish you and your baby a beautiful breastfeeding experience.

1

THE SCIENCE OF BREASTFEEDING: WHY BREASTFEED?

We have often wondered why some mothers don't breastfeed. From our point of view, breastfeeding seems like the natural continuation of the relationship begun in the womb. Perhaps some women aren't convinced that breastfeeding makes a difference. As you will learn in chapter 1, it does; and the benefits extend to mothers as well as to infants. We believe that once you understand the benefits of breastfeeding, you will find a way to do it. Many modern Americans believe that formula is a close second to human milk. As you will learn, it isn't. As you read, you'll sense our passion for breastfeeding; it comes from our years of experience in our pediatrics practice and lactation consulting, where we've seen how much better breastfeeding is for babies and mothers. Deciding to breastfeed is the single most important brain- and body-building gift you can give your child. Here's why!

1

Why Breast Is Best

IN THE EARLY DAYS of learning to breastfeed, there may be times when you feel like tossing in the nursing bra and reaching for a bottle. You may be tempted to believe those advisers who suggest that formula feeding is easier or just as good. Or you may worry that you're "not the type of mother" who succeeds at breastfeeding. Yet when you consider how breastfeeding benefits your baby, your family, and yourself, you will find the determination you need to overcome any obstacles and master the womanly art of breastfeeding. This chapter describes some of the innumerable ways that breastfeeding builds healthier brains, healthier bodies, and healthier families.

WHAT'S IN IT FOR BABY?

How would you like to give your baby a gift that could raise his IQ; cut medical bills; make your baby's eyes, heart, intestines, and nearly every other organ work better; reduce the risk of life-shortening, debilitating diseases such as diabetes; and help your baby avoid many of the common complaints of infancy, such as ear infections, tummy upsets, even diaper rash? What's the magic gift that can do all these things? Your milk!

You can make your baby's life that much better simply by choosing to breastfeed.

Brighter Brains

Your baby's brain grows more during infancy than at any other time, doubling its volume and reaching around 60 percent of its adult size by one year. As with every system in the body, the better you feed the brain, the better it can grow. Breast milk is the best food for developing brains, and a flurry of brainy breast-milk research is now confirming what nursing mothers have long suspected: breastfed babies are smarter. Back in 1992, a headline in *USA Today* boasted "Mother's Milk: Food for Smarter Kids." Many recent headlines have renewed interest in the fact that breastfeeding is an important and often overlooked way to give a child a head start. Scientific studies on the influence of breast milk on intellectual development conclude:

- Children who were breastfed score higher on cognitive and IQ tests in school than children who were formula fed.

- The intellectual advantage gained from breastfeeding is greater the longer the baby is breastfed.

YOUR MILK IS YOUR BABY'S MEDICINE

"Let food be your medicine," wrote Hippocrates, known as the father of modern medicine. These words may not have been written specifically about breast milk, but they are accurate in their description of it. We would upgrade this wisdom to: "Let mother's milk be baby's medicine." Besides being the best preventive medicine for just about any disease, breast milk can also help cure an illness once it has started. This is particularly true of diarrheal diseases. The low mineral content of breast milk enables inflamed intestines to absorb the water in breast milk very efficiently. In addition, human milk contains anti-inflammatory substances and immune factors that help heal intestines rather than irritating them further, as formula would. This is why it has long been noted that not only do diarrheal illnesses occur less frequently in breastfed infants, but in addition, if they do occur, breastfed babies experience less dehydration and recover more quickly than formula-fed babies.

Other curative properties of breast milk come from the one million white blood cells contained in each drop of milk, which is why it can be appropriately called white blood (see page 9). Breast milk has long been observed to help heal superficial infections such as conjunctivitis. Try squirting some in the eye of a baby with conjunctivitis. (Express milk into a cup and use an eyedropper if your aim isn't so good.) It really helps.

The enteromammary immune system (the gut-brain connection) is another way mother's milk protects as well as nourishes her infant. When an infant is exposed to a germ, mother is often exposed to the same germ. But in the first six to nine months of life, the infant's ability to make antibodies to fight that germ is limited. So the mother makes these germ fighters for her baby, and these antibodies travel to her milk and are delivered to her baby. This system is especially helpful in fighting intestinal germs. Even when a baby contracts a germ — say, at day care — the baby "exposes" mother's breasts to that germ through sucking, and within eight hours the breasts are able to make antibodies to that germ and offer them to the baby via the milk.

• Intellectual differences between breastfed and formula-fed children were once attributed to the increased holding and interaction associated with breastfeeding and to the fact that mothers who breastfed were better educated and/or more child centered. New research suggests these differences may actually be attributable to nutrients in breast milk that enhance brain growth.

For years, doctors told formula-feeding parents that by holding and interacting with their babies during feedings they could imitate breastfeeding, and their babies could then receive any intellectual and social benefits associated with breastfeeding. This was true to a point (it is better to hold the bottle and talk to your baby than to prop the bottle and walk away), but research is now showing that the smart stuff is in the milk, and it's not just the mothering that matters.

Smarter fats. As we emphasize in our book *The Omega-3 Effect,* one key ingredient in breast milk is a brain-boosting fat called DHA (docosahexaenoic acid), an omega-3 fatty acid. DHA is one of several fats that have gotten a lot of attention as true health foods. DHA is considered a vital nutrient for the growth, development, and maintenance of brain tissue.

DHA and other fats in breast milk contribute directly to brain growth by providing the right substances for manufacturing myelin, the fatty sheath that surrounds nerve fibers, insulating them so that these pathways can carry information. As you will learn in chapter 4, a mother should supplement her diet with DHA-rich foods such as salmon and tuna or take a daily DHA supplement.

Breast milk's role in the development of high-quality myelin and brain cells may play a role in the prevention of multiple sclerosis — for both the baby *and* the mother. (In the July 2017 issue of *Neurology,* researchers showed that breastfeeding has a dose-related effect on the risk of multiple sclerosis — women who breastfed for a cumulative total of fifteen months or more were half as likely to develop MS compared with women who breastfed for four months or less.) The symptoms of multiple sclerosis are caused by myelin breakdown, and researchers speculate that a deficiency of omega-3 fatty acids in the myelin sheath makes the sheath more vulnerable to premature degeneration.

Also, breast milk is rich in cholesterol; formula contains none. Cholesterol provides basic components for building the brain and manufacturing hormones and vitamin D. (Higher dietary cholesterol at the stage of fastest brain growth — what a smart idea!) Studies show that during the first year, exclusively breastfed infants have higher blood-cholesterol levels than formula-fed babies do. Depriving infants of sufficient amounts of this brain nutrient at a critical stage, as you do when you feed your baby formula, seems like a dumb idea.

BRAIN FATS VERSUS BODY FATS

In his book *Smart Fats,* Dr. Michael Schmidt points out that the type of fats needed to make a large body are different from those needed to make a large brain. Cows, for example, give milk to their calves that is high in saturated fats that encourage rapid body growth, but cow's milk is low in the fats that support rapid brain growth. The milk of each species is tailored toward the survival mechanism of that species. The calf runs for survival. This is why a calf's body grows rapidly in the first six months while its brain grows slowly. Human beings must depend on their wits, so in human infants the brain grows quickly. To nourish this faster brain growth, human milk is rich in special long-chain polyunsaturated fatty acids (known as LC-PUFAs, pronounced "elsie-poofas") but low in saturated fats. A human baby's brain triples in size during the first year; but compared with the calf's, the body's growth is relatively slow.

Smarter sugars. The predominant sugar in breast milk is lactose, which the body breaks down into two simpler sugars, glucose and galactose. Galactose is a valuable nutrient for brain-tissue development. Anthropologists have demonstrated that the most intelligent species of mammals have greater amounts of lactose in their milk, and, not surprisingly, human milk contains one of the highest concentrations of lactose of any mammal's milk. Cow's milk and *some* cow's-milk formulas contain lactose, but not as much as human milk does. Soy-based and other lactose-free formulas contain no lactose at all, only table sugar and corn syrup. As we'll later discuss, lactose also promotes intestinal health.

Smarter connections. Brain cells, called neurons, resemble miles of tangled electrical wires. During the period of rapid brain growth in the first two years of life, these neurons proliferate and connect with other neurons to make circuits throughout the brain. The more circuits a baby's brain makes and the better the quality of these circuits, the smarter the baby. Every time a baby interacts with her caregivers, her brain makes new connections. Breastfed babies feed more often and are held more closely, allowing more skin-to-skin contact, so that each feeding is an opportunity to help the growing brain make the right connections, adding more circuits each time.

Leaner Adult Bodies

Breastfed infants become leaner adults. New research is discovering that leanness is associated with general health and well-being and with a lower risk of such diseases as heart disease, stroke, and diabetes. Studies have shown that children who were breastfed are less likely to be obese during adolescence and that longer periods of breastfeeding greatly reduce the risk of being overweight later in childhood. Since overweight children are more likely to become overweight adults, preventing obesity in childhood is important. *Lean* means having just the right amount of body fat for an individual's body type. In 1992 the DARLING (Davis Area Research on Lactation, Infant Nutrition, and Growth) study from the University of California at Davis compared the growth patterns of healthy breastfed and formula-fed infants and found that breastfed infants were leaner at one year of age than their formula-fed counterparts. Even plump breastfed babies gradually lose a lot of their adorable baby fat and eventually wind up leaner than their formula-fed peers.

Why this difference? The amount of fat and calories in formula is about the same as in breast milk. The answer lies both in the type of fat and in the feeding method itself. As we discussed before, breast-milk fats, which are high in omega-3 fatty acids, are healthful fats. Also, breastfeeding gives infants the opportunity to control their fat intake themselves. The fat content of breast milk changes during a feeding to meet the needs of baby. If baby is simply thirsty or just needs some comfort sucking as a pick-me-up, she sucks briefly for the foremilk, or low-fat milk that is stored right behind the nipple. If your baby is particularly hungry, she sucks longer, stimulating mother's milk-ejection reflex, and gets the higher-fat hindmilk. Contrast this with the formula feeders. Regardless of whether baby is hungry, thirsty, or just needs to suck for comfort, he gets the same amount of fat whether he needs it or not.

Also, the fat content of mother's milk changes as the baby grows. The older infant needs fewer calories per pound of body weight than does the younger one, so by a wonderful quirk of nature, the amount of fat in mother's milk gradually decreases to lower levels in the second half of the first year.

The satiety factor. Breastfed babies take smaller meals and eat more slowly. Eating patterns established in infancy reduce the tendency toward overeating later in life. Also, the high-fat milk that the baby receives toward the end of the feeding gives him a feeling of fullness. This and a satiety-producing hormone in the infant called cholecystokinin (CCK) condition the satisfied infant to stop eating. The breastfed baby himself controls how much he eats. You can't urge him to finish up the last half ounce at the breast the way a parent might when giving a bottle. A breastfed baby learns to trust his own signals about how much he needs to eat and when.

Better Eyes

Not only does breast milk build brighter brains and healthier bodies, it's valuable to baby's vision, too. Studies comparing breastfed and formula-fed infants show that visual development (visual acuity in particular) is better in breastfed babies. This finding is especially noticeable in premature infants. Again, the smart fat DHA may be one of the reasons. DHA is one of the prime structural components of the retina of the eye. As with all tissues, the better you feed it, the better it grows and functions. So the better you feed the retina, the better the vision.

More Engaged

Also, breastfed babies get more "face time," because they spend a greater part of their waking hours face-to-face with their favorite person in the whole world. Imagine implanting this lifelong skill of making eye-to-eye contact in infancy. Dr. Bill has noticed that breastfed babies talk to him with their eyes when he examines them.

Better Hearing

Not only do breastfed infants think, grow, and see better, they are also likely to hear better. Being able to hear well is necessary for language development, so this benefit of breastfeeding is very important. The reason breastfeeding promotes healthier hearing is that breastfed babies have fewer ear infections. Because breast milk is a human substance, babies are not allergic to it (but they can be allergic to cow's-milk protein or other proteins in mother's diet that piggyback into the breast milk). Allergies to soy or cow's-milk proteins can cause fluid to build up behind the middle ear. This fluid not only dampens the vibration of the eardrum, decreasing hearing, it also provides a culture medium for bacteria and thus is a breeding ground for middle-ear infections. A history of frequent ear infections is common in children who are experiencing language delays.

A Nicer Smile

Pediatric dentists report that breastfed babies have better jaw alignment and are less likely to need orthodontic work. The sucking action used in breastfeeding involves more complex motions of the facial muscles and tongue. This improves the development of facial muscles, jawbones, and palate, leading to better jaw alignment and more room for teeth. The tongue-thrusting action bottle-fed infants use to control the flow of formula can contribute to malocclusion. Experienced pediatric dentists are often able to tell whether or not a baby was breastfed by the shape of the mouth and hard palate. Thus a baby's breastfeeding efforts will be reflected in her face.

Better Breathing

Another benefit pediatric dentists have noticed is that breastfed babies develop a larger nasal space, which can lessen problems with snoring and sleep apnea later in life. Breastfed babies grow a rounder, U-shaped dental arch, whereas bottle-fed babies develop a narrower, higher, V-shaped arch, which not only contributes to the misalignment of teeth but also infringes on the nasal passages directly above the hard palate.

Better Hearts

Formula is cholesterol-free, but you won't find formula manufacturers advertising this fact, even though you might expect a low-cholesterol diet to be good for babies—after all, many adults concerned with good nutrition try to limit their cholesterol intake. The cholesterol that is naturally present in cow's milk is removed during the formula-manufacturing process and replaced with fats from plant sources. Cholesterol is not only present in breast milk in just the right amounts, it is also most likely there for a heart-healthy reason. Some heart researchers theorize, therefore, that a breastfed baby's liver learns to metabolize cholesterol better than a formula-fed infant's does. Breastfed babies may then have more healthful blood-cholesterol levels as adults and may thus enjoy a lower risk of heart disease. Supporting the heart-healthy theory, studies show that although breastfed infants tend to have higher blood-cholesterol levels than formula-fed babies do, adults who were formula fed as infants tend to have higher blood-cholesterol levels and are more likely to have atherosclerotic plaque, which can lead to heart attacks.

Breastfeeding has an additional perk for infant hearts: the resting heart rates of breastfed babies are lower. The significance of this is unclear, but it could be a situation similar to the lower heart rate in the physically fit body of an athlete. A lower resting heart rate is an indicator of overall physical and emotional health.

Intestinal Health

Breast milk is known as the "easy in, easy out" food. It's easier to digest and makes easier-to-pass stools. In fact, breast milk contains enzymes that help babies digest their meals from the breast. Whey, the predominant protein in breast milk, forms an intestines-friendly, soft, easy-to-digest curd, unlike the rubbery, harder-to-digest casein curd formed in the digestion of most formulas. Tiny tummies like breast milk. It's digested more quickly and is less likely to come back up. It doesn't leave permanent stains on clothes, either.

While all babies spit up a bit, some regurgitate excessive amounts of milk because of a condition called gastroesophageal reflux (GER). Normally, the circular band of muscle where the esophagus joins the stomach acts as a one-way valve, keeping milk, food, and stomach acids from backing up into the esophagus when the stomach contracts. When it doesn't do its job, acids enter the esophagus, resulting in an irritation that adults would call heartburn. In many infants, it takes six months to a year for this muscle to mature enough to prevent this regurgitation, or reflux. GER occurs less often in breastfed infants because breast milk is emptied twice as fast from the stomach and because breastfed babies tend to eat smaller meals that are more appropriate in size. It's less likely to be regurgitated than slow-to-digest formula, with its tough casein curds.

Breast milk is friendly to immature intestines. The cells of the intestinal lining are tightly packed together so that potential allergens cannot seep through into the bloodstream. But in the early months, the lining of the baby's immature intestines is more like a sieve, allowing potential allergens to get through, which sets the infant and child up for allergies and infections. Breast milk contains a special protein called immunoglobulin A (IgA), which acts as a protective sealant in the digestive tract. Allergens and germs can't get through as easily. Breast milk also contains a special substance called epidermal growth factor (EGF), which promotes the growth of the cells lining baby's intestines as well as other surface cells, such as the cells of the skin.

Since formula does not provide this protective coating, it's easier for allergens to pass through into the bloodstream, causing a condition known as leaky gut syndrome. This is part of the reason for the higher incidence of allergies in formula-fed infants. By the second half of the first year, the intestinal lining matures enough to prevent these leaks (a developmental process called closure).

Breast milk produces caregiver-friendly stools. Unlike the stinky stools of a formula-fed baby, the stools of a breastfed infant have a not unpleasant buttermilk-like odor. In watching moms and dads change the diapers of a formula-fed baby, we have noticed that their facial expressions generally reflect reactions that range from mild aversion to downright disgust. Because the odor of breast-milk stools is not offensive to most parents, changing the diaper of a breastfed infant is not an unpleasant task (which is fortunate, because young breastfed babies have several bowel movements a day). When the baby looks at the face of the diaper-changing caregiver and sees happiness rather than disgust, he picks up a good message about himself—perhaps a perk for building self-esteem.

Breast milk helps better bugs live in the bowels. Intestines are healthier when you can keep the right bugs in your bowels, and that's exactly what breast milk does in your baby's bowels. The intestines contain healthful as well as potentially harmful bacteria. The healthful bacteria, known as bifidus bacteria, do good things for the body in return for a warm place to live. They manufacture vitamins and nutrients and keep the harmful bacteria in check. Breast milk promotes the growth of healthful bacteria and inhibits the growth of harmful ones. The high level of lactose in breast milk particularly encourages the growth of the healthful resident bacteria *Lactobacillus bifidus*.

Reduced Risk of Diabetes

Breastfeeding, plus the delayed introduction of cow's milk, reduces the risk of juvenile-onset diabetes. In addition, researchers have documented a lower insulin release in breastfed infants compared to formula-fed infants. This preventive effect is particularly important for those who have a family history of diabetes.

Immunities

Your milk, like your blood, is a living substance. In the Koran, mother's milk is called white blood. A drop of breast milk contains around one million white blood cells. These cells, called macrophages (literally "big eaters"), gobble up germs.

Colostrum, the "supermilk" you produce in the first few days (see page 44), is especially rich in IgA, just at the time when a newborn is most susceptible to germs. Colostrum also contains higher amounts of white blood cells and other infection-fighting substances than does mature milk. Think of colostrum as your baby's first important immunization.

Filling the gap. Throughout the first six months, your baby's ability to produce his own antibodies to germs is somewhat limited. His immune system doesn't click into high gear until the second half of the first year. The maternal antibodies a baby receives through the placenta provide protection for a while, but antibodies gotten through the placenta are gradually used up during the first six months. Around six months of age, the influence of mother's antibodies is waning and baby's own antibodies are not yet at high levels. During this time, human milk's germ-fighting antibodies and white blood cells provide what's missing and protect baby from many of the germs in his environment.

The immune-boosting effects of breast milk are the reason behind the medical truism that doctors make their living on formula-fed infants. Studies comparing exclusively breastfed infants with formula-fed babies have shown that breastfed babies have lower rates of virtually every kind of infectious disease. This is all because of the protective effect of mother's milk, which can't be duplicated by factory-made formula.

Mother continually updates baby's immune protection. Because mother and baby are so close to each other, mother is exposed to the same environmental germs that a baby comes in contact with. The baby's immune system is too immature to respond quickly to germs, so mother's milk comes to the rescue. The mother's more mature immune system makes antibodies to the germs to which she and baby have been exposed, and this army of infection fighters enters her milk and eventually her baby.

**IMMUNIZE YOUR BABY EVERY DAY!
BREASTFEED**
Motto of the International Lactation
Consultant Association

Healthier Skin

Many pediatricians who have developed a sharp eye and keen sense of touch over years of examining babies report that they can often tell by the look and feel of an infant's skin whether the baby is breastfed or formula fed. The skin of a breastfed baby often has a softer, smoother feel. There is also less delineation where the fat under the skin ends and the underlying muscle begins. The skin of formula-fed babies tends to be rougher, with dry, often sandpaper-like patches. Breastfed babies feel more solid. Researchers report that the subcutaneous fat in breastfed and formula-fed infants actually has a different composition.

Since skin is primarily made of fat, these "fat feel" differences may be the result of the more healthful fats in human milk, especially DHA. The higher concentrations of healthy omega-3 fatty acids in breast milk may give the skin layers a healthier structure. In our pediatrics practice, we often prescribe for older children a diet high in omega-3 fatty acids (including wild salmon and omega-3 supplements) for treatment of eczema and dry, scaly skin conditions. Human milk provides this naturally for babies. We have noticed infants' dry skin and eczema markedly improve following supplementation of the mother's diet with omega-3 fatty acids—namely, from fish and flaxseed or flax oil. Epidermal

growth factor (EGF) in human milk may also make the skin healthier.

Breastfed babies also enjoy a lower incidence of eczema, since they are protected from allergies by breast milk's various immune factors. Because these babies avoid early exposure to foreign proteins, such as cow's-milk protein and soy, their skin is less likely to erupt in irritating and ugly rashes.

Better Taste

Try the taste test. Sample a bit of breast milk (that is, if it's currently available in your home) and compare it with formula (if that's available in your home). Your tongue and nose will instantly tell you why babies prefer the real thing. Breast milk, because of its high lactose content, tastes fresh and sweet, unlike canned formula. Babies are born with a sweet tooth—the taste receptors for sweetness on their tongues are highly developed, so there's a perfect match between the milk and infant gourmets. The more appealing, sweeter taste of breast milk may be why some breastfed infants refuse to take formula.

Healthier Children and Adults

Derrick and Patrice Jelliffe, pioneers in breastfeeding research, stated that breastfed infants are "biochemically different." This difference in body chemistry may be the reason they are healthier. There is evidence that breastfeeding protects babies against a great variety of illnesses, and in some cases this protection extends even beyond the time babies are nursing. While babies are breastfeeding, they have fewer and less serious respiratory infections, less diarrhea, and less vomiting. When breastfed babies do become ill, they are less likely to become dehydrated and less likely to need hospitalization. They enjoy protection from rotavirus (a type of respiratory infection), meningitis, infant botulism, and urinary tract infections. In developing countries, where there may not be safe water or good medical care, the protection that breastfeeding offers against cholera, various kinds of parasites, and other serious infections helps babies born in poverty to stay healthy. Researchers have also found that as children grow, having been breastfeed as an infant is associated with a reduced risk of juvenile diabetes, childhood cancers, and digestive disorders, including ulcerative colitis and Crohn's disease.

Many parents are relieved to learn that breastfed babies are less likely to become victims of sudden infant death syndrome (SIDS). There are many ways in which breastfeeding could influence the incidence of SIDS. One recent theory suggests that infants who die of SIDS may sleep too deeply and fail to awaken if they stop breathing for a moment or two, as babies often do when they're sleeping. Breastfed babies sleep less deeply and thus may be more likely to wake up if there is a problem with their breathing. Breastfeeding's protection against infection may also help to lower the SIDS risk. (For more information about breastfeeding and SIDS protection, see AskDrSears.com.)

Breast milk's influence on health probably reaches even further than researchers have dared to imagine, but studies of factors that affect the development of disease in adults seldom ask their research subjects about how they were fed as infants (and many adults would have trouble giving a reliable answer to the question). But new studies of what is in breast milk suggest that this living biological fluid carries substances that are critical to the optimal development of many systems in the body. This early development may very well affect the progress of many diseases throughout life. Will breastfeeding protect your baby against a heart attack, a stroke, or cancer later in life? We believe it might, though this can't

be known for certain. In the meantime, the evidence is overwhelming that babies get a head start when they begin life at their mother's breast and that the benefits of breastfeeding increase the longer they stay there. There are hundreds of substances in breast milk that aren't in formula, and we don't yet understand how these many elements work together for babies' optimal development. Human milk is a complex and constantly changing dynamic substance, one that can never be completely duplicated in a laboratory.

I LOVE M.O.M.

The longer you breastfeed, the lower your baby's incidence of just about every illness. Now, thanks to new and exciting research into milk-oriented microbiota (appropriately known as M.O.M.), we

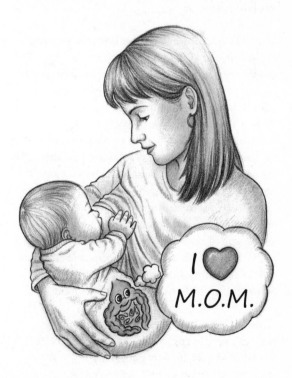

know another principal reason why. In fact, M.O.M. is the single most important nutrient influencing the transformation of the immature gut garden in the hours, days, and weeks after birth. More fascinating, this early activity in baby's gut may lead to lifelong health benefits by decreasing the incidence of illnesses related to immune imbalance, such as allergies. Moms, get ready to learn how your milk helps grow your baby's newborn gut garden. And the healthier the garden grows, the healthier your baby is likely to be—for life.

The microbiota, also called the microbiome, is the community of bowel bugs, primarily bacteria, that grow up in a baby's gut and reside within the lining of the gut throughout life. In return for free food and a warm place to live, they do good things for baby's body. Think of your bowel bugs, or microbiome, as your immune network. Seventy percent of your immune system resides in your gut.

Mother's microbiome. Better bowel bugs build a better immune system for your baby. During pregnancy, mother's vaginal microbes undergo healthful growth. Mother's birth canal gets populated with healthful bacteria that she will share with her baby. These beneficial bugs increase in number to benefit mother's health and the health of her baby, who will soon pass through her probiotic-rich birth canal. As Dr. Martin Blaser said in his brilliant book *Missing Microbes*: "These early lactobacilli, which bloomed in mother's vagina during pregnancy, now set up residence and begin to bloom in baby's intestinal tract." Some microbiome-knowledgeable hospitals now swab a surgically birthed baby with microbe-rich vaginal secretions from the baby's mom.

Growing your baby's early gut garden. The healthier the gut garden, the healthier the baby. But what grows a healthy gut garden? A healthy microbiome. What do you need to grow a healthy

garden? Food and fertilizer. What is the best food and fertilizer for baby's growing gut garden? You guessed it: your milk.

MOTHER'S MILK MAKES THE BEST MEDICINES

For decades, pediatric research has shown that breastfed newborns—especially premature newborns—who receive their mother's milk (real food, with the right intestinal bacteria) are not only more likely to grow up smarter, they are also more likely to have healthier immune systems than formula-fed babies. Breastfed babies enjoy fewer "itis" illnesses, such as allergies and eczema, and are much less likely to get the sometimes fatal newborn intestinal inflammation called necrotizing enterocolitis. Here's a bit of baby-gut-bug data: a day's worth (one quart) of mother's milk can nourish baby's gut to the point where it grows ten trillion resident gut bacteria.

The protective aspect of breastfeeding cannot be overstated. When mother is exposed to an environmental germ potentially harmful to her baby, Dr. Mom—baby's earliest pharmacist—naturally makes antibodies against the germ and dispenses this "medicine" by way of her milk. In this way, mother's breast milk helps protect her precious newborn just as baby's first immunizations do. Following is a list of some of the immune protectors that mother manufactures and gives to baby in her milk. As we go through each item, you will understand why, in many cultures, mother's milk is upgraded to the medically appropriate label white blood.

White blood cells. The list of natural immune-strengthening biochemicals in breast milk is growing, but they include, to name a few, secretory IgA, lactoferrin, lysozyme, mucin, cytokines, insulin growth factors, interleukins, interferon, tumor necrosis factor, and prostaglandins. A 2014 study from Brigham and Women's Hospital of Harvard Medical School (incidentally, the hospital where our first baby, now Dr. Jim, was born) showed that the intestinal microbiome of breastfed babies recovered more quickly following antibiotic treatment. When they need antibiotics, preterm babies, those most vulnerable to infections, get the biggest benefit from mother's milk.

Oligosaccharides. M.O.M. seals a leaky gut. A baby's intestines are, shall we say, babylike. The intestinal lining is very permeable, and it leaks because the immature cells of the lining are not yet close enough to one another. Think of this lining as similar to millions of tiny tiles on a floor or countertop, but with gaps between them. Artificial food, germs, and environmental chemicals can therefore "leak" through the immature gut. The last thing you want in a precious newborn adapting to our germy world is leaks in the lining of the intestines, one of the major entry points for harmful bacteria.

Enter Dr. Mother Nature, baby's earliest gastroenterologist. The tiles start closing tightly together faster in breastfed infants than they do in formula-fed babies, a protective gut change called closure. Mother's milk contains natural nutrients called oligosaccharides that help a baby's immature intestinal-lining cells mature and stop leaking.

MOTHER'S MILK — BABY'S FIRST H.M.O.

A nutrient called human milk oligosaccharides (H.M.O.), one of the most significant in mother's milk, has puzzled nutritionists for many years. Since it is indigestible by infant intestines, it was wrongly disregarded for many years as not useful because "it provides no food for baby." This was the erroneous conclusion of formula makers, or would-be breast-milk duplicators, who justified leaving it out since it "wasn't really baby food." How wrong they were! It may not directly feed baby, but H.M.O. is the best food for nourishing baby's growing gut garden, especially the healthful bacteria known as bifidus, or BIF. BIF is higher in breastfed babies because BIF's favorite food is H.M.O.

Historically, formulas haven't included H.M.O. Some formula companies are now putting H.M.O. into formula, but they are still uncertain which type to put in, and those made in the factory may be structurally different from those mother makes in her milk.

A tale of two nipples. The formula-fed baby sucks from an artificial nipple that has been cleansed and sterilized, so not only does it not feel soft, like mother's nipple, it also does absolutely no good in growing a healthy microbiome. The breastfed baby, by contrast, sucks from the nice, soft, familiar nipple of mother, where, thanks to Dr. Mother Nature, the two bacteria that the microbiome loves — bifidobacteria and lactobacilli — reside. These bacteria help break down the lactose sugar in milk, producing lactic acid, which is why they are classified as lactic acid bacteria.

BABY'S GROWING GUT GARDEN BEGINS AT BIRTH

The first stop on baby's microbiome health tour comes when baby passes through the vaginal canal and picks up a healthy dose of (primarily) lactobacillus bacteria. The next stop comes when baby lies skin-to-skin and cheek-to-breast with mother during their first embrace, delivering a welcome dose of good bugs. The final stop comes when baby ingests mother's microbial milk, ingesting another dose of healthful bacteria. Previously thought to be sterile, this milk is now known to be a rich source of protective bacteria for the immune system growing in baby's little gut.

A few years ago, we had the honor of speaking at an international breastfeeding conference in Australia. Two of the other speakers were Nils and Jill Bergman, authors of *Hold Your Premie.* One of the most important bits of information they imparted was that unless a medical complication occurs, a baby should pass through the birth canal and be immediately placed on mother's abdomen, where he will instinctively inch his way toward the breast. Next, baby rests cheek-to-breast and gradually finds the nipple, as if some inherent GPS guides him toward M.O.M. Mother shares the healthy bacteria around her breasts to help quickly fertilize baby's immature gut garden and protect him from intestinal infections. Imagine following the rite of passage through mother's birth canal, experiencing skin-to-skin contact, and taking the first sucks and swallows. M.O.M. says to baby, "Happy microbiome birthday, baby!" and a growing community of gut-brain bugs celebrate.

DON'T BATHE THE BABY

The discovery of M.O.M. has led hospital nurseries to change their policies. Unless a medical complication demands it, baby is not briskly wiped off, quickly taken over to a warmer, and given to mother only after he is nicely clean and wrapped. Think about it. There's no M.O.M. there.

Instead, the newly-born baby, calm and, because he hasn't been wiped off, not crying, is quickly placed on a better "warmer" — mother's abdomen and breast. This should happen whether the birth is vaginal or surgical. Yet one more piece of evidence that this is the warmer where baby belongs is the fact that the temperature of mother's breasts increases one to two degrees immediately after birth.

SMELL AND TELL

You can often tell by the smell of your baby's bowel movements whether your infant's microbiome likes what you are feeding him. Pediatricians have long appreciated that the nature and smell of stools from breastfed infants is so much nicer and that the daily movements are more numerous. Credit this pleasant diaper perk to the fact that breastfed infants enjoy a smarter microbiome. And when breastfed babies are weaned before their time and switched to formula, the pleasant poop downgrades to... well...you parents know the rest.

"HAPPY MILK"

Watching our own eight babies breastfeed, we saw how happy, calm, and peaceful they became right after feeding. We used to joke, "Looks like he just got a tranquilizer!" But it's no joke: babies do get a dose of a natural biochemical tranquilizer triggered by breastfeeding. We call breast milk happy milk because it contains the unique food that baby's microbiome loves, human milk oligosaccharides. Picture the microbiome saying, "Yum — our favorite food is coming. Let's thank our host by making some feel-good biochemicals [called metabolites] that make him feel satisfied." This magical medicine the microbiome makes — and that the brain loves — is a natural mood mellower called gamma-aminobutyric acid (GABA).

WHAT'S IN IT FOR MOTHER?

By providing milk from your breasts, you're guaranteeing the best nourishment for your baby. But breastfeeding is not just more healthful for babies. It's more healthful for mothers, too. During breastfeeding, you give your baby ideal nourishment and nurturing, and as "payback," your baby, in effect, gives something back to you. You tap into a design for mothering and nurturing your baby that is tested and true—as old as time itself. Breastfeeding will make it easier to care for your baby, and it will make it easier for you to know and understand your baby. It will affect the way you listen to your child, the way you communicate, and the way you respond for many years to come. This will make disciplining your child easier as she grows, and it will help you feel good about parenting.

Breastfeeding is, after all, more than a way of delivering food. When you breastfeed, you continue the oneness that you and your baby experienced during pregnancy. Your body continues to provide nourishment, a warm touch, comfort, and safety, just as it did when baby was inside you. This relationship is unique, a different journey for each mother and baby.

Faster Postpartum Recovery

Breastfeeding helps your body recover from pregnancy more quickly. The baby's sucking stimulates the release of the hormone oxytocin, which causes your uterus to contract and return more quickly to its prepregnant size. This hormone is a natural version of the synthetic one (Pitocin) that obstetricians often give women immediately after birth to help contract the uterus and expel the placenta.

Faster Weight Loss

When compared with formula-feeding moms, breastfeeding mothers have an easier time losing weight postpartum. Making milk uses up fat stores from pregnancy. In one study, breastfeeding moms showed more fat loss and larger reductions in hip circumference by one month postpartum than nonbreastfeeding moms. In another study, breastfeeding women tended to lose more weight

three to six months postpartum than formula-feeding mothers did, even though the breastfeeding moms were consuming more calories.

Hormonal Health

Lactation is a natural part of a woman's reproductive cycle, along with ovulation, menstruation, pregnancy, and childbirth. Good things happen throughout your body when baby sucks at your breast. The hormones released by sucking (prolactin and oxytocin) influence the overall balance of many of your other hormones and keep estrogen levels low, which may affect the development of certain cancers. Mothers report that breastfeeding is a pleasant, sensual experience. They enjoy the closeness, the skin contact with the baby, and pleasurable feelings from the nipple stimulation. These good feelings may originate in part with the hormone oxytocin, which is released during breastfeeding to stimulate the milk-ejection reflex. Oxytocin is released also during childbirth and during sexual intercourse. It acts as a bonding hormone; the good feelings it creates during important interpersonal acts such as breastfeeding and sex help to build the strong human relationships that nurture babies and keep families together.

Relaxation

Not only does breastfeeding benefit mother's body, it helps mother's mind, too. The same hormones that help make milk help a mother feel peaceful. When mothers sit down to breastfeed, they may find themselves drifting off to sleep. If they've been feeling stressed or harried, breastfeeding brings a sense of contentment and relaxation. This may be prolactin at work, since prolactin is known to be one of the body's stress-fighting hormones, and research has shown that breastfeeding mothers are more tolerant of stress. There is also a sleep-inducing protein in breast milk that may help baby into dreamland. When you watch a breastfeeding pair, you will notice that, as the feeding progresses, mother mellows and baby drifts peacefully to sleep, as if both have been given a natural tranquilizer— which is in fact what happens. Martha found the relaxing effect of breastfeeding especially helpful when she was having a tense day. She would enjoy breastfeeding the baby because it helped her calm down. Breastfeeding is a particularly relaxing perk for mothers who work outside the home. One mother in our pediatrics practice told us, "When I come home after a busy day at work, breastfeeding my baby helps me unwind better than a cocktail would."

Reduced Risk of Breast, Uterine, and Ovarian Cancers

Breastfeeding reduces the risk of breast cancer, especially premenopausal breast cancer, by as much as 25 percent, depending on how much time the woman spends breastfeeding during her lifetime. Breastfeeding is also associated with a lowered risk of uterine and ovarian cancers. The cancer-lowering effects of breastfeeding are thought to be the result of the lower estrogen levels that occur during lactation. The less estrogen available to promote the growth of the cells lining the breasts, uterus, and ovaries, the less risk there is of these tissues becoming cancerous.

Less Osteoporosis

Women who have breastfed are less likely to suffer hip fractures in the postmenopausal years. Women who have not breastfed have a four-times-greater chance of developing osteoporosis than women who have breastfed do.

Natural Child Spacing

The same hormones that make milk also suppress ovulation and menstruation, provided that you

feed by the rules. For a discussion of breastfeeding and fertility, see chapter 3.

Easier Discipline

Breastfeeding is an exercise in baby reading. One veteran disciplinarian told us, "I can tell my baby's moods by the way she behaves at the breast." Discipline 101 begins with becoming an expert on your baby, knowing how to read her cues and respond appropriately, and this is where breastfeeding shines. You learn not only to understand your baby's signals when you breastfeed but also to trust them. A prominent psychotherapist once revealed this observation to us: "Breastfeeding mothers are better able to empathize with their children." The ability to get behind the eyes of your children and see things from their viewpoint is one of the keys to shaping their behavior appropriately. More than milk flows into the baby when you breastfeed. An infant who is on the receiving end of nature's best nurturing learns to trust his caregivers, which is the basis of learning to respect authority. The breastfeeding pair develops a mutual sensitivity that helps the mother convey to the child the behavior she expects and helps the child behave accordingly. With breastfeeding you enjoy the concept of *mutual giving:* mother gives the best start to baby; baby gives the best start to mother.

Reduced Cost

A year's worth of the cheapest store-brand powered formulas can cost about $1,600. But that number rises to as much as $3,163.86 when you use ready-to-feed formula. Now add the expense of buying and cleaning bottles, nipples, and tote bags as well as the medical costs for more frequent doctor's visits, and you'll see that breastfeeding is a nutritional bargain. It does cost slightly more to feed a breastfeeding mother than a woman who is not lactating, but these food costs are negligible compared with the price tag on formula feeding. Doctors estimate that an increase in frequency and duration of breastfeeding could save $13 billion per year in medical costs in the United States. Another US estimate found that if 90 percent of infants were exclusively breastfed for six months, we could save about $3,140 per infant. A similar study found a savings of $9,042 per mother if more mothers breastfed for at least one year.

GREAT INGREDIENTS IN THE RECIPE FOR BREAST MILK

Each species of mammal makes a unique kind of milk that can satisfy all the nutritional requirements of its offspring at the beginning of life. This milk, like blood, has specific qualities that ensure the survival of the young in its particular environment. This principle is known as biological specificity. Mother seals, for example, make a high-fat milk because baby seals need lots of body fat to survive in cold water. Since brain development is crucial to the survival of humans, human milk is high in nutrients for rapid brain growth.

No matter what animal it comes from, milk contains the basic nutritional elements of fats, proteins, carbohydrates, vitamins, and minerals. Let's look at each one of these nutrients in human milk and compare them to the same nutrients in formula or cow's milk so you can further appreciate how your milk is custom-made to meet the needs of your baby.

Fabulous Fats

Human milk is rich in the essential fatty acids needed for optimal human brain growth. Not only do breastfeeding babies get the right kind of fats, they also get the right amount. The fat content of your milk changes during a feeding, at various times during the day, and at various stages as your baby grows, according to the energy needs of your baby. At the start of a feeding, your foremilk is low in fat. As the feeding progresses, the fat steadily increases until baby gets the "cream," the higher-fat hindmilk. After baby gets sufficient hindmilk, baby stops eating and radiates that contented look. During growth spurts, your baby nurses more frequently, and because of the shorter intervals between feedings, he receives milk with a higher fat content, which supplies the energy he needs to grow.

> TO NOURISH AND PROTECT ARE THE GOALS OF EVERY MOTHER. BREASTFEEDING DOES BOTH.

Not only does baby get the right kind of fat in just the right amount, but in addition, most of the fat in breast milk is absorbed, so baby gets more healthful fats with less waste. Breast milk contains an enzyme called lipase that helps digest fat, so more energy is available to the baby and less fat is eliminated in the stools. Formula and cow's milk do not contain this enzyme, and the baby's intestines — the body's food judge — may not be able to digest all the fat in formula and cow's milk. So the excess fat passes into the stools, giving them an unpleasant odor — unlike the acceptable milder smell of breast-milk stools.

Specific Proteins

Remember the curds and whey in the nursery rhyme "Little Miss Muffet"? Curds and whey are the two types of milk protein. The whey is the easy-to-digest liquid portion, and the curd is the casein protein that forms a rubbery, harder-to-digest lump. Breast milk contains a much higher whey-to-casein ratio than most formulas and cow's milk do, so it's easier to digest. (Note that whey is the preferred protein for competitive body builders.) Breast milk's amino acids (the components of protein) supply the specific nutrients that babies need to build healthy brains and bodies, and research has shown that the amino acid taurine, which is present in much larger amounts in human milk than in cow's milk or formula, is especially important to brain growth. Breast-milk protein is almost completely absorbed, so there is less waste and less strain on the digestive system. The excess protein in formula and cow's milk, on the other hand, creates extra work for the intestines and kidneys, a phenomenon known as metabolic overload.

Sweeter Sugars

How sweet it is! Taste infant formula and compare it with the sweeter taste of breast milk. Human milk contains more lactose than formula does, and it is not only sweeter but also better suited for brain growth. Lactose is an intestines-friendly sugar for babies. In infant formulas, some or all of the sugar comes from highly processed table sugar or corn syrup.

A CASE OF INDIGESTION

In the early months, baby's developing intestines are not mature enough to digest milk or formula completely. To facilitate digestion, mother's milk contains biochemical digestive aids called enzymes. You can recognize an enzyme by the suffix *-ase* at the end of its name. There are: prote*ase* for proteins, lip*ase* for lipids (fats), amyl*ase* for sugars, and many others. The type and amount of these enzymes in mother's milk automatically change according to baby's nutritional needs. Factory milk is deficient in these enzymes, accounting for frequent indigestion in formula-fed infants.

More Usable Vitamins and Minerals

No factory can make minerals and vitamins as well as mom can. On paper the vitamin and mineral profiles of breast milk and formula may look the same—or it might even seem that formula contains more of some nutrients—but charts and comparisons can be deceiving. Mommy-made nutrients are better because of their high bioavailability, which means more of the vitamins and minerals that are in human milk get absorbed by the baby. What counts is not how much of a nutrient is listed on the Nutrition Facts label on a can but how much of that nutrient is absorbed through the intestines into the bloodstream. What counts is how much is available to the body—thus the term *bioavailability*.

The three important minerals calcium, phosphorus, and iron are present in breast milk at lower levels than they are in formula, but in breast milk these minerals are present in forms that have high bioavailability. For example, 50 to 75 percent of breast-milk iron is absorbed by the baby, but as little as 4 percent of the iron in formula is absorbed into baby's bloodstream. To make up for the low bioavailability of factory-added vitamins and minerals, formula manufacturers raise the concentrations. Sounds reasonable: if only half gets absorbed by the body, put twice as much into the can. This nutrient manipulation may, however, have a metabolic price.

Baby's immature intestines must dispose of the excess, and the unabsorbed minerals (especially iron) can upset the ecology of the gut, interfering with the growth of healthful bacteria and allowing harmful bacteria to flourish. This is another reason formula-fed infants have harder, unpleasant-smelling stools.

To enhance the bioavailability of nutrients, breast milk contains facilitators—substances that enhance the absorption of other nutrients. For example, vitamin C in human milk increases the absorption of iron. Zinc absorption is also enhanced by other factors in human milk. In an interesting experiment, researchers added equal amounts of iron and zinc to samples of human milk, formula, and cow's milk and fed them to human volunteers. More of the nutrients in the human-milk sample got into the bloodstream than did the nutrients in formula and cow's milk. In essence, breast milk puts nutrients where they belong—in baby's blood, not in baby's stools.

Other Good Things Too Numerous to Mention

Each year scientists discover more health-promoting substances in human milk that can only be mommy-made, not man-made. The late Dr. Frank Oski, world-renowned pediatrician, former professor of pediatrics at Johns Hopkins University School of Medicine, and our friend, was a longtime advocate of the importance of breastfeeding. He once told us, "When researching the difference between human milk and formula, I discovered that there are over four hundred nutrients in breast milk that aren't in formula." As always, mother knows best.

QUESTIONS YOU MAY HAVE ABOUT GETTING READY TO BREASTFEED

WORRIED ABOUT BREASTS SAGGING

I'm expecting my first baby and I'm concerned that nursing may make my breasts sag. Will it?

Pregnancy, not breastfeeding, is what causes breasts to change. The hormones of pregnancy enlarge your breasts and stretch your skin as your body prepares to make milk whether or not you choose to give that milk to your baby.

Throughout a woman's life, her breasts change. The breasts of a young woman who has never been pregnant have a contour that is closer to the "ideal" in our culture. (Barbie was never pregnant.) But most women's breasts don't ever look like the ideal. Maternal breasts take on a more generous, rounder shape. Breasts change again as your baby weans. Some women feel that their breasts are fuller after pregnancy and breastfeeding, and some feel that they are smaller or lower. So while it's almost certain that your breasts will change because of childbearing, it's difficult to predict how they will change. Heredity and aging also affect the shape of your breasts and the ways in which they change. And, as one experienced breastfeeding mother put it, "In the end gravity gets us all."

BREASTFEEDING AS PREVENTIVE MEDICINE

Breastfeeding has been shown to lower the incidence and/or severity of the following childhood and adult diseases and conditions:

Appendicitis	Inguinal hernia
Asthma	Juvenile rheumatoid
Breast cancer	arthritis
Childhood cancers	Leukemia
Crohn's disease	Multiple sclerosis
Colitis	Orthodontic problems
Diabetes	Osteoporosis
Ear infections	Respiratory illnesses
Eczema	Sudden Infant Death
Gastroenteritis	Syndrome
Gastroesophageal	Urinary tract infections
reflux (GER)	Vision problems
Heart disease	Whooping cough

FRIENDS COULDN'T BREASTFEED

Some of my friends had so much difficulty breastfeeding that they eventually gave up. I'm eight months pregnant and I'm worried. How can I prevent the same thing from happening to me?

Believing that you won't be successful breastfeeding can become a self-fulfilling prophecy. Most likely your friends weren't successful because they got a poor start and didn't know where to go to get the help and information they needed. To avoid following the same path, first surround yourself with women who have breastfed successfully, so you have some role models. Find a breastfeeding support group and attend a series of meetings in your later months of pregnancy. Take a breastfeeding class, which will prepare you for the first days of nursing and teach you what to do if you have problems. Even before Delivery Day, contact a professional lactation consultant and arrange for her to visit you in the hospital for a hands-on demonstration of techniques for getting started. (Some hospitals provide this; some don't.) Veteran mothers have dubbed breastfeeding a confidence game. Convince yourself that you will be successful, and you will be.

PREPARING NIPPLES PRENATALLY

Is there anything I should do to prepare my nipples before my baby comes?

Lactation specialists believe that women do not need to do anything to prepare their nipples for breastfeeding. Sore nipples are avoided by using careful positioning and latch-on techniques when you begin to breastfeed rather than by following specific rituals before birth.

Once upon a time, pregnant women were advised to toughen their nipples by going without a bra for part of the day or by wearing a nursing bra with the flaps down and exposing the nipples to the air and the light friction of clothing. This isn't necessary, and, in fact, most mothers find this irritating, especially during the final months of pregnancy. Avoid using soap on your nipples and areolae while you are pregnant or nursing, as this can dry the skin and predispose your nipples to cracking. Daily breast massage will help you become more appreciative of your breasts. If you have not grown up in a breastfeeding family or been around many breastfeeding mothers, you may need some practice being comfortable with handling your breasts.

However, if you seem to have flat or inverted nipples, there are specific suggestions for you in chapter 2 (page 47).

KEYS TO SUCCESSFUL BREASTFEEDING

In all our years of helping mothers and babies enjoy breastfeeding, we have noticed that mothers who do the following are more likely to breastfeed successfully:

Attend La Leche League meetings or participate in other breastfeeding support groups. These groups discuss breastfeeding and parenting topics at monthly gatherings. They have lending libraries and are a wonderful source of information and support for breastfeeding mothers. Group leaders, besides having practical breastfeeding experience, have special training in helping new mothers with common concerns about breastfeeding and child care. Leaders are available by phone between meetings to answer breastfeeding questions.

KEYS TO SUCCESSFUL BREASTFEEDING (continued)

Surround yourself with supportive friends.
Nothing divides friends like differences of
opinion about child rearing and baby feeding.
Surround yourself with friends who inspire
confidence and affirm your choices in parenting
and infant feeding. Remember that you are likely
to get the most negative advice from mothers
who have either never breastfed or weren't
successful at it. Even a subtle put-down, such as
"maybe you don't have enough milk," can trigger
feelings of inadequacy. You'll think you don't
have enough milk even when you do. Don't let
anyone sabotage your breastfeeding relationship,
especially in those early weeks of getting started.

Take a breastfeeding class. Instruction in
breastfeeding is often part of the package in
hospital childbirth classes. Many hospitals also
offer separate breastfeeding classes, which
provide more detailed information than a
childbirth instructor can cover in part of a
session. The breastfeeding friends you meet in
this class can be a valuable support group.

Visit educational websites. Consult sites that
are sponsored by state and local health
departments, the Special Supplemental
Nutrition Program for Women, Infants, and
Children (WIC), the US government, the
American Academy of Pediatrics, the World
Health Organization (WHO), or a lactation
consultant. Avoid those sponsored by formula
companies. A few reputable sites are: La Leche
League's LLLI.org, WomensHealth.gov/
Breastfeeding/, BreastfeedingOnline.com,
KellyMom.com, and our own website,
AskDrSears.com. These sites offer articles,
discussions of current hot topics, handouts, and
links to local resources. Some sites also have
videos that will show you proper latching

technique and how it should look when an
infant is sucking correctly.

Contact a professional lactation consultant.
Prior to giving birth, or at least within the first few
days postpartum, contact a lactation consultant
and arrange to have a hands-on demonstration of
proper positioning and latch-on technique in case
you are not blessed with one of those newborns
who just naturally does it right. A lactation
consultant has received special training and
certification in helping new breastfeeding
mothers, and she may be an experienced
breastfeeding mother herself. The skills of a
lactation consultant are especially helpful if your
baby has sucking problems or some condition that
complicates breastfeeding. A lactation consultant
will usually have the initials CLC (Certified
Lactation Consultant) or IBCLC (International
Board Certified Lactation Consultant) after her
name. (You should be able to obtain the name of a
lactation consultant through your childbirth class,
health-care provider, or obstetrical hospital. Or go
to Ilca.org.)

*With our first baby, I knew nothing about
breastfeeding other than that it was good for baby,
and I was committed to giving my baby the best. I
assumed it would be natural, easy, and instinctive
and that my baby would just automatically know
what to do. What a difficult awakening I was in for.
On the third day, my milk came in, my breasts were
engorged, Jacob could not latch on, and he went
eight hours without feeding, mostly crying in fits of
frustration. My breasts ached, and my nipples bled.
I called a lactation consultant who came over and
found a screaming baby and a desperate mom and a
dad sitting on the bed with all our baby books and a
Bible. She got Jacob to latch on. He got five minutes
of sucking and promptly fell asleep. She told me not*

KEYS TO SUCCESSFUL BREASTFEEDING (continued)

to give up and give him a bottle lest he not want to return to the breast. She instructed me on how to pump and how to use hot and cold compresses, and she offered us her home phone number, which I used frequently over the ensuing weeks. She charged us $50. We would have paid her $500! Without knowing the benefits of breast milk and having the lactation consultant's help, I could not have gotten through this time. Others told me, "Some babies just can't nurse," or "Maybe you're not making enough milk because you're small breasted," or "Formula has everything that breast milk has with just some extra water" (a pediatrician told me that).

Choose health-care providers who are knowledgeable and supportive about breastfeeding. When making the rounds to choose a doctor for your baby, look for a health-care professional who is knowledgeable and supportive of breastfeeding and not someone who just pays lip service to "breast is best." Ask what percentage of mothers in the practice breastfeed. For how long does the doctor recommend breastfeeding? Is there a lactation consultant in the practice or one with whom the doctors in the practice work closely? What would this doctor recommend if your baby wasn't gaining enough weight on your milk? (The answer should include more suggestions than just "supplement with formula.")

Choose your birthing environment wisely. Mothers who have had a stressful and traumatic labor and delivery have a higher incidence of breastfeeding problems. Mothers who have had a cesarean birth also have a higher incidence of unsuccessful breastfeeding, primarily because the babies and mothers are more likely to be separated after birth. Anything you can do to increase your chances of having an uncomplicated and satisfying childbirth experience increases your chances of having a satisfying breastfeeding relationship. Unless a medical complication prevents it, choose an LDR room (mother labors, delivers, and recovers in the same room). This is the birthing environment that is most likely to get you and your baby off to the right breastfeeding start. Consider employing the services of a professional labor support person — a woman trained in either childbirth instruction or midwifery who can be with you throughout your labor and encourage you to respond to your body's signals. Studies have shown that mothers who have labor support progress better in their labors and have a more satisfying birth, which sets the tone for how they get started with breastfeeding.

Reinforce the infant's instinct to efficiently latch on. A good latch is one of the most important keys to successful breastfeeding. For breastfeeding to be a pleasant experience for you and an adequate source of nourishment for baby, it's important that baby maintains and practices efficient sucking habits in the first week, before a vicious cycle of sore nipples, insufficient milk, unhappy baby, and unhappy mother develops. In our experience, most breastfeeding problems stem from poor positioning and latch-on. You can reinforce the infant's instinct to latch, with a wide-open mouth, beyond the nipple and on to the milk ducts that collect under the areola by placing your infant skin-to-skin and allowing him or her to use reflexes to root around and find the nipple.

Think you can. As we will repeatedly emphasize, breastfeeding is a confidence game. Just as your body grew your baby, your breasts will deliver milk. Have confidence that your body will work for you and your baby.

KEYS TO SUCCESSFUL BREASTFEEDING (continued)

Make a commitment. In most circumstances, successful breastfeeding comes down to the fact that a mother who is intensely committed to giving her baby her milk will find a way to do it. She'll seek the support and information she needs and will get help with any problems she encounters. It's true that some medical situations can make breastfeeding very challenging, and we don't mean to suggest that if you don't succeed at breastfeeding it's your own fault. Keep in mind, though, that what you need most to breastfeed your baby are the five *c*'s: a class, camaraderie, consultants, confidence, and commitment.

BREAST SIZE

I have small breasts. Will this prevent me from nursing successfully?

Not at all. Size has nothing to do with how much milk you will produce. The size of the breast is determined primarily by the amount of fat in the breast and not by the amount of milk-producing tissue. Even though your prepregnant breasts may have been small, they will enlarge considerably during pregnancy and may even grow by another cup size or two within the week after birth. In our experience, women with small-to-medium-size breasts usually have an easier time with positioning and latch-on. While the size of a mother's breasts bears no relation to the amount of milk she can produce, some mothers store more milk than others. But when mother's storage capacity is less, babies adjust by nursing more frequently. Mothers with large, pendulous breasts may need some special techniques for positioning and latch-on, since baby seems buried in the breast (see chapter 3). Chances are great that your breasts and your baby will make a good match.

> *The newborn baby has only three demands. They are warmth in the arms of its mother, food from her breast, and security in the knowledge of her presence. Breastfeeding satisfies all three.* — *Dr. Grantly Dick-Read, author of* Childbirth Without Fear

A TALE OF TWO MILKS: NATURAL AND ARTIFICIAL

Nutrient/Factor	Breast Milk	Formula	Comment
Fats	• Rich in brain-building omega-3s, namely, DHA	• Contains DHA that comes from an algae source. DHA in formula may not work the same way as it does in breast milk	Fat is the most important nutrient in breast milk; the absence of cholesterol in formula, a vital nutrient for growing brains and bodies, may predispose a child to adult heart and central nervous system diseases
	• Automatically adjusts to infant's needs during feedings, depending on the time of day and baby's age	• Doesn't adjust to infant's needs	

A TALE OF TWO MILKS: NATURAL AND ARTIFICIAL (continued)			
Nutrient/Factor	**Breast Milk**	**Formula**	**Comment**
	• Rich in cholesterol • Nearly completely absorbed because of fat-digesting enzymes	• No cholesterol • Not completely absorbed because it lacks enzymes	
Protein	• Soft, easily digestible whey • More completely absorbed; higher in the milk of mothers who deliver preterm • Contains lactoferrin for intestinal health • Contains lysozyme, an antimicrobial that stops germs from growing • Rich in brain- and body-building protein components • Rich in growth factors • Contains sleep-inducing proteins	• Harder-to-digest casein curds • Less completely absorbed; more waste; harder on kidneys • No lactoferrin or only a trace • No lysozyme • Deficient or low in some brain- and body-building proteins • Deficient in growth factors • Does not contain as many sleep-inducing proteins	Infants aren't allergic to human protein
Carbohydrates	• Rich in lactose • Rich in H.M.O. (human milk oligosaccharides), which promote intestinal health	• No lactose in some formulas—although some have lactose, others replace it with corn syrup and sugar • Some formulas are deficient in oligosaccharides, and although some do have them, they may not be as good at promoting intestinal health, since formulas do not have the type found in human milk	Lactose is considered an important carbohydrate for brain development: studies show the level of lactose in the milk of a species correlates with the size of the brain of that species
Immune boosters	• Rich in living white blood cells—millions per feeding—that fight infections	• No live white blood cells—or any other cells: dead food has less immunological benefit	When mother is exposed to a germ, she makes antibodies against that germ and gives these antibodies to her infant via her milk

A TALE OF TWO MILKS: NATURAL AND ARTIFICIAL (continued)			
Nutrient/Factor	**Breast Milk**	**Formula**	**Comment**
	• Rich in immunoglobulins	• Few immunoglobulins and mostly the wrong kind	
Vitamins and minerals	• Better absorbed, especially iron, zinc, and calcium	• Less well absorbed	Vitamins and minerals in breast milk enjoy a higher bioavailability—that is, a greater percentage is absorbed: to compensate, more are added to formula, which makes it harder to digest
	• Iron is 50 to 75 percent absorbed	• Iron is 5 to 10 percent absorbed	
	• Contains more selenium (an antioxidant)	• Contains less selenium	
Enzymes and hormones	• Rich in digestive enzymes, such as lipase for fats and protease for proteins	• Processing kills digestive enzymes	Digestive enzymes promote intestinal health and nutrient absorption; hormones contribute to the overall biochemical balance and well-being of baby
	• Rich in many hormones: thyroid, prolactin, oxytocin, and more than fifteen others	• Processing kills hormones, which are not human to begin with	
Taste	• Varies with mother's diet	• Always tastes the same	By taking on the flavor of mother's diet, breast milk shapes the tastes of the child to family foods
Cost	• Around $600 a year in extra food for mother	• Between $1,600 and $3,100 for formula alone	Breastfeeding families save $1,000 to $2,500 per year, and often much more in medical bills, since baby stays healthier; in addition, employed breastfeeding mothers miss less work
		• Cost for bottles and other supplies	
		• Lost income when baby is ill	

II

The Art of Breastfeeding: How to Breastfeed

Breastfeeding is a learned art, and it's a rather simple one—otherwise, the human race would not have survived. But it isn't as simple as it might seem. You can't just put a lactating mother and an eager baby together and expect that the milk will always flow and baby will always grow. You need to know what you're doing to get off to a good start at breastfeeding. Mothers who help their babies learn efficient latch-on in the first week not only give their babies more milk but also experience fewer problems. In this section you will learn the trick of the trade. Tips such as the lower-lip flip can make the difference between pain-free and uncomfortable feedings. You'll also learn how to have confidence in yourself and your milk supply and how to distinguish between advice that helps you breastfeed and advice that sabotages your breastfeeding relationship. Finally, you will learn a valuable lesson in Parenting 101: how to take care of yourself. Babies are happiest when mothers are happy, too.

2

Getting Started

SUCCESSFUL BREASTFEEDING doesn't just naturally *happen*. While babies come with built-in instincts to seek the breast and suck and new mothers have breasts full of milk, getting the two together requires that both learn and practice new skills. When you and your baby get a good start at nursing in the early days, the milk will soon flow and baby will grow. Careful attention to positioning and latch-on will make the difference between a pleasant beginning to your breastfeeding experience and one in which your baby struggles while you worry.

During the first few months, you will spend more time feeding your baby than on any other kind of care, so it's worth investing some time up front in learning to breastfeed efficiently. The baby will get more milk, and you are less likely to experience problems with sore nipples and engorgement. Both of you will enjoy the time spent feeding. This chapter contains some time-tested step-by-step techniques that will help you and your baby get started.

FIRST MEETING

Unless a medical condition prevents mother and baby from being together, introduce your baby to your breast just minutes after birth. Drape baby over your chest, tummy-to-tummy, cheek-to-breast, skin-to-skin. Your helpers can cover baby with a warm towel, and your body heat will keep him warm better than any elaborate hospital equipment.

Both mother and baby benefit from being in contact — or being skin-to-skin — immediately after birth. Studies show that early-contact newborns learn to latch on more efficiently than babies who are separated from their mothers. This is a time when baby will usually be in a state of quiet alertness, the optimal behavioral state for interaction with you. Her eyes are wide open, she is attentive, and she is instinctively programmed to connect with you. So give her your full attention. Gaze into her face and let her hear the voices that she has been hearing all these months.

This is a special time, and it is important to instruct your caregivers to delay all hospital routines such as eye drops, weighing, and bathing while you get to know your baby over the next hour or two. In fact, the bath can wait even longer (see below).

Remarkable films of newborns after birth have shown that babies draped over their mother's abdomens make stepping and crawling motions, using their rooting reflex to move toward the breast and find their target (the round, dark areola) with minimal assistance. We call this instinctive discovery self-attachment. As you hold

BABY'S FIRST BATH CAN WAIT

Generally, newly born babies don't need a bath for a few days. The vernix (white coating) they're born with is a clean, protective "salve" for the skin; it protects by fighting infections and keeping baby warm. It also helps the skin continue to grow and develop. Bathing and removing this coating also increases the risk that the baby will get too cold and/or develop low blood sugar (hypoglycemia). Becoming cold increases the chances that your baby will need to be taken from you and placed under a warmer, and low blood sugar increases the chances that the baby will need to be fed supplemental foods. In addition, a baby who doesn't have to work to stay warm and maintain sugar levels has more energy to effectively breastfeed. Another benefit of vernix is that, because of powerful pheromones, it helps the baby pick up the scent of the mother's breast, locate the nipple, and latch on correctly. Therefore, keeping this amazing vernix coating in place helps mother successfully breastfeed by preventing separation and supplementation and by improving the baby's ability to nurse. So yes: the bath really needs to wait.

your baby skin-to-skin against your body, be patient—let your baby move at her own pace, and let her root around and use her reflexes to find the nipple over the next thirty minutes or so. If baby is too sleepy, you may guide her movements so that she can find and nuzzle at your nipple. Just relax and enjoy each other. Don't rush the breastfeeding. This first meeting is not a time to practice everything you'll learn later in this chapter. *Introduce* your baby to the breast. This is a time for her to discover where her food will come from, not a time to fill her tummy. Newly born babies often just lick the nipple at first.

When they latch on, they take a few sucks, pause, and then may lick the nipple again or resume gentle sucking. Sucking in irregular bursts and pauses is the usual pattern for the first few hours, sometimes even the first few days.

This first nursing is important for several reasons. Sucking is good for the newly delivered baby. Crying is not. Sucking eases the tension that has built up during the stress of labor and birth. And sucking is a familiar behavior, so it helps baby adjust to her new environment. (Babies make sucking motions in the womb, and some suck their fingers and thumbs; one of our babies was born with a pink hickey on his wrist!) Although you may think that there is little or nothing in your breasts, your baby is getting colostrum: thick, yellowish "supermilk" (see page 44) that delivers concentrated germ-fighting ingredients and also has a laxative effect, helping baby clear the meconium from his intestinal tract.

Infant sucking is also good for mothers immediately after birth. Stimulating the nipples triggers the release of oxytocin, which makes the uterus contract. This helps control postpartum bleeding and hastens the return of the uterus to its prepregnant size. Breastfeeding frequently in the first hours and days after birth will also help your milk "come in" sooner.

This first lesson in breastfeeding teaches baby to whom she belongs. She settles in and learns that she can feel comforted and secure in this new world. After an hour or two, expect baby to fall asleep. While you may still be ecstatic (or stunned) from bringing a new life into the world, it's also a good time for you to succumb to sleep. As you doze off, picture your baby nursing at your breasts. Filling your brain with pleasant nursing pictures will get your milk flowing.

FIRST FEEDINGS

You can practice skin-to-skin contact and self-attachment often in the days after birth to

HOW THE BREASTS MAKE AND DELIVER MILK

Understanding how your breasts produce milk and how you can get them to work better for you will help you appreciate the wonderful womanly art and science of breastfeeding. The lactation system inside your breast resembles a tree. The *milk glands* make milk. Milk travels from these glands down through the *milk ducts* (the branches). These ducts twist like the roots of a tree, then collect and spread out beneath the nipple and areola. Finally they empty into the openings on your nipple, which can number anywhere between four and eighteen. The milk ducts located beneath your nipple and areola expand and fill with milk during feedings. To empty these full milk ducts effectively, your baby's gums must be positioned *over* them so that her jaws compress the ducts where the milk is pooled. If baby sucks exclusively on your nipple, only a little milk will be drawn out and your nipple will be irritated unnecessarily. Remember the golden rule of effective latch-on: *Babies feed on areolae, not nipples.* Baby must have enough of your areola in her mouth all the way around the breast to get the milk out.

Your baby's sucking stimulates nerves in your nipple that send messages to the pituitary gland in your brain to secrete the hormone prolactin. Prolactin surges encourage continued milk production, which goes on around the clock. As your baby continues sucking, the sensors in your nipple signal the pituitary gland to secrete another hormone, oxytocin. This hormone causes the elastic tissue around each of the many milk glands to contract, squeezing a large supply of milk through the milk ducts and out the nipple. This is called the milk-ejection reflex, or MER. The milk may come out so fast that it leaks out the side of your baby's mouth. If you were pumping or expressing by hand, you would see the milk spray out in every direction.

The first milk your baby receives at each feeding is the foremilk, which is thin, like skim milk, because of its low fat content. As baby continues to suck, more oxytocin brings on phase 2 and produces the later milk, called hindmilk, which is much higher in fat and slightly higher in protein and therefore helps baby gain weight and helps baby's tummy feel full. Consider this creamier hindmilk "grow milk."

The more milk removed from your breasts, the more milk your body makes to replace it. Frequent removal of milk from your breasts by your baby or by a pump will stimulate your body to produce additional milk. This is how mothers produce enough milk for twins or even triplets. When your baby reduces her breastfeeding, your body responds by cutting back on milk production.

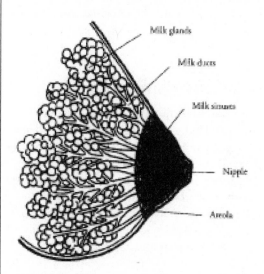

Milk glands

Milk ducts

Milk sinuses

Nipple

Areola

Anatomy of the breast.

FREE FORMULA — NOT FOR BREASTFEEDING BABIES

It's very tempting in the middle of the night for a dad or grandmother to give a fussy baby a bottle of formula rather than wake a tired new mother. It's also easy to blame breastfeeding for baby's fussiness and decide that giving formula will fix the problem. That's why formula companies like to get free samples into the hands of breastfeeding families. In fact, studies have shown that mothers who receive formula samples in a hospital discharge pack are likely to be less successful at breastfeeding and to wean earlier than mothers who don't receive free samples. Discharge packs for breastfeeding mothers should contain helpful information on breastfeeding—not products that sabotage it.

reinforce your baby's instinctive abilities to latch on and suck correctly. The baby latching efficiently will prevent or minimize problems with sore nipples and engorgement, and your baby will be able to get plenty of milk at your breast.

We encourage first-time breastfeeding mothers to seek hands-on help from a professional lactation consultant within the first few days after birth. Reading or even watching videos about positioning and latch-on and trying to translate what you learned into what you do can be a lot harder than having someone there to help you, and it's a lot easier to maintain efficient positioning and latch-on from the beginning than it is to correct inefficient latching or the resulting poor sucking habits days or weeks later. In fact, it's wise to line up a lactation consultant prior to delivery. Most maternity hospitals now have lactation consultants on staff, or you can get a referral from your obstetrician, La Leche League leader, or childbirth-class instructor.

Feeding in the Sitting Position

Settle yourself comfortably. One of the first lessons in mothering is that for baby to be comfortable, mother must be comfortable, too. You need to be relaxed so that your milk-ejection reflex can function. Since baby may want to nurse a long time once she is latched on, you don't want to be trapped in an uncomfortable position. You may feel most comfortable learning to breastfeed if you are sitting up in a chair that has arms. A rocking chair is fine. Place a pillow behind your back, on your lap, and under the arm that will support the baby. If you are sitting in a chair, use a footstool to raise the level of your lap so you don't have to strain your back and arm muscles to bring your baby closer to your breast. (If you are sitting in bed, use several pillows behind your back to help you sit up straight. Use another pillow for support under your knees as well as pillows in your lap and under the arm that is holding baby.)

Think nourishing thoughts. Now that you have prepared your body to breastfeed, prepare your mind. Anticipate the feeding and imagine your nourishing milk flowing from your breasts into your baby. Take a few deep breaths and focus on your precious little one.

Position Baby Comfortably: The Cradle Hold

Newborn babies feed best when they are awake and alert. Undress your baby down to her diaper to promote skin-to-skin contact. If baby is sleepy this will encourage her to wake up and nurse. Talk to her, stroke her skin. Bring her gently from a horizontal position to a vertical one while calling her name. Repeat this several times until she is alert and ready to eat. Now get ready to position her at your breast in the cradle hold.

1. Place the pillows. Raise baby to the level of your breast (i.e., up to the "table") by using pillows under your arms and in your lap. If you are sitting in a chair, place a footstool under your feet. Nestle baby in your arm so that her neck rests at or near the bend of your elbow, her back rests along your forearm, and her buttocks are in your hand. Be sure baby's head is a bit higher than her tummy. Let the pillow(s) on your lap support your arm and baby's weight. If baby rests too low on your lap, she will pull down on your breast, causing unnecessary stretching and friction on the nipple. You want to bring baby up and in toward you rather than lean forward toward her.

2. Place baby straight on. Turn baby's entire body sideways, so she is facing you tummy-to-tummy, face-to-breast. Her head should be lined up with her body, not arched backward or turned sideways. Baby should not

have to turn her head or strain her neck up or forward to reach your nipple. (Try swallowing a sip of water while your head is turned to the side or looking up at the ceiling. Swallowing is much easier when you hold your head straight. This is true for nursing babies, too.) Don't let baby's body dangle away from yours. Head, shoulders, and hips should be in line with each other.

3. Tuck away the arms. As you turn baby on her side, facing your breast, tuck her lower arm down along the side of her body so it doesn't get trapped uncomfortably between the two of you and get in the way of your pulling baby in close. If her upper arm is flailing around and getting in the way, hold it down with the thumb of the hand that is holding her buttocks.

4. Bend baby. Wrap your baby's body around you and anchor her in close to you. Try having your

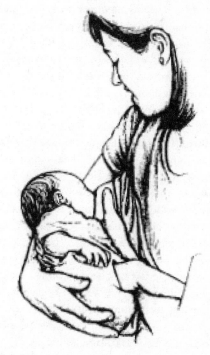

Cradle hold

opposite arm (the one that will be supporting the breast) between her legs, with her upper leg resting on top of your arm and her lower leg tucked between your arm and the pillow. This keeps baby from dangling and stretching and wiggling out of position. Wrapping baby around you in a curved position relaxes baby's entire body, which also relaxes her sucking muscles. She'll do her best latching on and sucking in this position. When babies stretch and extend their bodies, they're more likely to latch on to the nipple tightly and suck with a clenched jaw. (Ouch!) If keeping your baby relaxed and bent is difficult in this position, use the football hold described on page 39.

Present Your Breast

First express several drops of milk from your nipple by firmly rolling your thumb and fingers together down over the areola toward the nipple. Then when you present your breast, you have a few options. If your baby has been latching on and sucking well when you've practiced skin-to-skin self attachment, you can simply keep letting him go to breast with the two of you positioned for comfort. If baby seems to need more guidance (or your nipples are getting sore), you can help him by supporting the weight of your breast (to keep it off his chin) with your hand on your chest wall underneath your breast, thumb on top. This is called the C-hold. You can also try the U-hold, where your thumb is on one side of your breast and fingers on the other side. Another hold sometimes seen is the scissors hold, or cigarette hold, in which the nipple is centered between the index and middle fingers. However, if you use this hold you must make sure that your fingers are well off the areola so that they are away from the area where baby needs to latch on. The hold you choose depends on which way baby is coming to breast. By

experimenting with different holds you'll learn what works best.

Make a Sandwich

For babies who don't have a good instinctive latch, here is a more detailed approach. Using the C- or the U-hold, move your thumb and forefinger together so that they can shape the areola into an elongated "sandwich." Your fingers should be off the areola, or at least one to one and a half inches from base of the nipple.

If your forefinger still seems to get in the way of baby's lower lip when you're forming the sandwich, you can try the "teacup hold." Pull your forefinger back, closer to your thumb, keeping your other fingers extended, and compress pushing forward, so that it looks like you are holding a pinch of skin as you would a teacup. This makes the nipple and areolar area smaller so that baby can get more of the areola into his mouth. You can use this handy pinch of skin to move the breast and line up the nipple-areolar area with baby's mouth.

Another variation of the sandwich is to hold your breast well back on the areola with your fingers underneath and thumb on top. Press in with your thumb and fingers while at the same time pushing back toward your chest wall. This elongates and narrows the areola, which enables baby to latch on more easily. Note that the position of your hand must change as outlined above based on the type of hold you use.

Once your baby is in position and you have your breast in place, use your milk-moistened breast as a teaser and lightly brush your baby's lower lip downward to encourage her to open her mouth wide, as if yawning. Tickling the lower lip works like magic for getting baby's mouth to open wide. She'll look like a baby bird opening its mouth wide for food and then quickly closing.

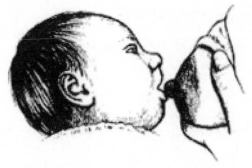

Presenting the breast

Latch-On

Even though it takes a lot of space to describe the next steps, they happen quickly. Don't be put off by the detailed descriptions. We have included a lot of detail, trying to be as clear as possible about things that are best taught in person. Once baby learns efficient latch-on, you won't have to consciously go through all these steps. It will just happen naturally.

1. Put baby on breast. As your baby opens her mouth wide, aim your nipple at the roof of her mouth, upward toward her palate, and with a *rapid arm movement* (remember this as R-A-M) pull her in very close to you. You want her to take the breast just as her mouth is open to its widest point. Remember to *pull baby in* toward you quickly but gently. You are actually putting the baby on the breast. This is opposite of bottle feeding, in which the bottle is put into the baby's mouth. "RAM baby on" may sound a bit extreme (and it *can* actually startle a sensitive baby), but it helps you remember the two important components of effective latch-on: *moving your arm,* not your body, and *doing it fast!* If you lean your breast forward toward baby, you'll wind up sitting hunched over your baby with a sore back at the end of the feeding. We like this term because most new mothers are timid with

this step and do not pull their babies in closely enough or quickly enough. You can't be passive and expect baby to do the moving. If you move your arm in too slowly or hesitate even a bit, baby's mouth will be closing again as she takes the breast, causing her to slurp (or "spaghetti suck") just the nipple into her mouth, stopping short of the desired position over the areola and milk ducts.

2. Feeding on the areola. Remember the golden rule of latch-on: *Babies feed on areolae, not nipples.* Your baby's gums should bypass the base of the nipple and encircle *at least* a one-inch radius of your areola as you quickly pull her onto the breast. Remember, the milk ducts collect pooling milk beneath the areola, back from the nipple, and baby has to compress these ducts with her tongue, pushing against her palate, in order to get enough milk. If you pull baby on quickly enough when her mouth is wide open, her gums will close far back on your areola, not on the nubbin of your nipple, where all the nerve endings are. When your baby is latching on correctly and suckling efficiently, you should not feel painful pressure on your nipple.

3. "Open wide!" The most important part of latch-on is getting baby to open her mouth wide enough. You can help your baby open her mouth wider by using the index finger of the hand supporting your breast to press firmly down on your baby's chin as you pull her onto the areola. Don't be afraid to press firmly. You won't hurt baby, and it may take firm pressure to overcome her resistance if she wants to latch on the way she learned in utero—i.e., by sucking on her tiny fingers. While you both are learning, you may need someone else to help you with this step. Talk your baby through this important latch-on step ("Open, Susie, open"). If pressing down on baby's chin makes her angry (or she goes for your finger), use the "lead with the baby's chin" approach: tilt

SIGNS OF EFFICIENT LATCH-ON AND SUCK

How do you know if you've got this latch-on business right? Eventually you will know that your baby is latched on and sucking efficiently by the way it feels. If you have a lactation consultant helping you, pay close attention to how your nipple feels after the two of you have gotten the baby latched on well. Also pay attention to how the sucking feels on the areola, how it draws out the milk from those deeper structures. There is the certain feel of a solid, secure connection between baby's mouth and your breast—that's what latch-on is! When baby is not securely latched on to the areola, the painful sensations in your nipples will register "Red alert! Poor latch-on." You then take the baby off and start again. Here are other easy-to-identify "look-and-listen" signs of efficient latch-on:

- You see the pink of baby's lips. This tells you that baby's lips are turned outward rather than tucked tightly inward.
- There is a tight seal between the baby's mouth and the areola. Baby has a good mouthful of breast.
- When baby is sucking, you see not the base of your nipple but only the outer part of your areola. Much of the areola (at least a one-inch radius) is inside baby's mouth. No leaking from the corners of baby's mouth occurs. Also, there are no clicking sounds, which babies make with their tongues as they suck with a poor latch-on.
- You do not see dimpling (the middle of baby's cheeks caving in) during sucking. Dimpling indicates a loss of suction, caused by incorrect latch-on and a poor seal on the breast.
- You observe the "ear-wiggling sign." During active sucking and swallowing, the muscles in front of baby's ears move, indicating a strong and efficient suck that uses the entire lower jaw.
- You hear baby swallow. During the first few days after birth, baby may show five to ten consecutive sucks before you hear a swallow. (You may have to listen carefully.) Once your milk has increased in volume, you should hear a swallow after every suck or two, especially after the milk-ejection reflex is triggered.
- You can see baby's tongue between the lower lip and your breast when you carefully pull the lower lip aside to take a look. If baby is latching on efficiently, the tongue will be out over baby's lower gum, forming a trough around the nipple and cushioning pressure from the jaw. Hurrying the latch-on before baby's mouth is wide open and the tongue is down and forward results in baby gumming the nipple, leading to sore nipples and inefficient milk delivery. Instead of hurrying latch-on, wait for baby's mouth to open wide and watch for the tongue to drop down so that the breast doesn't get pushed away by the tongue's forward thrust.

her head back slightly as you pull her on chin first. This encourages her mouth to open wider. For a more complete description of this technique, see the reversed cradle hold, page 41. Also see laid-back nursing, which helps babies open wide (page 39).

4. Lower-lip flip. Many babies develop the habit of tight-mouthing the nipple with lips pursed inward, causing a pinching sensation. This can lead to sore nipples and insufficient milk delivery. When baby takes the breast, her lips should turn out in a fishlike position to encircle the areola. If the tongue can come forward. Or slip a finger in to pull the lower lip out. Since it is often difficult for mother to bend over and see the position of baby's lower lip (it's easier in the football hold than in the cradle hold), someone else can do the lower-lip flip for you. Eventually, you will know what it feels like when baby's lips and jaws are properly positioned over your areola, and you will be able to do the lower-lip flip yourself as soon as your nipple gives you the uncomfortable message that baby isn't on right.

Once you do the lower-lip flip, you should sense immediate relief from the discomfort. If your baby does not cooperate or the lower-lip flip doesn't bring relief, break the suction by gently wedging your index finger (keep your fingernails short) between her gums and start again, remembering to press firmly down on her chin. If baby is still tight-mouthing you, causing a pinching feeling, repeat the lower-lip flip and be sure her lips are turned out, especially the lower one. When the lips are well flipped out, get your hand back in the position of supporting the breast.

During efficient latch-on, the tip of baby's nose touches the breast, but the sides of the nose are clear for breathing. If baby's nasal openings seem to be buried in the breast, pull baby's bottom toward you or lift up your breast a bit and you'll change the angle just enough to clear the nose. Don't just press down on your breast to clear baby's nose, as this could disturb the seal of a good latch-on.

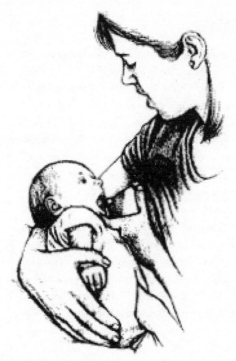

Open wide

you pull down gently on baby's lower lip, you should see her tongue cupped under the breast, positioned over the lower gum. If your baby's lower lip is tucked inward, she can't position her tongue or her gums effectively to get milk from the reservoirs beneath the areola. While she is latched on, use your index finger to press firmly down on her chin (as described above). This will usually evert the lower lip, or flip it out, so that

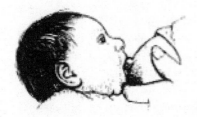

Lower-lip flip

Lower lip in correct position

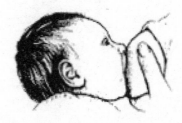

Lower lip in wrong position

NIPPLE NUISANCES

As you and your baby are learning to breastfeed, watch for and correct these common latch-on nuisances:

- *Hanging on nipple.* If baby's head is not facing the breast straight on or if baby's body dangles away from your body during nursing, baby pulls on the nipple, which can cause painful nursing, cracked nipples, and insufficient milk delivery.

  Corrective measures: If using the cradle hold, wrap baby in close around you. Be sure baby's head lines up with his body and his mouth is right at your breast level. Elevating baby on another pillow should help. If baby is a habitual dangler or back archer, use the football hold to get more control over his body.

- *Sliding down onto the nipple.* You will recognize this problem not only by the pain you feel while nursing but also by the temporary indentation you'll see at the base of your nipple just after

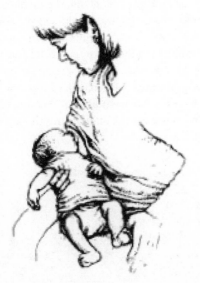

Wrong! Dangling from the breast

baby comes off the breast. Gumming the nipple is what happens when baby slides down from the areola onto the nipple or turns the lips inward tightly during sucking.

  Corrective measures: Try the lower-lip flip to correct this. Press firmly down on the chin with your index finger as you latch your baby on again. Reposition baby correctly at the breast whenever baby starts to slide down onto the nipple.

- *Nipple slurping.* When baby slurps the nipple into her mouth without opening wide, she stops short of the desired position of gums over the areola. The tender nipple skin takes a beating that could be avoided with better latch-on.

  Corrective measures: If baby slurps the nipple in as soon as you use your breast to tease open her lips, break the suction and start over, holding her off and slowing her down until her mouth opens wider. Brush baby's lips with your index finger instead. Once her mouth is wide open, pull baby on quickly so that her gums and lips bypass the nipple. Babies tend to do this when they are so hungry they don't want to wait for guidance. Watch for earlier ready-to-eat cues.

- *Nipple yanking.* Baby tosses her head back and forth while latched on, causing her gums to come down onto the nipple with painful pressure. Baby does this if impatient for milk to flow or if her tummy is cramping.

  Corrective measures: First, try switching to the other breast; the milk flow will likely be faster, which will satisfy the baby. If this is unsuccessful, use the football or reversed cradle hold so that you can steady baby's head. You can also steady baby's lower jaw by sliding the hand that is supporting the breast forward a bit,

NIPPLE NUISANCES (continued)

bringing your thumb and forefinger to either side of baby's jawline.

- *Tight-mouthing the nipple.* Sometimes babies will turn their lips tightly inward around the nipple, an annoyance that can create sore nipples and inadequate milk delivery. **Corrective measures:** Use the lower-lip flip. Gently break the suction and start over, being sure baby goes onto the breast with his mouth open wide.
- *Baby struggles to grasp the nipple.* Some babies just can't seem to get enough breast in their mouths, perhaps because their mouths are

small, mother's nipples are large, or her breasts are engorged. A baby having this problem will cry in frustration or seem confused as he moves his head back and forth right in front of the breast, desperate to latch on.
Corrective measure: Make a "sandwich." Holding your breast well back on the areola with your fingers underneath and thumb on top, press in with your thumb and fingers while at the same time pushing backward toward your chest wall. This elongates and narrows the areola to enable baby to latch on more easily (see page 34).

Even if you have to start over several times to get baby to latch on correctly, hang in there. This is good target practice and helps baby learn to get it right. Consider this your first opportunity to discipline (that is, teach and guide) your child.*

Other Nursing Positions

Besides the cradle hold, four other helpful breastfeeding positions are: laid-back nursing, the football hold, the side-lying position, and the reversed cradle (also known as the cross-cradle) hold. The football and the side-lying positions are especially useful in the early days of recovery from a cesarean birth, when you may not want to lay baby over your tender incision, even with the protection of a pillow. The reversed cradle hold is a good training hold to use in the short term while you and your baby are learning latch-on.

---

* *In teaching breastfeeding techniques to nurses and interns, we used to make latch-on rounds in the maternity ward. After simply pressing down on baby's chin and using the lower-lip flip, mothers would exclaim, "It doesn't hurt anymore! It feels right!" The students dubbed this teaching session "Sears lower-lip rounds."*

Laid-back nursing. This position helps baby remember and rehearse the self-attachment he discovered right after birth (see page 29). Lie on your back on a couch, recliner, or bed. (Be aware that a couch or recliner can present a safety concern because of the crevices between cushions if you and baby fall asleep.) You should be semi-reclined, or you can even lie almost flat. It helps to put some supportive pillows under both arms as well as under your head. Next, if you want baby to self-attach using his rooting and stepping-crawling reflexes, place him tummy-down on your abdomen. Otherwise place baby directly on your breast and help him latch on. Baby's body can be vertical or angled toward the middle, but usually his entire body is resting on yours. You and baby can be dressed or bare-chested in this position. When bare-chested, you are engaging in skin-to-skin contact, or "kangarooing." This is considered the ideal position for practicing self-attachment and serves as a powerful tool that reinforces baby's instinct to open wide, latch correctly, and suck efficiently.

Football hold. Try this hold with babies who have difficulty latching on and those who arch their backs, squirm, and frequently detach themselves from the breast. It is also useful for sleepy, small, or premature babies—it helps them stay awake. This position is also especially helpful for managing overactive letdown (choking or sputtering on a fast milk flow), particularly if you hold the baby at ninety degrees or are semi-reclined. Another benefit of this position is that you get a good view of baby latching on to the breast, while your hand at the nape of his neck gives you control of what he's doing with his head. The football hold naturally bends baby at the waist, which helps relax a baby who tends to tense his muscles. If his body is relaxed, he'll latch on better.

Sit up in bed or in a comfortable armchair and position one or more pillows at your side or wedge one between you and the arm of the chair. Place baby on the pillow to have him up at breast level along the same side as the breast you're using. Cup the *nape of his neck* in your hand and have his legs

angled upward so they are resting along the pillow supporting your back or against the back of the chair. Avoid holding the back of baby's head, as this stimulates some babies to arch away from the breast. Be sure that baby does not push his feet against the back of the chair, causing him to arch his back. Pull baby in close to you using the latch-on technique described above. Once baby is sucking well, you can wedge a pillow up against the hand holding baby to help keep him in close. Lean back and relax. Avoid the tendency to lean forward, hunched over the baby.

Side-lying position. The side-lying position is basically the same as the cradle hold except that baby and mother lie on their sides facing each other. For complete comfort, place two pillows under your head, a pillow behind your back, another under your top leg, and a fifth pillow tucked behind your baby. Five pillows sounds like a lot, but remember a golden rule of nursing: *If mother is comfortable, baby is likely to be more comfortable, too.* (Once you try this, you may find yourself sleeping with a pillow tucked behind your back long after your baby has weaned.) Have your baby on his side facing you and nestled in your arm. (If you're recovering from a cesarean, someone will need to help you get baby's mouth lined up with your nipple.) Use the positioning and latch-on techniques described in the cradle hold. This

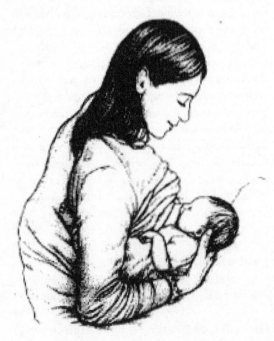

Football hold

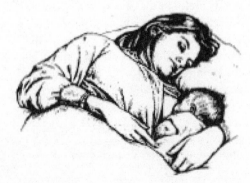

Side-lying position

position is good for night feedings and nap nursing (see chapter 9). Unless you need to lie down during feedings for physical reasons, the side-lying position is not the best to start with, since in this position you are less able to maneuver baby's head to guide his latch-on. It's best to use this position after good latch-on habits are established.

Reversed cradle hold. A reverse of the cradle hold, this across-the-body position allows better visibility of baby's mouth during latch-on and better control of baby's head. It's a good alternative to the football hold if your baby needs extra support during latch-on but you like the maternal feelings that come from having baby across your body.

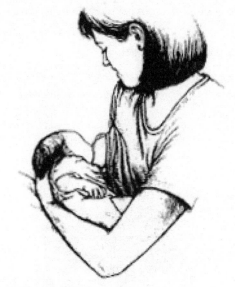

Reversed cradle hold

- Starting with a pillow in your lap, hold baby as you would in a cradle hold, then switch arms. With one hand, hold baby by the back of his neck just below the ears. He should be on his side and facing you, *his nose lined up with your nipple.* His mouth will be off-center as you start but centered after latch-on.

- With your free hand, make a "sandwich" (see page 34).

- Next, tilt baby's head back slightly, then use your breast to touch his lower lip and encourage him to open his mouth. When he opens wide, pull him in quickly, "landing" the breast on his lower jaw and tongue first, then "rolling" him the rest of the way on. The breast usually ends up pushing his mouth open wider, so that he gets a big mouthful of breast.

- If your breasts are engorged or tight, you may need to use the sandwich during the entire feeding; otherwise, baby may "slip" down to the end of the nipple. Once your breasts are soft or baby has a solid latch-on, you may try to release the sandwich and switch your arms back to the regular cradle hold.

HELPING YOUR MILK-EJECTION REFLEX (MER)

Once your baby is latched on and sucking, your nipple will send signals to your brain that stimulate the release of oxytocin, which triggers the milk-ejection reflex. This causes cells in the milk glands to squeeze out milk and send it down the ducts to your nipple. This milk contains more fat than the milk stored in the milk ducts between feedings. The MER is crucial to successful breastfeeding. It's what delivers the goods! A good MER is necessary for baby to thrive. Without it the baby receives mostly foremilk, which does not satisfy baby's hunger and doesn't provide adequate calories for growth. When a mother feels she "doesn't have enough milk," it may be that her MER isn't releasing enough milk.

Mothers experience the milk-ejection reflex as a feeling of fullness or a tingling sensation that occurs thirty to sixty seconds after baby starts sucking. A mother may notice it several times during the feeding. Because of the downward flow of this creamier milk and the sense of release that accompanies it, this sudden outpouring of hindmilk is also called the let-down reflex, though lactation consultants prefer the term milk-ejection reflex.*

Mothers experience the MER differently, and the sensation may change from one stage of breastfeeding to another, or it may be different from one baby to the next. Some mothers, especially first-time mothers, may not notice a sensation in their breasts. Here are other ways to tell that your milk-ejection reflex is working:

- Watch for a change in the rhythm of baby's sucking. Baby's sucks will deepen in response to the increased milk flow, and you will hear more swallowing, maybe even gulping of milk.
- Some mothers will leak or spray milk from the other breast, especially in the early weeks of breastfeeding.
- You may see milk leak from the sides of baby's mouth if he is having trouble keeping up with the flow.
- During the first days postpartum you'll notice uterine contractions, called afterpains, when the MER is triggered, especially if this is not your first baby.
- Thinking of your baby or just getting ready to nurse triggers leaking.

---

* *Bill comments: I prefer the more accurate term milk-ejection reflex instead of let-down reflex because of an embarrassing incident that occurred in my first week of medical practice. One day while making hospital rounds, I entered the room of a new mother breastfeeding her baby and asked if she was having any problems. She confided, "Yes—I haven't experienced any letdown." Having no idea what she was talking about, I assumed she was referring to depression, so I began counseling her about postpartum depression. Later that day, after asking Martha about the term letdown, I learned that my patient was referring to her breasts, not her mind. At that point I realized that in all those years of medical training, I had been taught nothing about how the breasts make milk (perhaps it was not considered scientific enough). Later, when I became a teacher of young pediatricians, I resolved that this pathetic lack of knowledge about such a valuable human function would not taint the next generation of physicians, especially my sons Dr. Bob and Dr. Jim, who have now joined me in my pediatrics practice.*

- You feel at peace and relaxed during breastfeeding (oxytocin and prolactin bring a feeling of well-being).

Appropriate, pain-free nipple stimulation triggers oxytocin release. A baby who is not latched on efficiently and not sucking correctly may not consistently stimulate mother's milk-ejection reflex, perhaps because nipple pain will inhibit MER. There's a difference between *making milk* (which is automatic) and *giving milk* (which is influenced by the interplay of many endocrine and emotional factors). Stress, for example, can release the adrenal stress hormone epinephrine, which can constrict the blood vessels around the milk glands, reduce the blood circulation to these glands, and thereby reduce the milk-ejecting effect of oxytocin on these glands.

Think Baby — Think Milk!

Events that the brain associates with breastfeeding can also affect the MER. Dairy cows may let

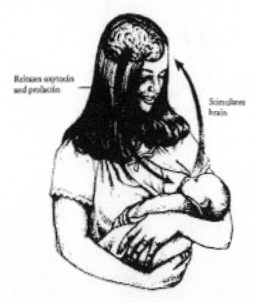

Releases oxytocin and prolactin

Stimulates brain

The three b's of breastfeeding: baby, brain, and breast

MASSAGING YOUR MER

Giving your breasts just the right touch can help trigger your MER, especially if your breasts are engorged, your nipples are sore, or your baby is impatient.

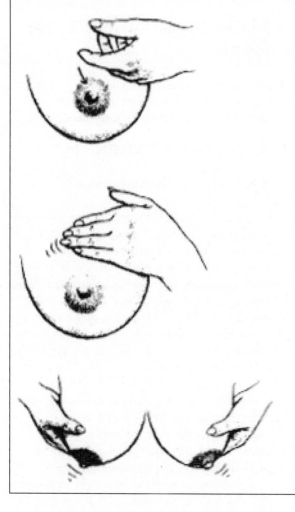

1. Apply a warm compress to your breast, such as a warm towel or cloth diaper soaked in warm water. Then, with your fingertips, stroke from the top of the breast down and over the nipple, using a light feather touch. This helps you relax and helps stimulate your oxytocin.

2. Using a motion similar to the one you use when examining your breasts, massage the milk-producing glands and ducts by pressing the breast firmly with the flat of the fingers into the chest wall, beginning at the top and working in a spiral down toward the areola. Massage in a circular motion a few strokes at a time before moving to another spot.

3. While leaning forward, gently shake your breasts, allowing gravity to encourage the stimulation to release milk.

down their milk when they line up to get into the milking barn or when the farmer washes their udders. Their bodies recognize what's about to happen. Similarly, in human mothers, the sight, sound, or scent of the baby may trigger the MER. Or it may kick in when you pick up your baby and head for your favorite nursing chair. In some women the MER is a conditioned response, accounting for the leaking that occurs just at the sight, sound, or thought of their babies. However, fear, tension, pain, fatigue, stress, distraction, or embarrassment can keep your milk-releasing hormones from operating. After all, if something in your immediate environment is not right, your body wants you to flee, not settle in for a long and comfy feeding. So when mother is upset, her milk-release mechanism may be upset, too. This brain-breast link is why mothers may find their MER does not operate as freely during stress or an emotional crisis, such as a move, illness, death in the family, or something as normal as holiday busyness.

Now, don't jump to the conclusion that you won't be able to nurse your baby successfully if your life is stressful, if troubling things are happening around you, or if you're just plain too "nervous." Mothers with all kinds of temperaments and personalities have breastfed through all types of crises. Most of the time, if you just put your baby to the breast, your body will respond by releasing milk. If it doesn't, take a few relaxing breaths and concentrate on your baby—those beautiful eyes, those round cheeks, that adorable smile. Touch his hair or stroke his soft skin. Remember that you nourished your baby in your womb for nine months and now your breasts are filled with milk that will nurture your baby outside the womb. You might imagine waterfalls or fountains of milk to help your milk flow. Or picture the triangle of breastfeeding: baby, brain, breast. Imagine your baby's sucking your breast sending messages to your brain, and the milk-producing hormones traveling back to your breasts and causing the milk glands to squeeze down and eject the milk into the milk-collecting reservoirs and into baby. Many mothers can testify to the strong emotional link between brain and breast by the fact that they begin leaking milk while just thinking about their babies even though they may be miles apart.

Before I had my baby, I had visions of how wonderful it would be to breastfeed. Matthew would latch on right away and everything would be perfect. Wrong! It's important to be realistic and not expect everything to go just as planned. It takes patience. Don't give up if it's difficult at first. Relax and have

confidence in yourself—and get support. It will happen. It just might not happen exactly as you planned.

QUESTIONS YOU MAY HAVE ABOUT GETTING STARTED

Here are some questions you may have as you and your baby are working on getting off to the best start in your breastfeeding relationship.

MATURE MILK "COMING IN"

When will my mature milk come in?

Your milk "comes in" in several stages. You begin to make colostrum during pregnancy, and you may even experience a bit of leaking during the final months before delivery. Colostrum is the thick, creamy, yellow "supermilk," small in volume but power-packed with nutrients and immunity builders. The amount of colostrum you produce in a single feeding is measured in drops, not ounces; it's the perfect amount for a newborn. It's best to nurse your newborn baby frequently whenever she shows hunger cues so she gets as many of the nutrient-rich drops as possible. Sleepy babies may need mom to offer the breast every two to three hours or be fed hand-expressed colostrum. Mothers who have breastfed infants previously tend to produce more colostrum.

Protein-rich, low-fat colostrum prepares baby's intestines for the milk feedings that will soon follow. Colostrum helps establish the growth of helpful bifidus bacteria in the intestines as well as acting as a laxative to facilitate the passage of meconium. Think of your colostrum as a superfood, particularly rich in infection-fighting antioxidants such as vitamin A, vitamin E, and carotenoids. In fact, the high beta-carotene content in colostrum accounts for its yellowish color. Be proud of this nutrient-rich colostrum you produce.

Over the next week, your breasts make a gradual transition from producing colostrum to making mature milk. The amount of fat, carbohydrates, and calories gradually increases in the milk, and you produce more of it. Your milk, therefore, becomes more filling for baby. It may take as long as two weeks after birth for your milk to change from the yellowish white color typical of early milk to the bluish white of mature milk. You will know when your mature milk "comes in," sometime between the second and fifth day, as your breasts seem to increase two cup sizes overnight. How soon this happens depends upon many factors: your previous nursing experience, how tired you are from the birth, how quickly your baby learns to latch on, and how frequently and effectively baby sucks. To get your milk to come in sooner and better, do the following:

- Plan for a satisfying birth experience.
- Room-in with your baby immediately after birth.
- Encourage early, frequent, unrestricted feedings.
- Consult a lactation consultant in the first day or two.
- Avoid supplementation unless medically necessary.
- Don't worry, and be confident!

SUPPLEMENTAL BOTTLES AFTER BIRTH

My baby is two days old, and I have been advised to offer a bottle after each feeding in case I don't have enough milk. Is this okay?

No, it's not okay. Supplementing breast milk with water and/or formula can sabotage breastfeeding, even if the formula is given via spoon or syringe. Water quenches an infant's thirst, and formula will make baby feel full and make him want to nurse less. If the supplement is given with an artificial nipple, it can also confuse his sucking, so that when he is offered the breast he won't know how to make it work. And babies can quickly learn to prefer the easier way the artificial nipple works. Studies have shown that supplementation, especially in the first few days after birth, negatively influences the duration of breastfeeding and can also lead to childhood obesity.

Besides interfering with the baby's learning process at the breast, offering supplementary bottles messes with mother's mind. Suggestions from well-meaning health-care providers, friends, and relatives that include "in case you don't have enough milk" plant the seeds of doubt in your mind, and one way or another, they can keep you from making enough milk. These first few days after birth are a time when mother and baby are working hard at breastfeeding. When people suggest that your milk supply is inadequate, you may be quick to conclude that baby's fussiness or wakefulness or sleepiness (or anything else your baby is doing) is your fault. If baby nurses for a long time, you worry that he is just not satisfied. If baby nurses for a short time, you're concerned that there isn't enough milk in your breasts to keep him interested. Doubt produces confusion about how to interpret baby's cues and worries about his being hungry. Supplementary bottles look like the solution to your dilemma, but depending on supplements will make it impossible for you and your baby to develop breastfeeding harmony. Eventually you *won't* have enough milk.

As much as possible, surround yourself with people who support and trust breastfeeding and who make you feel more confident. This will help you avoid the inadequate milk supply–inadequate mother syndrome. If you run into difficulties, get help from a reliable source and solve the problems.

NIPPLE PREFERENCE AND NIPPLE CONFUSION

Beware of nurses bearing bottles. It's customary in some maternity wards to set a bottle of formula or glucose water on the bedside table of the breastfeeding mother. This happens in hospitals where the staff is not very knowledgeable and not very supportive about breastfeeding. That innocent-looking little bottle gives big, bad messages: "You won't make enough milk"; "This will prevent your newborn from starving"; or "Breastfeeding is tricky—you need this bottle for insurance." This bottle appears at the worst possible time—when mother is unsure of herself and vulnerable to suggestions that she might not make enough milk for her baby.

Bottles bring more than just mental confusion for mom. There are some basic differences between breastfeeding and bottle feeding, so that giving bottles often leads to the breastfeeding-sabotaging conditions known as nipple preference and nipple confusion. Some babies learn to prefer the rubber nipple, especially if mother has flat or inverted nipples or they've just imprinted on the rubber nipple and prefer it for that reason. But some babies develop sucking problems. This happens because babies suck human nipples differently from the way they suck rubber nipples. When baby latches on to the breast, he opens his mouth wide and draws the very stretchable human nipple and areolar tissue far back into his mouth. The tongue holds the breast tissue against the roof of baby's mouth while forming a trough beneath the nipple and areola. The lower jaw compresses the underlying milk ducts, while the tongue rhythmically "milks" the breast with a wavelike motion from front to back, drawing the milk from the areola and the nipple. Since the nipple is far back in the mouth, it is not compressed, so it can't get sore. While learning to latch on, baby must coordinate tongue and jaw movements in a sucking motion that's unique to breastfeeding.

Babies suck from a bottle entirely differently. Thanks to gravity, milk flows from a bottle so easily that baby does not have to suck "correctly" to get milk. He doesn't have to open his mouth wide or turn out his lips to form a tight seal. The bottle nipple does not need to be far back in his mouth, and the milking action of the tongue is not necessary. As a result, baby can lazily gum the nubbin of rubber and suck with only his lips. Also, when sucking on an artificial nipple, baby thrusts his tongue upward, using his tongue to stop the flow of milk if it comes out too fast. Milk flows from the bottle whether or not baby sucks, so there are no pauses for rest during bottle feeding. This is why lactation consultants advise against bouncing between breastfeeding and bottle feeding during the first three to four weeks, when baby is learning efficient latch-on. Supplements, if medically necessary, can be given in ways that don't involve artificial nipples.

The different tongue action during bottle feeding explains why sometimes a baby who gets bottles soon after birth ends up moving his tongue at the breast in a way that pushes the breast nipple out of his mouth. When you compare the illustration of sucking at an artificial nipple with the illustration of sucking at the breast, you will see that if baby starts to suck from the breast the same way he does from the bottle, the tongue and the gums will traumatize mother's nipple. And because the bottle-sucking technique won't get much milk out of the breast, baby starts to think the bottle is easier and balks at taking the breast. Mixed feedings can confuse the newborn. By giving baby supplemental bottles at the time he is learning to latch on efficiently to the breast, you run the risk of causing nipple confusion or a preference for bottles, resulting in sore nipples or in baby eventually refusing the breast. The mother-infant pairs most at risk for these problems include mothers with short, flat, or inverted nipples and babies who have short tongues, noticeably retracted chins, or a condition known as tongue-tie (see page 72).

Believe that you can make enough milk for your baby, and you will.

Mixing feeding methods can confuse the newborn because the way babies suck at the breast and the way they suck on the bottle are entirely different. Also, if you give your baby regular feedings of formula, he will not want to nurse at the breast as often, and your breasts won't make as much milk. Your milk supply won't meet baby's demands, and you'll come to rely on formula—permanently.

SHORT, RETRACTING, INVERTED, OR FLAT NIPPLES

My nipples don't stick out as much as I think they should. Will I be able to breastfeed successfully?

Yes, you can breastfeed, even if your nipples are short, retracting, flat, or inverted—if you believe you can.

If you're wondering whether your nipples are inverted, gently compress the areola between your thumb and forefinger. A nipple that is normal will protrude. Flat nipples don't do anything at all. A dimpled or inverted nipple will retract. It's not unusual for one nipple to be flat or inverted and the other to be normal. Truly inverted nipples that prevent successful breastfeeding are rare. Remember, it's how they function, not how they look, that matters. A nipple can actually appear normal but invert when the areola is compressed.

Learn the golden rule of latch-on: *Babies feed on areolae, not nipples.* How much your nipple protrudes is not a predictor of your success at breastfeeding. A baby who latches on and sucks can stimulate and draw the nipple out, making it just the right size and shape. In addition, there are techniques and devices that can help you get him started if baby balks at first. If you work closely with your baby in the first days after birth and give him lots of opportunities to practice nursing, he will figure out what to do, and the two of you

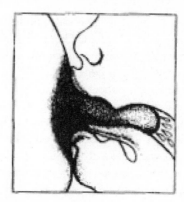

How baby sucks from the breast

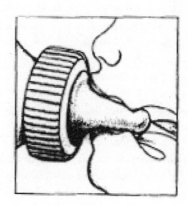

How baby sucks from the bottle

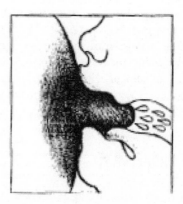

Nipple preference causing sore nipples

will go on to breastfeed long and happily. Remember, your baby doesn't know any other nipples, so he can't compare—*unless* someone gives him a bottle or pacifier!

Indeed, worrying about the adequacy of your nipples may zap your confidence. If you believe your nipples will keep you from breastfeeding, they probably will—because you won't make the effort to do what it takes to solve any problems that occur. You'll just feel that your attempt to breastfeed was doomed from the start. If you have confidence in your ability to breastfeed, you will also confidently seek solutions if you encounter difficulties. You may also find it reassuring to know that lactation consultants frequently remind mothers who are worried about their nipples that "babies *breastfeed,* not nipplefeed." So if you believe that you have problem nipples, *don't worry.* First of all, there are a couple of things that nature does to improve matters. Throughout pregnancy the nipples are growing and may evert or get longer, especially in the third trimester. Also, a natural birth experience that minimizes the use of medication results in an alert baby who sucks well. This is the best remedy for inverted nipples. As a matter of fact, after-birth sucking stimulates your nipple-erection reflex, which makes the nipple more flexible and easier to latch on to. Finally, stimulate the baby's natural instincts to latch on correctly by practicing lots of skin-to-skin contact in the hours and days after birth, maximizing mother-baby togetherness. So with this in mind, you can just wait until after the birth to see how your baby latches on. But you also should be prepared and familiarize yourself with the tools available as well as some strategies used to manage short, flat, retracting, or inverted nipples.

NIPPLE MANAGEMENT

Prenatally, apart from seeing a lactation consultant for evaluation and using a new tool called a supple cup (see below), there is little you need to do. In the past, it was common practice to recommend nipple-stretching exercises and/or breast shells. Today, nipple exercises are never prescribed by knowledgeable health-care providers, and although some mothers do find breast shells helpful postnatally, they are rarely used prenatally: in addition to simply being ineffective, prenatal breast-shell use may actually reduce a mother's likelihood of breastfeeding successfully. There is proof that a supple cup, however, will pull the nipple out after a few weeks of use. Used correctly, supple cups can be very effective. They can be used before becoming pregnant or in early pregnancy (less than twenty weeks), late pregnancy (more than thirty-eight weeks), and early postpartum, while colostrum is present. Pregnant mothers should only use them with the guidance of their obstetrical health-care providers. In addition, supple cups should not be used by women at risk of preterm labor, and if you notice uterine contractions associated with their use, they should be discontinued. They come in various sizes and need to be fitted to your erect nipple.

After birth, there are many techniques and tools you can use to help your baby latch on to your breast.

- Practice skin-to-skin contact frequently. Since your baby's sucking may be all that is needed to stimulate your nipple-erection reflex and draw your nipples out, connecting skin-to-skin is the best way to ensure the baby latches on correctly. It's helpful to work hard at getting your baby to latch on well during the first and second days after birth, before your milk changes from colostrum to mature milk.
- Line up the services of a lactation consultant and get hands-on consultation on the first day after birth. Often, teaching baby adequate positioning and latch-on is all that is needed to draw out flat or inverted nipples. Again,

remember that babies feed on areolae, not nipples.

- Use the "sandwich" technique to get more breast tissue into baby's mouth (see page 34).
- Prevent and treat engorgement promptly, because it tends to exaggerate nipple flatness or inversion and makes latch-on more difficult. The best way to prevent engorgement is to feed frequently and help baby latch on deeply. Express the milk by hand after feedings if baby's sucking is not doing enough to relieve the engorgement. If baby is still acting hungry, supplement with the expressed milk as needed.
- During the first days after birth, use a breast pump on low suction to draw out your nipples. The high-quality electric pumps that are available in maternity wards in most hospitals will do the best job with the least trauma to your nipple.
- Try a supple cup. Center it on the nipple and apply it for five to ten minutes before nursing your infant.
- Try wearing breast shells designed for flat or inverted nipples between feedings or for thirty minutes before feedings. Breast shells are made of plastic. They have two parts: a back with a hole through which the nipple can protrude and a rounded dome that fits inside your bra. Pressure on the shell from your bra against the areola gradually stretches out adhesions and allows the nipple to protrude. Be sure to wash these shells with soap and hot water between feedings and discard any milk that collects in them. Note that shells come with two types of backs; the one with the larger hole is meant for treatment of sore nipples. Be sure to use the back with the small hole, which fits close to the nipple base so that pressure on the areola will work.
- Shield your nipple. If baby is still having difficulty latching on, with the guidance of a lactation consultant, try using a silicone nipple shield. The shield stimulates the roof of baby's mouth (the S-spot), which triggers the sucking reflex.

Flat or inverted nipples don't last forever. As baby learns to latch on and suck well in the first week or two after birth, most mothers find that they no longer need exercises, shells, or pumps, as baby's own sucking does a very good job of shaping the nipples. Don't worry. Work with baby to get a good latch-on, and he will do his job of drawing out your nipples to just the right shape and length so that he can get all the nourishment he needs.

SLEEPY BABY

Our two-day-old baby falls asleep after a few sucks or a few minutes after I put him to the breast. Why isn't he more interested in nursing?

Many babies, and their mothers, need to "sleep it off" for a few days following the excitement of birth. Baby may be tired or overwhelmed or still under the influence of medications used during labor and delivery. After another day or two, expect that baby's nursing will improve. Babies are born with plenty of fluid and fat reserves (that's why they look so puffy) to tide them over until they're in the mood to feed and your milk is more abundant. Here is what to do to help baby awaken and feed more eagerly:

- Try to wake baby during REM sleep. This lighter stage of sleep is recognized by fluttering eyelids, sleep grins, clenched fists, and limbs that are not limp. A baby in deep sleep is harder to rouse.
- Encourage baby a bit. Undress both of you from shoulder to waist and place baby skin-to-skin against your tummy and breast while you drape a lightweight blanket over baby's exposed back and head. Your own body heat will keep him warm enough (a mother's skin temperature

automatically goes up a bit while breastfeeding) but not so toasty that he falls asleep.

- If that doesn't work, hold baby upright and talk to him to encourage him to open his eyes.
- Instead of using the usual bending cuddly positions (which relax babies), straighten out his body and extend his arms, both postures that perk up the brain.
- Stroke the palms of his hands and soles of his feet to help him wake up.
- Pat baby's face with a cool washcloth.
- Hand-express a few drops of colostrum, your "supermilk." Using your moistened nipple, tickle his lower lip to stimulate him to open his mouth. While you feed him, encourage baby to continue to nurse with a bit of gentle chatter. If he nods off, stroke his legs or pat his back.
- Get in the habit of switching breasts as soon as baby begins to fade. Rouse him with a burping session or a brief back rub on the way to the other breast. This is called switch nursing.
- If baby drifts off after only a few minutes of sucking, take him off the breast and help him wake up again before latching him on to the other side. Wake him up several times if you have to, until he has nursed well for ten or fifteen minutes. When baby is done nursing, let him simply rest at your breast and lick your nipple, actions that get the milk-making hormones flowing.

While conventional wisdom says, "Let sleeping babies lie," this advice does not always apply to breastfeeding newborns. Sleepiness interferes with the usual law of supply and demand in breastfeeding, so if your baby continues to be too sleepy to nurse well beyond the second or third day postpartum, you will most likely need to pump your breasts for a few days and offer your baby your expressed milk via a feeding syringe (see page 142), a cup, or finger. Your lactation consultant can explain how to do this. Even though the word *schedule* is usually not a part of

successful breastfeeding, with sleepy babies you will have to take the initiative and schedule the feeding routine for a while rather than wait for baby to cue. Wake baby up every two to three hours during the day and set your alarm so that baby goes no longer than four or five hours between feedings at night.

UNINTERESTED BABY

I couldn't wait to breastfeed, but my day-old baby isn't at all interested in feeding. I'm feeling rejected!

You've read the breastfeeding books, taken breastfeeding classes, and have a picture in your mind of your baby eagerly awaiting your milk. You picture yourself and your baby as a happily nursing pair. Then, still high from the excitement of birth, you put your baby to the breast for that long-awaited first real feeding—and nothing happens. Baby looks around a bit, takes a few licks, indulges in a bit of a snooze, awakens, and you try again. Still nothing happens. Discouraging thoughts enter your mind. You may even feel as if your baby is rejecting you. You remember one of your friends complaining about having a baby who "wouldn't nurse." Is that going to be my baby, you wonder? Am I going to be one of those breastfeeding failures?

Don't be discouraged: your baby will nurse. As with the sleepy baby, some babies just take a while to want to feed. The first key to overcoming this problem is not to let baby's lack of interest in breastfeeding carry over into your attitude. Don't allow yourself to become discouraged. Your milk is the best nutrition for your baby, and as your baby's mother, you shouldn't let his seeming lack of interest in the breast keep him from having this wonderful start in life.

This doesn't mean that you will have to force your baby to breastfeed. Battles over breastfeeding will only make you tense and worried. That anxiety will transfer over to your baby, and he may be even less interested in breastfeeding than before. Your job is to make milk and woo your baby to the breast by making nursing a pleasant experience for you both.

As you begin each feed, manually express a few drops of milk. Then use your milk-moistened nipple to stroke his lower lip, all the while talking him into nursing by saying, "Open...open." Once your baby gets a taste of the sweet, rich milk, he'll be more eager to nurse. Try nursing in the laid-back or side-lying position and let baby fall asleep at your breasts while snuggling and licking your nipple. (This should be a pleasant experience for you, too.) Manually express a little bit so he starts to lap up the milk that drips from your nipple. Put a diaper under his head to catch the drips. Be patient. Enlist the help of a lactation consultant, and remember that you are in charge. With patience and persistence on your part, breastfeeding will soon be working well.

BREASTFEEDING AFTER A CESAREAN

I'm scheduled for an elective cesarean section. Will I need extra help breastfeeding?

Yes, you will need extra help, since you'll be doing double duty: healing yourself and feeding your baby. Try these time-tested helpers for successful breastfeeding following a surgical birth:

- Pain suppresses milk production and makes it harder for you to enjoy your newborn. To decrease postoperative pain, talk to your anesthesiologist about using medications that will help you feel the most comfortable yet alert after the surgery. Discuss with your doctor the use of patient-controlled analgesia (PCA), in which you administer your own pain-relieving medication as you need relief. This medication is safe for your breastfeeding baby.
- Ask your lactation consultant or attending nurse to show you how to breastfeed in the laid-back, side-lying, and football positions. These positions keep baby's weight off your incision.
- When nursing in the side-lying position, comfortably surround yourself with pillows. Place one or two pillows between your back and the side rail, another pillow between your knees, a pillow under your head, and one behind baby. To support your incision while lying on your side, wedge a tummy pillow (a small foam cushion or even a folded bath towel) between the bed and your abdomen. In the laid-back position, pillows need to be under your head and both arms.
- Have one of your attendants (either the nurse or your partner) bring baby to you and help you position his body and mouth for latch-on.
- Be sure your partner watches how the professionals help you breastfeed. Encourage them to demonstrate how to help you in the hospital and later on at home, especially with the lower-lip flip (see above).
- As much as possible, arrange to keep your baby with you in your room after a cesarean. Get help from dad, grandma, or a friend—someone who can be with you much of the time in the hospital and lend a hand with the baby.

Depending on the type of anesthesia and your recovery time, it may take a bit longer for you to begin breastfeeding and for your colostrum to change to mature milk following a surgical birth. This may be a direct result of the surgery, or it may be because mothers who have cesareans have fewer opportunities for early and frequent breastfeeding. The good news is that studies show that mothers who have a surgical birth are just as successful at breastfeeding as mothers who deliver vaginally, as long as their commitment to breastfeeding remains high.

3

Common Concerns Breastfeeding Mothers May Have

AS YOU AND YOUR BABY GROW together in your breastfeeding relationship, you both will continue to encounter new joys and challenges. Each time you solve a problem, you draw closer to your baby and become more of an expert in breastfeeding. The following are the most common challenges and problems you may face.

FEEDING FREQUENCY

How often and how long should I feed my baby?

Frequently, frequently, frequently! Those are the magic words for successful breastfeeding. Both experience and research have shown the following benefits when infants enjoy frequent, unrestricted breastfeeding.

- Infants grow better—they *thrive.*
- The fat and calorie content of mother's milk is higher.
- Mothers experience less engorgement and fewer breast infections and sore nipples.
- Frequent feedings are most important in the first three months of life.

Watch your baby, not the clock. Breastfeeding is a harmonious relationship, not a mathematical exercise. One breastfeeding mother put it this way: "I don't count the number of feedings any more than I count the number of kisses." It's the frequency of breastfeeding more than the duration of individual feedings that stimulates your milk-producing hormones.

The storage capacity of breasts varies from mother to mother. Mothers with a lower storage capacity simply need to feed their infants more frequently. Each mother-infant pair enters into a continual, mutual negotiation about when to nurse, so that mom's supply equals baby's need.

Babies' feeding patterns are as varied as their personalities. Early in your breastfeeding relationship you realize that the term *schedule* has absolutely no meaning for the breastfeeding baby, certainly not during the first month. The only schedule your baby will have, and should have, is her own. One of the most beautiful and natural biological negotiations is between a mother and her nursing baby working together to get the law of supply and demand in breastfeeding working comfortably. Again, listen to your baby's cues and watch your baby, not the clock.

In the first few days, most babies suck in varying intensities, intermittently, and for long periods of time, some even for as long as an hour. Newborns will often fall asleep during a feeding and then wake up in an hour and need to feed again. The duration of the feeding often depends upon baby's sucking style. Little "gourmets" suck gently and leisurely, stopping to savor the moment and look around. "Barracudas" get down to business quickly and feed ravenously.

WHAT THE EXPERTS ADVISE

Once upon a time most health-care providers were lukewarm about breastfeeding. Because of the decades of research on the health advantages of breastfeeding, health-care providers now actively encourage mothers not only to breastfeed but also to think of this relationship in terms of years rather than months. The American Academy of Pediatrics currently recommends exclusive breastfeeding for about six months, followed by supplementary breastfeeding as complementary foods are introduced and continuation of breastfeeding for one year or longer as mutually desired by mother and baby. So when a well-meaning friend or relative admonishes you, "What? You're still nursing?" you can reply that the medical profession is on your side.

As for the length of feedings, ignore the old but still sometimes given advice "Begin with three minutes on each side and gradually increase the length of feedings by one minute each side up to ten minutes." Neither babies nor experienced breastfeeding mothers wrote these restrictive rules. Three minutes per side may not even allow enough time for your milk-ejection reflex to operate. Normal newborns can take up to an hour to get a full meal. You will notice that the length of most feedings varies from fifteen to forty-five minutes, with the average feeding lasting around thirty minutes. The longer and more frequently a baby nurses in the early weeks of breastfeeding, the more milk you will produce. Within a month or two, once mother and baby have worked out a mutually satisfying, harmonious routine, most babies can get all the milk they need within the first ten minutes of a feeding. Yet some babies still linger at the breast and luxuriate in comfort sucking. This is good for them—and good for mother's milk supply, too.

Restricting the length of feedings was once thought to prevent sore nipples. Lactation consultants have long known that positioning and latch-on problems, not frequent feedings, cause sore nipples. If your nipples are getting sore, you need to change the *way* your baby is nursing, not how often or how long he feeds.

Another myth is that frequent feeding can cause painful engorgement. Research shows just the opposite. The more a mother restricts the frequency and length of breastfeeding or encourages her newborn to have long stretches of sleep, the more likely she is to get engorged.

Realistically, expect your baby to breastfeed every two to three hours for the first few weeks. Some babies need to cluster-feed, meaning feed every hour or so during a portion of the day, such as late afternoon and early evening. We have noticed that babies who thrive (meaning grow to their fullest potential) will breastfeed eight to twelve times a day in the first few weeks. Once your milk supply is well established, the frequency of feeding may drop to about eight times in twenty-four hours. But the frequency may increase again with growth spurts or when an increase in milk volume is needed.

Frequent versus spaced feedings is a hot topic among baby-care advisers. Proponents of spaced feedings (we dub them baby trainers) try to sell scheduled feedings as a way of getting babies to fit more conveniently into parents' lifestyle. Baby trainers advocate feeding even young babies no more than every three or four hours throughout the day. This advice can lead to undernourished babies as well as to the end of breastfeeding. Both experience and science have proved that spaced feedings are not right for the great majority of babies and that babies who feed frequently grow better and cry less. In short, *frequent feeders thrive.*

Frequent feeding is biologically correct. Looking at nature gives us clues to how often human babies should breastfeed. Mother animals who are away from their young for an extended period of time (called intermittent-contact species) produce a milk that is very high in fat and calories so that offspring can thrive on infrequent feedings. Human milk is relatively low in fat and calories, an indication that humans are a continuous-contact species. The way the milk-producing hormones prolactin and oxytocin behave in the body further supports the idea that human babies should breastfeed frequently. The term *biological half-life* means the amount of time it takes the body to use up half of a given substance. Prolactin has a very short biological half-life, approximately half an hour; the half-life of oxytocin is even shorter, around four minutes. Since these milk-making hormones are released mainly when the baby sucks at the breast, frequent nursing is necessary to keep these hormone levels high. Research has also shown that the fat concentration of mother's milk is maximized when the time intervals between feedings are short. The longer and the more frequently the infant breastfeeds, the higher the fat content of mother's milk. Restricting the length and frequency of breastfeedings will limit baby's growth and mother's ability to make milk.

Nursing tip: *Finish the breast.* Let your baby determine when he is finished on the first side and ready to switch to the other breast. Babies get more of the creamier hindmilk if allowed to finish the first breast first.

How soon should I try to get my baby on a feeding schedule?

If you try to make a breastfeeding baby follow a schedule, you run the risk of causing problems in the breast and in the baby. Rigidly scheduled babies often don't gain weight adequately, and scheduling moms are more likely to become engorged, get breast infections, and have problems with their milk supply. Babies digest breast milk more rapidly than formula, so they feel hungry more often than formula feeders and need to be fed more often. Also, in the early months, babies have growth spurts around every three weeks, during which, just like teenagers, they need more food. Babies also enjoy periods of comfort sucking, when they are more interested in the feel than in the food. Sometimes babies are only thirsty and suck a little to obtain some of the watery foremilk. All these varied needs can be met at the breast, but not on a set schedule.

We prefer to use the less rigid term *breastfeeding routine* to describe the way a mother and baby work together to breastfeed successfully. Even better is *breastfeeding harmony,* a term that implies that baby's needs and mother's responses are in tune. In the early months of breastfeeding, it's important for every mother and baby to work out their own mutually satisfying routine, one in which baby gets enough milk and comfort at the breast and mother feels happy, rested, and relaxed as she meets her baby's needs. Keep working at following a routine that helps you both thrive. This is an ongoing process, since baby's needs change and so do mother's.

Should I nurse my baby on demand?

Instead of the term *demand feeding* we prefer *cue feeding*. *Demand feeding* sounds like something you do in a tyrant-slave relationship. While it is true that in the early months of feeding, mothers are givers and babies are takers, it's important that baby and mother eventually work out a mutually satisfying routine that respects the needs of both. On the other hand, it is okay for you to "demand" that your baby nurse if you are feeling full or if you think baby needs a nap. Just as there is a language of love, there is a language of breastfeeding, and learning to read and respond to baby's breastfeeding language is the first step in learning to know your child.

FEEDING CUES AND SIGNS OF BEING FULL

When babies are hungry, they are alert and may start looking for their food, licking their lips,

THE SCIENCE OF FREQUENT FEEDINGS

Both the baby and the breasts were designed for frequent feedings. Babies have tiny tummies, and breast milk is digested rapidly—a combination that necessitates frequent feedings. New research also suggests that frequent feeding during the first three months enables the breasts to continue an adequate level of milk production until weaning. Breastfeeding specialists have long observed that mothers who nurse less frequently or tend to follow a restrictive feeding schedule may produce adequate milk during the first few months but then often wean their babies early because they "didn't have enough milk."

According to recent insights into milk production, here's what seems to happen. In the first few months, frequent feedings keep the level of mother's prolactin (the milk-making hormone) high. Because of frequent feedings, the milk glands mature, possibly by increasing the number and efficiency of receptor sites for prolactin within the breast. This renders the milk-making cells very sensitive to prolactin. Then, when prolactin levels diminish after the first few months of breastfeeding, these milk-producing glands can continue to produce sufficient quantities of milk, even with less

hormonal stimulation. The breasts, in effect, become more efficient at making milk. If there was not enough nursing in the early weeks to increase the number of receptor sites for prolactin (that is, if there were scheduled feedings with an emphasis on longer sleep periods), the breasts become less efficient at making milk as time goes on.

Further support for the importance of frequent feedings comes from studies that show that the more frequently babies feed and the more thoroughly the breasts are drained, the higher the fat content (and therefore the calorie content) of the breast milk. This accounts for the frequently inadequate weight gain of infants who are breastfed on a restrictive schedule. The longer a mother goes without nursing her baby, the lower the fat content of her milk.

On restrictive feeding schedules, too many babies don't thrive—and, all too often, neither do their mothers. Remember: this beautiful biological system of cue feeding worked for millions of years before clocks were invented or the new age of "baby trainers" promised to make breastfeeding conform to mother's convenience. Ignore the clock and go with the program that has proved effective.

making sucking sounds, and/or sucking on their fingers or toys. If these first cues are missed, their arms and legs start to move, their breathing becomes faster, and they start fussing. As a last resort, they cry. It is best if you feed your baby at the earliest sign of hunger whenever possible. If you think of the early signs of hunger as polite requests from your child for food, waiting until she is crying frantically would be similar to making baby scream, "I am hungry!" Crying without looking, licking, or sucking may indicate that the baby is tired, wants to be held, or is uncomfortable. So if you don't see specific feeding cues, you may want to try other ways to comfort your infant before attempting to feed.

When babies are full they will pull off, arching their backs and/or pushing away from the breast. Full babies are calm, their extremities are relaxed, and they may act sleepy or fall asleep. Other signs include slow or no suckling, open palms, sealing lips, and releasing your nipple.

GETTING ENOUGH MILK

I'm worried my baby isn't getting enough milk. What signs should I look for?

Rather than worrying and wondering about whether your breastfed baby is getting enough milk, check the following signs to be reassured that your baby is growing and thriving on your milk.

Weight gain. The most reliable sign, of course, is adequate weight gain, which for the average infant is four to seven ounces a week, or a minimum of one pound a month. Unless a special electronic scale is used, weighing baby before and after a feed "to see how much milk she's getting" is notoriously inaccurate. On a typical scale, the varying positions and movements of the baby can cause the readings to fluctuate a few ounces. After the first month or two of breastfeeding, you will automatically know that your baby is getting

enough milk, since your baby will look and feel heavier. Yet in the first several weeks, especially if you are a first-time mother, it is not easy to eyeball weight gain. This is why your doctor will check your newborn's weight a few days after you leave the hospital and perhaps again a week or two later.

Most infants, whether breastfed or bottle fed, will lose an average of 5 to 7 percent of their birth weight in the first days of life, largely because of the loss of excess fluid. How much they lose depends on the plumpness of the baby and individual variations in fluid retention as well as on how well they are nursing. In our experience, when mothers and babies share an uncomplicated birth and feed according to "the rules" (that is, frequent and unrestricted feedings with efficient latch-on), babies tend to lose much less weight. Babies who get off to a slow start at breastfeeding (either because of a medical complication or problems with latch-on) tend to lose more.

Number of wet diapers. A baby who is getting enough milk will have four to six wet diapers a

WEIGHT-GAIN CHECKUPS

Babies who are getting adequate amounts of milk will weigh within one or two ounces of their birth weights at their two-week checkups. Remember to ask the nurses at the hospital to tell you your baby's weight at discharge time; your doctor will want to know this figure at your baby's first checkup, since weight gain is measured from baby's lowest weight, not from the birth weight. If weight gain is marginal (four ounces or less per week), your doctor will continue to monitor your baby's weight. Be sure the same scale is used every time and that your baby is weighed naked. Also, ask that the scale be balanced; otherwise, the result can be off by several ounces.

day by the fourth day after birth (six to eight wet diapers if you're using cloth). Put two tablespoons of water on a diaper to learn what most newborn wet diapers will feel like. It's easier to evaluate the wetness of cloth diapers than superabsorbent disposables. And it may be easier to judge the wetness of a disposable by its weight than by the way it feels to the touch. After the first month or so, your baby's wet diapers will be even wetter — the equivalent of four to six tablespoons of water.

Color of urine. The color of the urine gives you a clue to whether baby is getting enough milk to keep him adequately hydrated. Pale or water-colored urine suggests adequate hydration; darker, apple juice–colored urine (after the first four days) suggests that baby is not getting enough milk. If your baby is not getting sufficient hydration, you may notice a "brick dust" residue on the diaper — the effect of urate crystals from overconcentrated urine (a normal finding in the first few days that should disappear after increasing baby's hydration).

Number and nature of bowel movements. If lots of stool comes out, lots of milk must have gone in. In the first few days, infants' stools gradually change from sticky black meconium stools to green, then brown. Eventually they become milk stools, which are the color of mustard, seedy, and the consistency of cottage cheese. Here's the progression:

- *Meconium stools.* These greenish black, tarlike stools are composed of a lot of debris from the fetal intestines. These stools can last a few days, until the gut is cleaned out. Frequent colostrum feedings speed this process.

- *Transition stools.* Brownish stools occur between days four and seven as the meconium is being completely expelled and mother's milk is increasing.

- *Milk stools.* These frequent mustard-colored, seedy, cottage cheese–like stools appear a day or two after mother's milk becomes mature.

While urine output tells you that baby is getting a sufficient quantity of fluid from the milk, stool output tells you about the *quality* of the milk — that is, whether baby is nursing well enough to get the high-fat hindmilk she needs to grow. Between week 1 and week 4, babies who are getting enough hindmilk will produce at least two to three yellow, seedy stools a day. Because breast milk is a natural laxative, some breastfed babies produce a stool with each feeding, which is a good sign that baby is getting enough milk. When a baby has only two or three bowel movements a day, expect to see a substantial amount in the diaper. After the first month or two, as the gut matures, the frequency of bowel movements decreases. At this stage, your baby may normally have only one bowel movement a day; some breastfed babies have one bowel movement every three to four days but are still getting enough milk. Some babies save up their bowel movements and have what is affectionately dubbed a "mud slide" once a week. As long as baby has an adequate weight gain and is not uncomfortable, this is normal for that baby.

If baby's stools continue to be dark, scant, or infrequent, baby may not be getting enough milk. By *getting enough milk,* we mean both getting enough *volume* and getting enough *calories.* Some babies get enough milk to keep them hydrated but don't nurse long enough or well enough to trigger mother's milk-ejection reflex, which brings them the creamier, high-calorie hindmilk. Babies who don't get enough calories (the creamier hindmilk) may still have a good urine output and appear adequately hydrated (the membranes of their eyes and mouth will be wet), but their weight gain will be poor, their skin will feel loose, and they will act unsatisfied. When week-old babies are not producing sufficient stools, it's time to take a close look at what's going on at the breast. Get help from a lactation consultant.

How your breasts feel before and after a feeding. Usually your breasts will feel fuller before and softer after a feeding. Most mothers will notice a milk-ejection reflex a few minutes after the feeding begins. If you don't feel any sensation in your breasts, watch your baby. His sucking will strengthen and you'll hear more frequent swallowing when the milk-ejection reflex increases the milk flow. Other signs that affirm that your baby is getting enough milk include seeing a few drops of milk leaking from the sides of her mouth and hearing her swallow after every one or two sucks. Baby generally *seems* content during and after a feeding. If you feel your baby sucking vigorously, hear her swallowing, notice your milk-ejection reflex, and see your baby drift contentedly off to sleep, chances are she's getting enough milk.

Nursing tip: *Don't worry about your milk supply.* Remember, breastfeeding is a confidence game, and nothing undermines a mother's confidence like being afraid her baby isn't getting enough milk. If your baby is producing enough wet diapers and bowel movements and is gaining weight, believe that she is getting enough. If you worry constantly about your milk supply, you'll be tempted to offer your baby formula supplements. If you offer supplements, your baby will nurse less at the breast. If your baby takes less milk from the breast, your breasts will make less milk, and then your fears about not having enough milk will become reality. The great majority of nursing mothers *make* enough milk, but some mothers may not *deliver* enough milk to their babies. A faulty delivery system is usually the result of inefficient latch-on, inefficient timing of feeds, inadequate support for breastfeeding, or an overly stressed and tired mother. Nurse your baby frequently throughout the day. Be sure she is latched on and sucking well, and you'll have nothing to worry about.

INCREASING MILK SUPPLY

Our one-month-old doesn't seem to be gaining as much weight as he should. How can I increase my milk supply?

Remember the three *b*'s of breastfeeding: breast, baby, and brain. To increase your milk supply, the breast needs more stimulation from the baby. Helping your baby and breasts work together to make more milk will require some adjustments in your brain, so that you can make breastfeeding a priority.

- *Increase feeding frequency.* Breastfeed your baby at least every two hours. Wake your baby up for feeding during the day if she sleeps more than two hours, and consider waking your baby for at least one extra night feeding. When we talk about the law of supply and demand in relation to breastfeeding, it may seem that we're implying that all babies demand what they need. But this is not always the case. Some babies, especially babies who fall asleep easily and those with mellow personalities, may not breastfeed as frequently as they need to without mother taking the lead. If this sounds like your baby, you need to offer the breast more often.

- *Nurse longer.* Don't limit the length of your baby's feedings to a predetermined number of minutes on each side. Allow your baby to finish the first breast before switching to the other side. This gives baby an opportunity to fill up on the high-fat hindmilk brought down by the milk-ejection reflex. If you switch your baby to the second side too soon, he'll fill up on foremilk from both breasts, which will satisfy his hungry tummy but may not give him enough calories to grow.

- *Use breast compression during feedings.* Breast compression can be used to increase the flow of milk and encourage your baby to feed more effectively. While baby is sucking, grasp your breast with your whole hand and gently squeeze until the sucking pauses. Then rest your hand and wait for the sucking to resume. Once it does, squeeze again until the sucking pauses once more. This is a very effective tool for helping infants gain weight and increasing milk supply because it makes it easy for baby to drink a lot of milk in a short period of time.

- *Try switch nursing.* Sometimes nursing longer (even with breast compression) doesn't work—perhaps because baby is too sleepy, a slow nurser, or gets frustrated that the milk is not flowing fast enough. If you find yourself in this situation, try switch nursing. First, watch your baby carefully. Let him nurse on the first breast until the intensity of his suck and swallow diminishes. Before he drifts off into comfort sucking, switch him to the other breast and encourage him to nurse actively until his sucking diminishes again. Then switch back to the first breast and, finally, finish feeding on the other breast. Rousing your baby by switching him back and forth encourages longer periods of active sucking and swallowing that will enable him to get more of the creamier, higher-calorie hindmilk. Switch nursing is particularly effective for sleepy babies who tend to drift off during feeding before they are able to get enough "grow milk." As an added trick to stimulate more enthusiastic feedings, burp baby just before you switch breasts (this method is also known as the burp-and-switch technique).

- *Try double nursing.* As an alternative to switch nursing, after you feed your baby to his satisfaction, hold him for a while instead of immediately putting him down to sleep. Hold or carry baby upright and awake for ten to fifteen minutes, allowing any trapped air bubbles to be burped up. This makes room for

---

COMFORT SUCKING

Besides delivering milk, your breasts deliver comfort. Many babies show two sucking styles.* In nutritive sucking, baby nurses with enthusiasm and vigor and efficiently milks the breasts. Nonnutritive sucking is characterized by short bursts of weaker sucking with pauses in between; the baby takes less milk and sucks mainly for comfort. Nutritive and nonnutritive sucking have been shown to facilitate milk digestion (sucking increases the enzyme lipase in the intestines) and infant weight gain. Again, babies do what they do for a biological reason. In general, the slower and stronger the suck, the higher the rate of milk delivery, which is why comfort sucking is usually rapid and weaker. Often when babies first begin feeding, they suck in short, rapid bursts, yet once milk begins to flow satisfactorily, their sucking changes to a slower pattern. As they are drifting off to sleep after feeding, babies will often flutter-suck, which is a rapid, quivering type of suck that usually lasts less than a minute.

---

* *Strictly speaking, "suck" refers to the action of the baby ("the baby sucks the breast"), and "suckle" refers to the action of the mother ("the mother suckles the baby"). Most breastfeeding writers now use these words interchangeably.*

---

more milk. Top him off by breastfeeding him on both breasts a second time. Double nursing, like switch nursing, stimulates more milk-ejection reflexes, thus increasing the volume of milk taken and the calorie content of your milk.

- *Undress baby during feedings.* Skin-to-skin contact helps awaken sleepy babies and stimulates less enthusiastic feeders. Also, partially undress yourself to increase the skin-to-skin contact. To prevent baby from getting chilled, place a blanket around his back.

- *Nap nurse and night nurse.* One of the most powerful ways to stimulate milk production is to follow the old adage "Take your baby to bed and nurse." This relaxes both you and your baby and stimulates longer and more frequent nursing. It also increases your milk-producing hormones. Prolactin levels go up when you sleep, and so do the levels of human growth hormone, which is believed to influence milk production, perhaps by working synergistically with prolactin (see page 63).

- *Sling feed.* Naturally, keeping baby inches away from his favorite cuisine will entice him to eat more. Wear your baby in a baby sling as often as you can between feedings. In fact, some babies tend to feed better and more often when on the move. The motion and rhythm of mom walking around helps baby stay alert for the task of sucking.

- *Get focused.* Take inventory of your lifestyle. Are there "drainers" in your life that zap energy that could be better spent in caring for yourself and your baby? Are you trying to do too much, so that you're not taking enough time for your baby? To make more milk for your baby, you have to make breastfeeding and taking care of yourself a priority. Delegate other responsibilities. Confer nonfeeding baby-tending chores and housework upon your partner. Your milk-making hormones can't perform to their fullest potential if you are stressed out by competing activities.

- *Get household help.* If you have a demanding toddler or preschooler, hire a teenager to come to your house after school to entertain that older child so you can sit and relax and nurse your baby. Get help with laundry, dishes, cooking, and cleaning.

- *Get rest.* To make more milk for your baby, you must make more energy for yourself. Treat yourself to exercise, a massage, a daily walk, a couple of naps a day—whatever you need to help you relax and focus on your number one priority: your baby. Relaxation reduces levels of stress hormones, allowing your milk-making hormones to work more efficiently and relax you even more. There are few daily jobs that have to be done by you, yet no one else can make milk for your baby. Sleep when your baby sleeps instead of using this time to "get something done." You *are* getting something done. You are doing the most important job in the world: mothering a human being.

- *No pacifiers, no bottles.* When there are concerns about weight gain, all your baby's sucking should be done at the breast. Bottles of formula will interfere with the balance between your milk supply and baby's needs. So will satisfying your baby's sucking need with a pacifier. If it is medically necessary to give your baby supplementary feedings, avoid using bottles. Use cups, syringes, or finger feeding instead (see page 142).

- *Think MER.* While you are feeding, stroke your baby and make sure she gets a lot of skin-to-skin contact—a practice called grooming. This will help your milk-ejection reflex. Sometimes it's not that you don't make enough milk but that the milk isn't getting to the baby. The milk-ejection reflex squeezes the milk you make out of the milk glands and down into the ducts under the areola, where it's available to the baby (see page 31). Between breastfeedings and immediately before a feeding, imagine your infant nursing at your breast and your breasts pouring out milk to satisfy your baby. Visualizing the milk flowing can actually help trigger your MER.

- *Think baby, think milk.* Breastfeeding is a confidence game. Trust that nature's system works. If you're nursing often enough and baby is sucking effectively, you will make enough milk. It's rare that a mother is unable to produce enough milk for her baby. And while it may seem to you that your life is stressful, mothers throughout history have breastfed their babies through war, famine, and personal tragedies. There's no reason to think that you won't succeed at breastfeeding.

- *Get professional help.* Contact a breastfeeding support group leader and/or a professional lactation consultant for tips on increasing your milk supply. A lactation consultant can also help you evaluate your baby's latch-on and suck so you can be certain that baby is nursing effectively.

- *Consider other remedies.* If despite these measures you are still struggling, it might be time to consider taking an herbal supplement or prescription medication that can treat low milk supply. See pages 111–113 for suggestions.

GROWTH SPURTS

Our three-week-old baby suddenly wants to nurse all the time. Does that mean I don't have enough milk?

No: this is a normal phenomenon. Most likely your baby is going through a growth spurt. These occur at around ten days, three weeks, six weeks, and three months of age. Think of these as *frequency days,* when babies want and need to nurse "all the time." Because of sudden growth, your baby's body suddenly needs more calories, so baby nurses more often. Keep in mind that when baby nurses more frequently he is getting more high-calorie hindmilk. So although the volume may be less, the higher caloric content will meet his needs. In addition, after a day or two of morning, noon, and night "marathon nursing," your body will be making more milk, and baby will resume feeding less often. It's the supply-and-

demand principle of milk production at work— only the demand part comes first, followed by the increased supply of milk. Most moms start out making, per day, about 500 cc of milk, or 16 ounces, the first week of baby's life, a volume that gradually increases via growth spurts to 1,000 cc, or 32 ounces, over the next six months.

Recognize these frequency days as nature's normal message: baby is telling your body that he is going through a growth spurt. When baby steps up his feedings, you need to cut back on your other commitments for a few days. Shelve the energy-draining activities (housework and so on) that can be put off for a while and conserve your energy for extra feedings. Just settle in and nurse your baby. Frequent feedings plus fatigue from too many other commitments lead quickly to exhaustion. Meanwhile, being exhausted will interfere with your body's ability to make more milk. Nature again to the rescue! The more often your baby nurses, the higher the level of milk-making hormones in your body. These will help you to relax during these potentially tiring days. Give yourself the opportunity to let biology work for you. This situation reinforces how important it is for new mothers to keep their lives very simple in the first few months. The stress of having pressing agendas can derail breastfeeding at times when you should be able to give all your energy to making milk for just a few days. A baby is a baby for a very short time, so take the time to enjoy all the nursing and all the holding. No one's life or growth is going to be affected if the housework doesn't get done.

SUPPLEMENTAL BOTTLES

My one-month-old doesn't seem satisfied after feeding. Should I give her a bottle?

Not necessarily. While supplemental bottles are less likely to cause nipple confusion at one month of age than in the first week, there are other

THE BODY CHEMISTRY OF BREASTFEEDING

When your body is allowed to do what it's designed to do, you enjoy better living and better health. Lactation is a prime example of this principle. One of the blessings of lactation is that it produces high levels of stress-relieving hormones at a time in a woman's life when she needs them.

The word *prolactin* means "supporting milk" because it promotes lactation. Prolactin concentration in the blood increases twentyfold during pregnancy and lactation. Levels are highest in the first ten days or so of breastfeeding, just at a time when new mothers need all the hormonal help they can get. When the baby nurses, prolactin levels go sky high, then gradually return to their high baseline levels until the baby nurses again. After peaking during the first days of nursing, baseline prolactin continues to be elevated during the first year. During the first three months, prolactin levels can be ten times higher in lactating women than in nonlactating women. Blood levels of prolactin diminish somewhat the longer breastfeeding continues, but the baby's sucking continues to cause a spike in prolactin levels even during the second year of nursing. In the nonbreastfeeding mother, prolactin returns to prepregnancy levels by two weeks postpartum.

Prolactin levels are significantly higher at night than during the day, and they increase during sleep. This biochemical quirk helps mother relax after daylong baby tending and may explain why many babies prefer night nursing, since mother may make more milk at night. It's interesting that studies have shown that prolactin levels may not increase when mothers just hold and play with their infants, but there is a striking increase within minutes after baby begins to nurse. The most powerful stimulus for keeping your prolactin levels high is frequent breastfeeding. To allow your natural hormones to work best for you, nurse your baby often throughout the day and at night.

The other hormone important to milk production is oxytocin. While prolactin release requires the stimulus of an infant's sucking, a woman's body can release oxytocin in response to her seeing, smelling, grooming, hearing, or just thinking about her baby. Oxytocin can be released as you are preparing to sit down with your baby to nurse, and it is the primary hormone behind the milk-ejection reflex. Oxytocin is released by the pituitary gland in the brain in response to sucking or other stimuli. The hormone causes the bandlike muscle around the milk-producing cells to contract, causing the ejection of milk into the ducts (hence the term *milk-ejection reflex*). Oxytocin contracts not only the muscle tissues around the milk glands but also the muscles of the uterus, accounting for the uterine contractions that most women notice while breastfeeding during the first few days after birth. Stress can inhibit the release of oxytocin, but oxytocin itself is associated with feelings of relaxation and well-being.

Not only does body chemistry support milk production for the baby, it also helps the mother. Compared with nonbreastfeeding mothers, breastfeeding women have decreased levels of stress hormones. Oxytocin also creates calm feelings that help mother and baby enjoy being together.

potential problems with them. While it may seem easier to reach for a bottle, doing so interferes with the balance between mother's milk supply and baby's demand. Baby fills up on formula and does not nurse as well or take as much milk at the next feeding. Your breasts get the message that they should make less milk. Meanwhile, because you gave the bottle, baby won't be hungry at his usual time, and you wind up skipping a breastfeeding, causing you to feel a bit engorged at first. But then your body will respond to this by slowing down its milk production, which lowers your milk supply. Soon your baby is getting two or three bottles a day, either because you don't feel you have enough milk or because you're off doing other things instead of focusing on your baby. Soon you have a diminished milk supply, diminished confidence, and premature weaning.

Immediately clicking into the bottle option keeps you from experimenting with feeding techniques that will work with your biology instead of against it. Rather than reaching for a bottle, reach into your breastfeeding bag of tricks and try the following.

Nursing for a few days. Perhaps your baby is going through a growth spurt and just needs a few days of increased nursing. Let her nurse longer at each feeding, and offer the breast more often — even if it seems like she just finished nursing a little while ago. She'll get more milk and more of the high-fat milk if you nurse more frequently. In addition, use breast compression if you need to increase your milk supply (see page 60).

Allow your baby to finish the first breast first before switching sides. This allows her to get the high-fat hindmilk. Switching sides too soon means she gets only the watery foremilk on both sides, which may fill her tummy without satisfying her appetite. Too much watery milk is

more likely to be produced when mothers watch the clock and change breasts at a specific time — say, after ten or fifteen minutes. So we suggest that you let the baby decide when the main course at the first breast is over before offering dessert on the opposite side. You can also offer the first breast a second time before switching if it doesn't feel empty. But if baby won't latch on or feed a second time, offer the opposite breast just in case the better milk flow will tempt her to eat a little more.

Take inventory of any recent changes in your lifestyle. Are there increased demands in your life that may be draining your energy or interfering with feeding according to baby's cues? Houseguests, holiday preparations, remodeling projects, and the like can distract you from feeding your baby as often as she wants to nurse.

Increase the length of some of your nursing sessions. Try nap nursing and night nursing in bed with your baby (see page 61).

Wear your baby. Perhaps your baby needs extra holding instead of extra milk. Try wearing your baby a couple of hours a day in a sling.

BABY PREFERS BOTTLE

My newborn seems to prefer the bottle to me. Is there something wrong with my milk?

Don't let this undermine your confidence in your breastfeeding abilities. You are making good milk, but your baby has learned to prefer the artificial nipple. With a bottle nipple, babies don't have to suck vigorously. They don't even have to open their mouths wide to take the artificial nipple. With the breast, they have to latch on well and work at it a bit to get the milk flowing. Nipple confusion and nipple preference are among the hazards of giving baby supplemental bottles during the early weeks of breastfeeding.

To correct this situation, start by practicing skin-to-skin contact and laid-back nursing, which promotes self-attachment. Stop the bottles. It isn't fair to expect a new baby to learn two different ways of sucking at the same time.* It also helps when you make it easier for your baby to get milk from your breasts. Faster milk flow is one reason babies learn to prefer the bottle: it dispenses immediate food, and babies don't have to elicit the MER, as they do at the breast. So humor baby a bit—show him that you can deliver instantly, too. Use a pump or hand-expression to get your milk flowing before baby latches on, and his first sucks will be well rewarded. In addition, if needed, you can start a feeding by giving baby a squirt of your pumped milk via syringe at the breast, so that each time he sucks, he'll get the idea and be encouraged to suck more (see page 142). In the long term, use the tricks listed in chapter 2 for encouraging your MER in order to increase your quick delivery of milk. Also, make breastfeeding a social interaction, with eye contact, skin contact, and lots of good feelings. As you woo your baby to the breast, you'll find that you no longer have to compete with the bottle, because your baby will absolutely prefer you to any other milk-delivery system.

WEIGHT GAIN (GROWTH PATTERNS)

How much attention should I be paying to my baby's weight gain?

Weight gain is determined by heredity and temperament as well as by diet, which is why there is such a wide variation in normal patterns of infant weight gain. Babies with different body types have different metabolic rates and therefore burn calories differently. Long and lean babies (we call them "banana babies") are hypermetabolizers. They burn off calories faster than the plumper "apple babies" and "pear babies." Banana babies are likely to grow more quickly in height than weight, so they normally plot above average in height and below average in weight on the growth chart. Apples and pears show the opposite pattern on the chart, usually showing gains in weight faster than in height. All these patterns are normal.

A baby's temperament also influences weight gain. Mellow, laid-back babies tend to burn fewer calories and therefore gain weight more quickly. Active babies with persistent, motor-driven personalities who always seem to be revved up usually burn more calories and tend to be leaner.

The frequency of breastfeeding also influences growth. Babies who are breastfed on cue and offered unrestricted feedings tend to grow better. Also, we have observed that infants who sleep next to mother and who enjoy the luxury of unrestricted night nursing tend to grow faster (see page 190). On the other hand, infants who are the product of "baby training" (parenting programs in which babies are fed on a schedule and encouraged to sleep through the night using variations of the "cry-it-out" method) often show delayed growth. Babies who are breastfed according to a parent-imposed and restrictive feeding schedule are not only likely to get less milk, but the breast milk they get will also have a lower level of fat and calories because of the longer intervals between feedings.

Breastfed and formula-fed babies grow at different rates. In general, breastfed babies tend to be leaner in the long run, which is healthier. In 1992, Dr. Kathryn Dewey of the University of

---

* *However, if you need to supplement your milk with formula for medical reasons, discuss with a doctor or lactation consultant alternative ways to offer it.*

California at Davis conducted a study comparing the growth patterns of normal, healthy breastfed and formula-fed infants. It was dubbed the DARLING study (for Davis Area Research on Lactation, Infant Nutrition, and Growth), and its results showed that breastfed and formula-fed infants grow at basically the same rate in the first few months, but between four and six months of age, formula-fed babies tend to gain weight faster than their breastfeeding peers, although length and head circumference were similar in both groups. After the first six months, breastfed babies tend to become leaner. Compared with their formula-fed friends, the breastfeeding infants in this study gained an average of one pound less during the first twelve months. The extra weight in formula-fed infants is thought to be the result of excess water retention and a different composition of body fat. Researchers in the study concluded that standardized growth charts are needed that will reflect the different growth patterns of healthy, normal breastfeeding babies. Today, such charts are available on the Centers for Disease Control website. These charts demonstrate the normal growth of infants: they are far superior to the older charts, which can make a thriving breastfed baby appear to gain weight poorly and should not be used to assess growth in breastfed infants. See CDC.gov/GrowthCharts for the latest guidelines (click on the WHO charts for babies between birth and age two and the CDC charts for children over the age of two).

While there is a wide variation of normal growth in breastfeeding infants, the following is a general guide to the growth of breastfed babies during the first year:

- 4 to 7 ounces a week from one week to three months
- Around 1 to 1 1/2 pounds per month from three to six months
- Around 3/4 to 1 pound per month from six months to one year
- Growth in length of about an inch a month during the first six months and around one-half inch a month from six months to one year

Another interesting finding from this study was that breastfed infants consume fewer calories than formula-fed infants—not because their mothers don't produce enough milk but because breastfed infants are more likely to self-regulate their calorie intake according to their individual needs. This ability to determine for themselves how much they eat is probably one of the reasons that infants who are breastfed are less likely to become obese later in childhood.

WEIGHING BABY

Should I buy a baby scale and weigh my newborn every day?

This is usually not a good idea. This custom is likely to cause you to focus so much on the scale that you forget to watch your baby for cues or fail to learn to recognize them. Worrying about daily weight gain may actually interfere with your milk supply. Babies normally don't show a steady weight gain. Instead, most babies grow in spurts with no change in weight for a day or two, and then they gain a couple of ounces the next day. It's best to watch your baby instead of the scale. Is he nursing eight to twelve times a day? Does he have sufficient wet diapers and bowel movements? Is he actively sucking and swallowing for fifteen to twenty minutes at every feeding? If you are worried about your baby's weight gain, take your baby to your doctor's office for a weekly weigh-in.

Unless a special electronic scale is used, weighing baby before and after a feed "to see how much milk he's getting" is notoriously inaccurate.

On a typical scale, the varying positions and movements of the baby can cause the readings to fluctuate a few ounces.

FATHER GIVING BOTTLE

I want my husband also to enjoy feeding our newborn. Is it okay for him to give our baby a bottle?

We discourage supplemental bottles, especially during the first month of breastfeeding, because of the risk of disturbing the biological harmony that mother and baby are working so hard to establish. Instead, encourage your husband to understand, respect, and support the uniqueness of the breastfeeding relationship.

Even though fathers can't supply baby's food in the preferred container, dads can "father-nurse." *Nursing* means comforting babies as well as providing food.* Fathers can enjoy the closeness that comes from soothing and comforting their babies. There are plenty of important ways for fathers to nurture babies besides feeding: wearing baby in a sling, playing with baby, giving baths, changing diapers, draping baby over his chest in the "warm fuzzy" position, walking and soothing baby to sleep after a breastfeeding session. And dads can look forward to feeding solids in about six months. Fathers of breastfed babies should not feel left out of the joys and responsibilities of baby care. (For more on a father's role in breastfeeding, see chapter 10.)

---

* *While we were on a speaking tour in Australia to promote breastfeeding, a grandmother (the mother of our host) offered to babysit our nine-month-old breastfeeding infant, Erin, during one of our evening talks. She inquired, "If she wakes up, should I nurse her?" The thought of this grandmother nursing our baby caught us by surprise, to say the least. We all had a good laugh when we realized that in Australia "nurse" means "pick up and comfort."*

EXTRA WATER

Does my breastfeeding baby need extra water?

Breastfeeding babies do not need extra water. Your breast milk contains enough water for your baby (around 90 percent of breast milk is water), even in hot, dry climates. The renal solute load, or concentration of solids, in breast milk delivers just the right amount of water to keep baby's body in physiological balance. The solute load of human milk is much lower than that of formula, because formula contains higher concentrations of salts and minerals. So not only is extra water unnecessary for breastfed babies, but giving bottles of water can also lessen the desire to breastfeed. This interferes with the balance between mother's milk supply and baby's demand. Bottles are also likely to cause nipple confusion and nipple preference. A baby who is too warm or thirsty but not hungry will satisfy his need for more water by feeding more frequently, but just enough to get the watery foremilk, not necessarily the creamier hindmilk. Breastfeeding babies are great self-quenchers of thirst, even in hot climates.

EXTRA VITAMINS

Does my breastfeeding newborn need extra vitamins?

Not usually. It does not seem logical that a milk that has been around for millennia and adapted for the survival of the human species would be deficient in any nutrients. Unless your baby has special nutritional needs, you don't need to give vitamin supplements. When fed by a healthy mother, a healthy, full-term baby who is getting enough breast milk does not need vitamin supplements. Premature infants usually do need vitamin supplements.

In the past, there was some concern about

possible low levels of various vitamins and minerals in breast milk. This led to the routine prescription of vitamin supplements for breastfeeding babies. Newer research has shown that sufficient amounts of iron, for example, are found in human milk in forms readily used by infants for at least the first six months. After six months, babies may need to be fed foods that contain iron. See AskDrSears.com/Iron for tips. Doctors routinely check a baby's hemoglobin during (or shortly before or after) the nine-month checkup.

However, vitamin D supplements, which are now routinely recommended by the American Academy of Pediatrics at birth, are controversial. Certainly they are necessary in the rare situations in which mothers and babies receive very little exposure to the sun, whether because of sunscreen usage, avoidance of the outdoors, or clothing choices that keep their skin covered nearly all the time. But mothers may opt to increase the amount of vitamin D in their milk by taking vitamin D supplements themselves, although pediatric health-care providers are often uncomfortable prescribing supplements to mothers. If you are a vegan—i.e., you eat no animal products at all—you may need to supplement your diet with a third nutrient, vitamin B_{12}. In any case, if you're concerned about your vitamin levels, it makes sense to ask your health-care provider to order a blood test (during pregnancy if possible) to help assess your baby's risk of a vitamin deficiency.

GIVING PACIFIERS

My baby nurses so often that my nipples are getting sore. Can I give her a pacifier?

Babies are born with an intense need to suck. Some infants even suck their thumbs in the womb. Babies not only suck for food, they also love to suck for comfort. Pacifiers are just that—

"peace makers"—but there is no more satisfying pacifier than mother's breast as baby nurses contentedly off to sleep following a feed. We discourage the use of artificial pacifiers in the early weeks while baby is learning to latch on at your breast. Pacifiers may also keep babies from nursing frequently enough to gain weight adequately. Some studies report that mothers who used pacifiers during the first six weeks after birth tended to wean their babies earlier.

Realistically, however, the human pacifier (mom) sometimes wears out. We suggest offering the baby an adult finger to suck on if mother's nipples are sore or her patience is wearing thin. Or try alternative methods of comforting your baby—walking, babywearing, patting her back, enjoying a "warm fuzzy" with dad. Realize, too, that there's nothing wrong with being a human pacifier. You want your baby to learn to seek comfort from people, not plastic.

LARGE BREASTS

I have large breasts. Are there special things I should do to make breastfeeding easier?

While babies can nurse quite efficiently from breasts of all sizes and shapes, you and your baby will both be more comfortable if you try these tips:

- Elevate your breasts to make it easier for your baby to latch on. You can use your hand to do this, but it is much easier to roll up a small towel or fold up a diaper to wedge under your breasts. Some mothers may prefer to purchase a breast pillow, which was specifically designed for this purpose.

- Throughout the feeding, support the weight of your breasts from underneath with the fingers and palm of your hand. This keeps the weight of the breast off the baby's chin.

- Use the nipple-sandwich technique (see chapter 2), which in effect presents baby with smaller breasts for more manageable latch-on.

- To keep from getting a sore back, use pillows to bring baby up to your breasts rather than leaning forward to feed baby.

- Take steps to prevent engorgement (see chapter 2).

- Wear a good supportive nursing bra for your own comfort. Large-size nursing bras are available online.

Some mothers have noticed that after weaning, their breasts actually become smaller than their prepregnant size.

READY TO QUIT

My baby is two weeks old, and breastfeeding isn't going well, to say the least. My nipples are sore, baby doesn't seem satisfied, and quite frankly, I'm not satisfied, either. Help!

Breastfeeding is meant to be a pleasurable experience; otherwise, the human race would not have survived. In our experience, breastfeeding nearly always works, providing the mother gets support and instruction during the first couple of weeks. In most cases, it's not the fault of the mother or the baby that breastfeeding isn't working. It's the support and instructional system that is failing. Try these suggestions:

Get help. Seeing a lactation consultant in the first few days of breastfeeding increases your chance of breastfeeding success, since positioning and latch-on techniques are the keys to establishing good milk production and delivery. If you're still having problems with breastfeeding at one or two weeks postpartum, see the lactation consultant again. Instead of just suffering, solve those problems.

Get rest. Cultures throughout the world have long recognized there is something magical about the first six weeks of life. Many cultures have a custom by which the mother is given lots of support and rest and is freed from all responsibilities except learning to care for and breastfeed her baby. Some cultures refer to this as the "one moon cycle," others as "the first forty days." Get help at home so that you can concentrate on feeding your baby. Getting help is especially necessary in large families, which is why Martha often advises breastfeeding mothers, "Don't take your nightgown off for at least two weeks." This is one of the high points of your life, when you should be free to do the job that no one else in the whole world can do as well as you: nurture yourself and nurture your baby. Your job is to make milk and delegate responsibility to others to make everything else. In the early weeks, don't expect to try to make milk for your baby and three meals a day for your family.

Be confident. Veteran mothers have long dubbed breastfeeding a confidence game. When you believe in your breasts, they will work for you. If you don't believe you can breastfeed, you set yourself up for all the problems that lead to failure. A doubt can become a self-fulfilling prophecy. Doubts about the ability to make milk are very common in the first week for first-time mothers, since in the first week of feeding it's hard to see anything happening. (Actually, even on the first day of breastfeeding, baby gets the small-volume but high-quality milk called colostrum.) Surround yourself with positive people, preferably those who believe in breastfeeding and who themselves have had successful breastfeeding experiences. If you didn't attend breastfeeding support group meetings during pregnancy, start going now. At these meetings you can talk about the problems you're having breastfeeding without anyone saying, "Are you sure you have enough milk?" or "Maybe you should give a bottle."

STRESSBUSTING

You can deliver enough milk to your baby even under the most stressful conditions. After all, for centuries mothers have successfully breastfed their babies during wars, famines, and floods. This is not, however, the kind of stress that gets to us on a day-to-day basis. The adrenal hormones that surge when you're overstressed can interfere with the hormones that make milk. Breastfeeding requires your body to be in hormonal balance. Chronic unresolved stress throws off the biochemical equilibrium of your body, which is why some women notice a reduction in their milk supply following a family crisis, such as illness or job loss, and why unhealthful reactions to the daily grind can zap a milk supply. Following are the stressbusters that we have found most effective when we counsel breastfeeding mothers.

1. Realize that you can't control situations, but you can control your reactions to them. Stress happens. Children get sick. People lose jobs. Some setbacks in life are beyond your control. Yet what is always within your control is how you react to these setbacks.

2. Focus on solutions, not problems. This destressor is especially valuable for breastfeeding mothers. If your milk supply suddenly dwindles or your nipples are sore, instead of filling your mind with "I can't do it" thoughts, believe in your body. It will work for you. Have a support group you can check in with when a problem pops up. Knowing whom to complain to keeps you from getting unhelpful advice.

3. Focus on the biggies and not the smallies. Don't miss sleep or waste energy over little annoyances that reduce your energy for making milk and caring for your baby. As the popular book title suggests, "Don't sweat the small stuff (and it's all small stuff)." Taking care of your baby is the "biggie" to focus on.

4. Feel good about yourself. Each day remind yourself that you are doing the most important job in the world: nurturing a human being. And you are doing what no one else in the whole world can do: make milk that is custom tailored to meet the needs of your baby. Each day (or even at each feeding) remind yourself that the milk you are giving your infant is going to make your baby smarter and healthier. The milk you are giving your baby is going to raise his IQ and lower the risk of every major illness. You're Dr. Mom. You are very important.

5. Learn to relax. Chronic, unresolved stress exhausts your brain's neurotransmitters, keeping you from feeling good and thinking clearly. Relaxation allows these neurotransmitters to recuperate from the exhaustion created by stress. Set aside some minutes each day for quiet time, whether it's soaking in a tub, taking a walk, or lying down. Giving birth and breastfeeding your baby helps you learn to tune in to your body. Now learn to tune in to your mind. You can do this easily by listening to music while you breastfeed. Music is thought to relax the mind and body by stimulating those "feel-good" hormones, endorphins. Relaxing your mind helps you make milk. Filling your mind with images of baby instead of disturbing thoughts gets your milk-making hormones flowing. As a bit of preventive medicine, as soon as you feel a disturbing thought coming on, quickly switch channels and fill your mind with positive thoughts before negative ones sink in.

STRESSBUSTING (continued)

6. Laugh and play a lot. There is a biochemical basis for the belief that laughter is the best medicine. It, too, stimulates endorphins. Hang out with people who know how to laugh. Rent funny movies; read joke books. Watch *I Love Lucy* reruns. Plan a fun party. Three enjoyable activities that have been shown to increase endorphins are exercise, laughter, and sex—all of which a breastfeeding mother can enjoy.

Get comfortable. Make feeding time special time. Play music to relax by. Choose a comfortable place in your home for breastfeeding and look forward to feeding time. If your nipples are sore, find ways to prevent soreness and treat them; pain or the expectation of pain can suppress your MER. Often, nap nursing—nursing while lying with your baby in bed—will relax you enough to trigger your MER, even if your nipples are sore. Or try the breathing you learned in childbirth class or other ways of relaxing. (For more on stimulating your MER, see chapter 2.)

Time is on your side. Certain anatomic quirks in newborns can make breastfeeding more challenging at the beginning. Baby's tongue may be relatively large compared to his small oral cavity or his jaw somewhat receded, so that baby has difficulty opening his mouth wide enough to grasp the areola as well as the nipple. As baby grows, the lower jaw moves downward. The tongue and the jaw protrude forward, and the oral cavity gradually enlarges, making latch-on easier and more efficient.

In our experience, once they get over the hump of the first few weeks, nearly all mothers and their babies are able to settle into a mutually pleasurable breastfeeding experience.

When I got discouraged I called a lactation consultant who reminded me that breastfeeding was the best gift I could give my baby. That did it for me! I realized that I had prepared the perfect nursery and layette, but that breastfeeding was more important than anything I could buy for her.

Nursing tip: *Prepare a nursing station.* Set up an area in your home as a nest for mother and baby, containing a rocking chair or other chair with arms at a comfortable height to support your arms for holding baby, a few pillows, a footstool, and a table to hold the things you'll want: a relaxing book, nutritious nibbles, a diaper and wipes, an extra T-shirt, and a glass of juice or water. Set up this station in your favorite room in the house, the one that gives you peace, quiet, and, preferably, a nice view. Listen to soothing music rather than watching a screen, which can be less relaxing and can keep you from tuning in to your baby. A nursing station helped Martha relax while breastfeeding our babies around all the activities of a busy family. Babies like a nice nest during feeding times, and so do mommies.

BABY PREFERS ONE BREAST

My baby prefers to nurse on one breast, and I'm looking a bit lopsided. What can I do?

It's usual for one breast to be more efficient than the other at storing and delivering milk. Babies soon learn which breast works best, and they prefer to go to that breast first. Sometimes there's no apparent reason why baby prefers one side. To keep your breasts from looking lopsided, try to begin each feeding and nurse more frequently on the less favored and often smaller breast. You may need to pump a few drops first to entice the one-sided nursing baby onto the disfavored breast. If baby still would rather fight than switch, don't worry as long as baby is thriving and getting most of the needed milk from one breast. Eventually, at least when you are finished nursing, your breasts will return to a more even size.

CLIPPING TIGHT TONGUES AND LIP TIES

My lactation consultant thinks that our newborn has tongue-tie. Could this interfere with nursing?

Yes. If the tip of baby's tongue is attached too tightly to the floor of the mouth, baby may not be able to extend the tongue over the gum and curl it into a trough underneath the nipple and areola for effective sucking. While in the past it has been customary to leave tight tongue tips alone because most loosen with time, Bill has for decades been clipping the frenulum (the thin membrane that attaches the tongue to the floor of the mouth) if it appears too tight and baby is not latching on well. These are the signs that the tongue is tight enough to warrant clipping: latch-on and sucking are painful to mother, or baby is not getting enough milk; the tip of the tongue doesn't extend past the lower gum; the tongue curls downward when baby cries, opens her mouth wide, or tries to suck (it should curl upward and form a trough). After this painless, thirty-second office procedure to release the tongue, mothers notice that latch-on is more effective and comfortable. In the early weeks, the frenulum is so thin that it's easy for your health care professional to snip with a scissors and usually yields only a few drops of blood or none at all. Here is the procedure Bill uses: while baby's mouth is wide open he holds the tip of the tongue with a piece of gauze (sometimes, if the mouth is open wide enough, holding the tongue is not necessary) and clips the frenulum back to the place where it joins the base of the tongue. Baby can go to the breast immediately for comforting. If your doctor or

lactation consultant feels that you are having breastfeeding problems caused by tongue-tie, get it clipped.

Lip ties, which occur when baby's lip is tied via a thin piece of tissue to the middle of the upper gum, can interfere with latching on, cause nipple trauma, and even cause cavities. The tissue causes the lip to curl inward, which can rub on the nipple and interfere with baby's ability to form a seal on the breast. Like snipping the frenulum, snipping the lip tie is also a simple procedure and is relatively bloodless and painless.

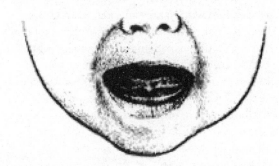

Tongue-tie

BREASTFEEDING AND FERTILITY

I've heard that breastfeeding can keep me from getting pregnant. Is this true?

We will answer this important question by referring to Sheila Kippley's book *The Seven Standards of Ecological Breastfeeding: The Frequency Factor.* The short answer to your question is that breastfeeding does not keep you from getting pregnant *unless* you practice what's known as "ecological breastfeeding," in which the mother meets her baby's needs for frequent suckling and full-time presence. A brief outline of the book will explain what the seven standards involve.

First standard: Breastfeed exclusively for the first six full months. Give your baby nothing but your milk, suckled only from your breasts. Give your baby no water bottles, no bottles of pumped milk, and delay starting solids until the age of six months or later. Exclusive breastfeeding is 98–99 percent effective in postponing pregnancy when (1) baby is less than six months old, (2) you have had no menstrual bleeding after the fifty-sixth day postpartum, (3) you truly follow exclusive breastfeeding, and (4) baby does not go more than six hours between feeds. This is the lactational amenorrhea method (LAM) of natural family planning.

Second standard: Pacify your baby at your breasts. Studies show that pacifier use is associated with an earlier return of menstruation. Comfort sucking, nonnutritive, gives babies the extra sucking they need and provides the extra hormone surge in mom that maintains natural infertility.

Third standard: Don't use bottles and pacifiers. This is implied in the first and second standards. We are repeating it here to reinforce the point that pumping your breast milk and giving it in a bottle will not have the same suppressing effect on your fertility-hormone levels.

Fourth standard: Sleep with your baby for night feedings. Extended breastfeeding infertility is associated with night feedings. Don't train your baby to sleep through the night. Nighttime breastfeeding maintains a steady milk supply and keeps your hormone levels primed for delayed ovulation. Sleeping with your baby is the key (see page 61).

Fifth standard: Sleep with your baby for a daily nap feeding. Avoiding fatigue will help your milk supply, which will help keep your fertility hormones suppressed. Babies need their naps, and so do mothers—there is nothing to feel guilty about ("But I could be getting so much done!") when you practice self-care. One of our favorite family sayings is "What a baby needs most is a happy, rested mother!"

Sixth standard: Nurse frequently day and night and avoid schedules. As we have already stated, it is the frequency of suckling that helps a mother breastfeed successfully. It is also what prolongs natural infertility after childbirth. Once again, studies show this, and personal experience in our family and in our practice bears this out. One thing is for sure: you learn to breastfeed in many different settings and circumstances.

Seventh standard: Avoid any practice that restricts nursing or separates you from your baby. Nature intends for mother and baby to be one, a biological unit. There is no reason to leave your baby at home. People got used to our showing up with our babies everywhere we went. (The nursery rhyme "Mary Had a Little Lamb" comes to mind.) This is countercultural in our society, where babysitters are the norm, so it is important to have support from family and friends.

To summarize: natural child spacing involves mother-baby inseparability. Frequent and unrestricted breastfeeding is a natural consequence of this inseparability, and the result is prolonged postpartum infertility and, most important of all, happier mothers and babies.

To learn more about ecological breastfeeding, to find support, to learn what comes next before you resume your periods, and to order the book, go to NFPandMore.org, a resource of Natural Family Planning International. Now is a good time to learn about natural family planning methods, which enable you to determine exactly when you are ovulating and could become pregnant.

LESS MILK DURING MENSTRUATION

My baby is only five months old. I just got my period and seem to be losing my milk. I really want to breastfeed for at least a year. What's happening?

Any change in hormones that affects your body often affects your milk supply. The hormones that trigger menstruation can cause mothers to feel anxious, restless, and experience a temporary decline in milk supply. The beginning of a menstrual period may also temporarily change the taste of breast milk, although many babies don't notice or seem to mind. After your period is over, your milk supply will return to normal. For a few days, baby may seem unsatisfied, and you may be tempted to wean or give a bottle, especially if you're feeling irritable and less confident than usual. Stick with breastfeeding until your period is over, and things will soon get back to normal. If supplements are needed temporarily, use your stored breast milk (see the discussion of building up a milk bank in chapter 7) and give it to baby in a cup so that baby doesn't get used to the bottle nipple.

Also, take the return of your periods as a cue to step up the frequency of breastfeeding, especially if your baby has begun solid foods, a recent change in lifestyle has caused you to extend the interval between daytime feedings, or baby is sleeping for longer stretches at night. Breastfeeding veterans have long considered the return of menstruation in the first six months a sign that baby is not breastfeeding frequently enough.

RELACTATING

I recently weaned my three-month-old, but she's become allergic to formula. How can I get my milk back?

You can get your body to produce milk again by allowing your baby to suck at your breast. How much milk you will produce and how soon depends on your baby's willingness to take the breast, how long it has been since you weaned, and your individual body's response. Relactation takes commitment and time. The best way to start is by gradually offering fewer bottles so that baby will be interested in having more suck time

at your breast. Also, until you see how much of your own breast milk you will be able to bring back, consider using donor milk to supplement it. Then use these strategies:

- As you discontinue the use of bottles, try alternative ways of delivering supplements, such as a nursing supplementer (also known as an SNS, or supplemental nursing system — see page 142) and finger feeding. Nursing supplementers generally work best with babies less than three months of age. Older infants can be too impatient to be satisfied with the slow drip of milk through the tubing. Use cup feeding instead.

- Woo your baby back to the breast. Some babies are reluctant to nurse at the breast after weeks of bottle feeding. Give baby lots of skin-to-skin contact. Wear her in the baby sling throughout the day and put her to the breast frequently while she's in the sling. Spending the day in a carrier close to your breasts gives baby a chance to rekindle her memory of breastfeeding. Revisit baby's favorite nursing environments, such as the rocking chair or your bed. Until she is willing to spend time sucking, use a breast pump to "wake up" your milk production hormones.

- Breastfeed your baby when she is most willing and eager to suck, such as before bed and upon awakening. Some babies take the breast better in a darkened, quiet room, some in the bathtub, some in the sling while mother is walking around the house.

- Sleep with your baby and nap nurse (see page 61).

- Don't plan on doing much else besides breastfeeding during the time you are working to get your baby to take the breast and to build up your milk supply. Spend all your time with your baby. Get lots of rest and take care of yourself, just as you did right after giving birth.

- Use the breast as a pacifier rather than using an artificial one. Baby may nurse willingly for comfort even when there is not much milk.

- If baby pulls away from the breast to protest the lack of milk, feed her first with a cup or bottle and finish the feeding at the breast. Feed frequently: you don't want her to get so hungry that she can't relax and suck. This behavior will diminish as your milk supply increases.

- Consult your health-care provider about using medications to help induce relactation.

- Watch your baby's diapers to be sure she is getting enough to eat. As she takes more of your milk, her stools will become softer and yellower.

- Read the section on breastfeeding an adopted baby (in chapter 11). If mothers who have never been pregnant or have never breastfed can make milk, so can you.

As a general guide, the time it takes to get your milk supply back will equal the amount of time that has passed since you weaned. If you weaned a month ago, it will probably take around a month to get your milk supply built up to the point where you can meet all baby's needs for nourishment at the breast. Don't be disappointed if you do not return to your previous level of milk production; giving your baby some of your milk guarantees her at least some of the benefits of breast milk and breastfeeding. Relactation is most successful if baby is three months of age or younger. After three months, relactation is still possible, but the older baby is, the less likely you are to produce enough milk to totally satisfy her nutritional needs. But even if you must supplement with hypoallergenic formula—or,

better yet, donor breast milk—you and your baby can enjoy your return to the closeness of breastfeeding. Focus on enjoying your baby, not just on how much milk you can make.

COLIC (A.K.A. THE HURTING BABY)

Our baby seems to be in pain, especially after I breastfeed. Is something wrong with my milk? Does she have colic?

There's nothing wrong with your milk, but it's possible that your baby is hurting because he is either (1) feeding too fast and furiously, (2) sensitive to something you are eating that gets into your milk (such as cow's milk and other dairy products), or (3) suffering from gastroesophageal reflux disease (GERD). First, remember that *colic* is a five-letter word meaning "the doctor doesn't know." Instead of calling it colic, we prefer to describe the baby who is painfully fussy as the *hurting baby*. This description motivates both the mother and the health-care provider to keep searching for reasons behind baby's complaints so the problem can be corrected. Here are some causes of fussiness to consider when your baby cries and complains after feedings.

Some babies feed so fast and switch from breast to breast so soon that they fill up on foremilk before they get the high-fat hindmilk, and foremilk contains higher concentrations of lactose. If the amount of lactose that arrives in the intestines is greater than the ability of the intestines to digest it, the excess lactose ferments, causing gas; bloating; watery, explosive, greenish bowel movements (this blowout may even occur during feedings); and a sore, red rash around the anus. This is enough to make anybody complain. These babies are not, strictly speaking, lactose intolerant; it's more a case of lactose overload. To correct the situation, mothers should feed baby on just one breast until he seems satisfied and decides

BURPING THE BREASTFEEDING BABY

You seldom see a baby being burped in non-Western breastfeeding cultures. The belief that babies need burping after feedings, or help "bringing up the wind," originated with the spread of bottle feeding. The faster flow of milk from bottle nipples forces babies to gulp air in between closely spaced swallows. Breastfeeding infants have fewer problems with air in their tummies. They can control the flow of milk at the breast, so they suck with a slower rhythm, which allows them to better coordinate breathing and swallowing. Also, breastfed babies tend to be fed in a more upright position and enjoy smaller, more frequent feedings, conditions that also lessen the swallowing of air. Yet even breastfed babies need to be burped occasionally, especially if they are fast feeders and/or mother has a strong milk-ejection reflex.

To lessen the likelihood that baby will swallow air at the breast, feed baby in an upright position (of at least a forty-five-degree angle). Help baby comfortably keep a tight seal during latch-on—and throughout the feed, if necessary—by supporting the weight of your breast and by wrapping baby around you rather than letting baby dangle away from the breast. Watch for signs that baby needs to burp during or after a feeding: she may balk at going to the other breast or she may squirm and grimace when you lay her down; there may be a pained expression on her face. Some babies are more comfortable if they burp when changing sides. Getting the air up makes room for more milk. This can help avoid large spit-ups when an air bubble gets trapped under the milk. If baby is content, the need to burp is past—if she even needed to burp at all. Don't feel you have failed if you don't manage to bring up a burp after every feeding. Babies often don't need to burp with snack-type feedings; after a big meal, it's usually worth putting in some patient effort

until baby burps. As babies get older and more proficient at feeding, burping becomes less of an issue. Try these burping positions:

- *Over-the-hand burp.* Sit baby on your lap and place the heel of your hand against her tummy, with her chin resting on the top of your hand. Lean baby forward, resting most of her weight against the heel of your hand to provide counterpressure on her tummy, and pat her on the back to move up the air bubbles.

- *Over-the-shoulder burp.* Drape baby way up over

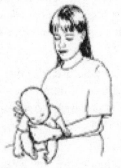

Over-the-hand burp

your shoulder so that your shoulder presses against her tummy, then rub or pat her back. Hold baby securely by hooking your thumb under her armpit. If she's on your right shoulder, do this holding with your right hand.

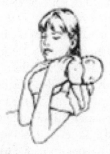

Over-the-shoulder burp

BURPING THE BREASTFEEDING BABY (continued)

- *Over-the-leg burp*. Drape baby over one thigh (legs crossed or spread) so that it presses upward against her tummy. Support baby's head with one hand while you pat or rub her back with the other hand.

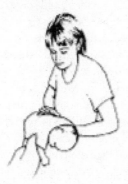

Over-the-leg burp

- *One-arm burp*. This position is particularly helpful when you're busy and baby needs to burp. Drape baby over your forearm so that your wrist presses against her tummy. You can simply stroll around the house and have one hand free. The only drawback is that spit-up may go on the floor or down over your arm.

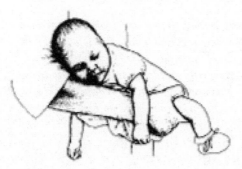

One-arm burp

- *Sling burp*. If the air just won't come up, place baby upright against your chest and wear her in a sling until the air comes up.

- *Nighttime burp*. Burping is often not necessary during night feedings, since babies feed in a more relaxed manner and therefore swallow less air at night. If a trapped air bubble seems to be causing nighttime discomfort, you can avoid sitting up and going through the whole burping ritual by draping baby up over your hip as you lie on your side.

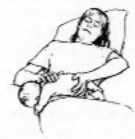

Nighttime burp

- *Knee-to-chest "burp"*. Sometimes babies need help getting air not only out the top end but also out the bottom. The knee-to-chest position helps baby pass excess gas.

to come off the breast by himself. Then offer the second side for however long baby is interested. In some cases, this problem can be attributed to an oversupply of milk: keep baby feeding at one breast only for a period of two to three hours, then switch to the other side for the next two to three hours. Soon your supply should settle down to match baby's needs.

Sometimes babies fuss after feedings because they get too much milk too fast as a result of an overactive milk-ejection reflex (see page 123). They gulp milk and swallow air, which can lead to uncomfortable tummies and colicky behavior.

Babies may also swallow air when they don't have a good seal on the breast. Be sure baby's lips are far back on the areola and you don't hear any clicking sounds that would indicate baby is breaking suction with each suck. Practice good burping technique and burp baby more frequently. See the box on page 76 for instructions.

Foreign proteins in mother's milk are a common cause of colic. The milk proteins in dairy products are the most likely and best-researched culprits. (See the discussion of food allergies, sensitivities, and intolerances, as well as what foods to avoid, in chapter 4 to learn how to track down the offending substances in your diet.)

Finally, one of the most common hidden medical causes of colicky behavior and night waking is a condition known as gastroesophageal reflux (GER), in which irritating stomach acids are regurgitated into baby's esophagus, causing pain that adults would call heartburn. Clues that your baby may suffer from reflux are painful bursts of night waking; fussiness, particularly after eating; frequent spitting up (though not all babies with

GER spit up regularly); frequent bouts of abdominal pain; frequent, unexplained wheezing and chest infections; and throaty sounds after feeding. If you or your doctor suspects your baby has GER, above all continue to breastfeed, since studies show that GER is less severe in breastfed babies. Medications prescribed to alleviate reflux symptoms act as antacids, and some cause the milk to empty faster from the stomach. Breast milk empties twice as fast from the stomach as formula does, so you're already ahead of the game if you're breastfeeding.

Try these other remedies to ease your baby's GER discomfort: feed your baby twice as often for half as long — small, frequent feedings help the stomach to empty even faster to lessen GER. Also, take advantage of gravity to hold the milk down by keeping baby upright and quiet for at least thirty minutes after a feeding. Discuss with your doctor the safest sleeping position for your baby if she has reflux. As the muscular valve between baby's esophagus and stomach matures (usually during the second half of the first year, which accounts for the observation that babies "walk away from the reflux"), this painful condition will subside. (For updates on GER, see AskDrSears.com/reflux.)

At age five months, and after four pediatricians, Jacob was diagnosed with gastroesophageal reflux. I am forever grateful I did not give up! The goal of one of Jacob's reflux meds was to help digestion, so he would not reflux. What could be better for him than the most easily digested food for babies... mom's milk! When the specialist first met Jacob, he was shocked to see him look so happy. He told me that most babies with that degree of reflux failed to thrive and were very sickly. I am convinced that Jacob did not fail to thrive because he was nursed.

III

Healthy Breastfeeding

The food you eat influences the milk you make. Breastfeeding may be just the motivation you need to upgrade your eating habits or continue the healthful eating you began during pregnancy. In this section you will get a crash course in nutrition and fitness. It's our wish that you will emerge from your breastfeeding relationship a healthier person. Many mothers tell us that breastfeeding their babies encouraged them to make healthful lifestyle changes. In this section we also tell you what to do if you get sick, if you must take medications, or if you experience a health problem related to breastfeeding. The good news, as you will learn, is that there are very few medications that you cannot safely take while breastfeeding and that nearly all breastfeeding problems can be solved or prevented entirely.

4

Nutrition and Fitness While Breastfeeding

DURING LACTATION, as during pregnancy, your body nourishes your baby's body. Just as your blood carried the nutrients your baby needed to grow and develop in the womb, your milk furnishes all the nutrients your baby needs after birth. Mothers all over the world make good-quality milk for their babies, many of them with less than adequate diets for themselves. But new insights into nutrition suggest that a nutritious diet for mother will make her milk even more nutritious and will help her cope with the stress of caring for a new baby.

A mother's body guards valuable nutrients during pregnancy and lactation. Calcium, for example, is absorbed more efficiently and less is excreted. There's no need to obsess about having to eat "just right" while breastfeeding. It's quite simple. In a nutshell, good nutrition while breastfeeding means eating foods that are good for you—and just a bit more than you would normally consume.

DR. BILL AND MARTHA'S TIPS FOR HEALTHFUL EATING WHILE BREASTFEEDING

Good nutrition and good sense go together. So turn on your "mommy brain"—that extra center in your brain that you grew while growing your baby in your womb. Yes, mommy brain is real. It's like a radar system implanted in your brain that helps you make the right decisions about what is best for your baby. Follow this commonsense logic:

- A breastfeeding mother needs to eat more of the nutrients her growing baby needs.

- A breastfeeding mother needs to eat less of the junk foods her growing baby does not need.

- A breastfeeding mother needs to eat more of the nutrients that give her mental and physical energy.

This follows the one simple piece of wisdom we mention throughout the Sears Parenting Library: **What your baby needs most is a happy, rested, well-nourished mother.**

So what "diet" should you be on while breastfeeding? Answer: the Real Food Diet. It's that simple.

THE NINE TOP NUTRIENTS YOU NEED TO EAT WHILE BREASTFEEDING

To best nourish your growing baby, consume *extra* amounts each day of the following nutrients in the quantities listed in the left-hand column.

Nutrients You Need	Best Food Sources
1,000 milligrams omega-3 DHA	Salmon, 6 ounces: 2,000 milligrams
25 grams protein	Seafood, yogurt, kefir
800 milligrams calcium	Kefir, yogurt, tofu, canned salmon
400 micrograms folic acid	Spinach, 1 cup: 260 micrograms Lentils, ½ cup: 200 micrograms
12 milligrams iron	Hawaiian spirulina, 1 teaspoon: 7 milligrams
1,000 IU vitamin D	Salmon, 6 ounces: 1,000 IU Sunshine
2 micrograms vitamin B_{12}	Salmon, 3 ounces: 4 micrograms Egg, 1 whole: 0.5 microgram
220 micrograms iodine	Salmon, 6 ounces: 100 micrograms Nori, 1 serving: 100 micrograms
300 milligrams choline	Salmon, 6 ounces: 190 milligrams Egg yolk, 1: 100 milligrams

TOP TWELVE FOODS

Food	Important Nutrients
Avocado	Thiamin, niacin, folic acid, fiber, protein, riboflavin, vitamin B_6, zinc
Eggs	Protein, vitamin A, riboflavin, vitamin B_{12}, folic acid
Fish (salmon, tuna)	Protein, niacin, vitamin B_{12}, zinc, iron, omega-3 fatty acids
Flaxseed and flax oil	Omega-3 fatty acids; seeds also rich in protein, fiber, thiamin, riboflavin, niacin
Kidney beans	Protein, fiber, thiamin, folic acid, calcium, zinc, iron
Lentils	Protein, fiber, riboflavin, vitamin B_6, folic acid, iron; intestine-friendly food
Nuts, raw	Protein, fiber, riboflavin, calcium, zinc, iron, vitamin E, healthful fats

TOP TWELVE FOODS (continued)

Food	Important Nutrients
Sweet potatoes	Fiber, vitamin A, beta carotene, vitamin C, riboflavin, phytonutrients
Tomatoes	Vitamin A, vitamin C, phytonutrients (especially lycopene)
Turkey, organic	Protein, niacin, vitamin B_{12}, zinc, iron
Whole grains	Protein, fiber, vitamin A, thiamin, riboflavin, niacin, vitamin B_{12}, folic acid, zinc, iron
Yogurt (plain, organic, whole milk)	Protein, calcium, zinc, folic acid, riboflavin, lactobacilli for colon health

HONORABLE MENTION

Food	Important Nutrients
Artichokes	Protein, fiber, vitamin A, vitamin C, thiamin, riboflavin, niacin, folic acid, calcium, zinc, iron
Broccoli	Vitamin A, vitamin C, folic acid, beta carotene, phytonutrients
Cantaloupe	Carotenoids, vitamin A, vitamin C, beta carotene
Chickpeas (especially tasty when made into hummus)	Protein, fiber, folic acid, vitamin B_6, calcium, zinc, iron
Oranges	Fiber, calcium, vitamin A, folic acid, vitamin C, carotenoids
Papaya	Fiber, vitamin C, folic acid, phytonutrients
Peanut butter	Protein, fiber, niacin, zinc, vitamin E
Pink grapefruit	Vitamin C, fiber, carotenoids
Soy nuts	Protein, folic acid, calcium, zinc, iron, vitamin E
Spinach	Vitamin A, folic acid, calcium
Sunflower seeds	Protein, unsaturated fats, fiber, niacin, folic acid, zinc, iron, vitamin E, selenium
Tofu (firm)	protein, fiber, vitamin A, thiamin, folic acid, calcium, zinc, iron, unsaturated fats, phytonutrients

You Don't Need to Count Calories During Breastfeeding

Eat smarter calories, not necessarily more calories. That is, instead of concentrating on the *number* of calories you eat, focus on their nutritional *quality*. Eat nutrient-dense foods, those that pack a lot of nutrients into each bite. For example, a palmful of nuts and a bagel may contain the same number of calories, but the nuts provide many, many more of the nutrients you and your baby need.

1. Go fish! A six-ounce fillet of wild salmon wins our nutrient-dense food award. (For a list of safe seafood sources as well as the nutritional profile of salmon, see AskDrSears.com/seafood.)

2. Go green! Try to eat one large plateful, or four fistfuls, of greens a day. Dark green vegetables such as broccoli, spinach, kale, chard, arugula, collard greens, and asparagus are good sources of the vitamins and minerals you and your baby need. And greens are a good nondairy source of calcium. As an extra perk, greens are high in fiber, which keeps things moving along, since postpartum mothers are often prone to constipation.

3. Go nuts! Nuts are one of Dr. Mother Nature's most balanced foods: they contain protein, fiber, and healthful fats. Nuts make a perfect snack because they enjoy what is called a *high satiety factor,* meaning it takes only a relatively small quantity to fill you up. Because nuts require lots of chewing, you get satisfied sooner and are unlikely to overeat. *Raw* nuts are an even more nutritious choice.

4. Enjoy avocados. Avocados win our most healthful fruit award because they are extremely nutrient-dense—rich in healthful fats, vitamins and minerals, and protein and fiber. Moreover, avocados—and guacamole—make nutritious additions to salads and omelets, and a half an avocado blends well into your daily smoothie.

5. Eat eggs. Besides salmon and avocados, eggs are some of the most nutrient-dense foods you can eat. For a mere seventy-five calories, you enjoy six grams of protein, many vitamins and minerals, and healthful fats. In addition, egg yolks contain choline, a valuable nutrient for baby's growing brain. In fact salmon and egg yolks are the best food sources of choline available. Egg yolks are also rich in the vision-building antioxidants lutein and zeaxanthin. Remember, the eye is part of the brain, so what's good for the brain is also good for the eye. We further advise that you enjoy the whole egg. Egg-white-only omelets are now going the way of the corded phone. An egg a day does not put on extra fat, nor, in most people, does it elevate cholesterol.

If by now you're wondering why our recommended foods are high in healthful fats, it's for three reasons: (1) your baby's brain needs them; (2) fats in foods are satisfying and add a tasty "mouth feel"; and (3) nearly all nutrition scientists are now teaching that you don't get fat by eating healthful fats—you get fat by eating junk carbs. A right-fat diet, not a low fat-diet, is what you and your baby most need.

6. Be berry, berry smart! Enjoy a cup (or two fistfuls) of an organic multiberry mix in your daily smoothie. They are full of fiber and antioxidants. Remember that blueberries are smartly called "the brain berry" because the blue skin is rich in the flavonoid anthocyanin as well as vitamin C, both of which help nourish the growing brain. In our medical practice we enjoy watching kids grow up saying, "Mommy, I want more brain berries!" Dr. Mom advises: "Put more color on your plate."

7. Eat yummy yogurt and kefir. Although you don't have to drink milk to make milk (after all, cows don't), dairy products are nutrient-dense and good sources of protein and calcium. While some mothers eliminate milk from their diets because they find that doing so helps their babies fuss less, breastfeeding moms can eat reasonable quantities of cheese, kefir, and yogurt with no effect on their babies. Yogurt contains more calcium and protein than a similar quantity of milk. And the potentially allergenic proteins in cow's milk become nonallergenic as the milk is fermented and made into yogurt. Choose yogurt and kefir that are

- organic;
- 100 percent grass-fed, if available;
- made from whole milk; and
- free of added sugar and artificial colorings.

8. Pour on the olive oil. Oh, olive oil! Indulge in extra-virgin olive oil, which is processed at a lower temperature and lower pressure than regular olive oil, thus preserving more of the olive's natural nutrients. Olive oil contains healthful fats and, when added to salads, increases the absorption of nutrients from the vegetables. Enjoy a tablespoon of olive oil a day mixed with balsamic vinegar.

EAT A RIGHT-FAT DIET

The worst nutritional advice ever fed to American mothers was that they should follow low-fat diets. Back to common sense:

- Baby's brain grows the fastest during the first two years, nearly tripling in volume.
- The number one nutrient in baby's growing brain is fat.

- Mother's milk naturally derives 40–50 percent of its calories from healthful fats.
- The quality of fats you consume makes a difference in the fat quality of your breast milk (the same cannot be said of proteins and carbohydrates). Eat healthful fats, and your milk will contain those healthful fats.

Therefore, it makes sense for mother to eat the smartest fats her baby's growing brain needs.

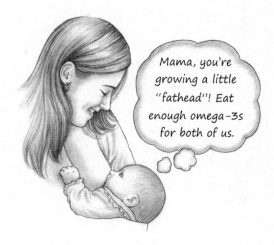

Mama, you're growing a little "fathead"! Eat enough omega-3s for both of us.

EAT AT LEAST 1,000 MILLIGRAMS OF OMEGA-3 FATS EACH DAY

Your daily dose of omega-3s can be in the form of safe seafood or omega-3 algae or fish-oil supplements. This one simple "oil change" can have a profound effect on your emotional health and the intellectual health of your baby. The latest research shows that omega-3 fats are the number one nutrient that a breastfeeding mother and her breastfeeding baby need in sufficient amounts.

SCIENCE SAYS: EAT MORE OMEGA-3S TO GROW A HEALTHIER BABY AND HAVE A HAPPIER MOMMY

Here's a summary of what science says:

- The longer a baby is breastfed, the higher his IQ is likely to be.
- Scientists believe this is attributable to a multitude of nutritional factors, including the high content of smart fats in breast milk, the healthier microbiome in breastfed babies (see page 12), and the better appetite-regulator mechanism that breastfed babies learn.
- Mothers who eat a lot of omega-3 fats during their pregnancies and while they're breastfeeding tend to have a lower incidence of postpartum depression. That makes sense, since a breastfeeding baby literally "sucks" omega-3s out of mom so that the little "fathead" will get sufficient omega-3s himself.

But this can leave mom with an omega-3 insufficiency if she isn't consuming enough omega-3s for herself *and* her baby. Because omega-3s are the most important nutrient for promoting emotional stability, an omega-3 deficiency is now thought to be one of the nutritional triggers of postpartum depression.

- The content of the smartest fat, omega-3 DHA, in the breast milk of North American mothers tends to be lower than it is in many other continents, where mothers typically eat a lot of seafood.
- Breastfeeding mothers who take omega-3 supplements have a higher content of the two smart fats, DHA and EPA, in their breast milk.

Wow! Looking at these studies may serve as a bit of encouragement for mothers who are tempted to wean early. Imagine that every time you breastfeed your baby, you are giving your baby a dose of "smart milk."

You may wonder how much omega-3 fat you should consume each day. Nutritional research reveals that the average American woman eats only around 150 milligrams of omega-3 DHA or EPA per day. We have thoroughly studied the nutritional requirements of breastfeeding mothers and have come up with this recommendation: breastfeeding mothers should eat at least 1,000 milligrams (one gram) of omega-3 DHA or EPA daily. Here's how to make sure you get enough omega-3 each day for you and your baby:

- Eat twelve ounces of safe seafood per week. Our top choice for the safest and most nutritious seafood is wild Pacific salmon. Eating six ounces of wild salmon twice a week will provide an average daily dose of 600 milligrams of DHA or EPA. (See AskDrSears.com/seafood for more safe seafood choices.)
- In addition, take 500 milligrams of omega-3 DHA or EPA fish oil or algae oil supplements daily.

Why do we say that wild Pacific or Alaskan sockeye or king salmon is the best choice? First of all, Alaskan seafood is grown wild in pristine waters. It's also reliably healthy because the Alaskan fishery authorities strictly enforce regulations to ensure safe seafood. In addition to containing high levels of omega-3s, salmon contains astaxanthin, one of nature's most powerful antioxidants, which balances your immune system and helps your body heal. (Yes, mom, you are still recovering from childbirth.)

VEGAN OR VEGETARIAN

If you're a vegan—which, we believe, is somewhat risky during pregnancy and lactation—or vegetarian, you must be extra vigilant about getting enough omega-3s in your daily diet. The levels of omega-3 fats tend to be lower in infants born to vegan and vegetarian mothers. You may be surprised by this, but we've consulted some of the world's foremost experts in omega-3 scientific research, whom we have listed in our book, *The Omega-3 Effect* (Little, Brown 2012). Pregnant mothers should not rely only on plant sources of omega-3s, such as flax. The reason is that the omega-3 fats in plants such as flaxseeds are biochemically different from those found in animal products.

Here's how we explain this difference to the vegan and vegetarian patients in our medical practice. The omega-3 fat in plants, called alpha-linolenic acid (ALA), while very healthful, is only eighteen carbon atoms long. We call ALAs "short guys." Yet your baby's growing brain likes the "tall guys," EPA and DHA (eicosapentaenoic acid and docosahexaenoic acid, twenty and twenty-two carbon atoms long respectively). When you eat the omega-3s found in seafood and sea plants, called algae, these "tall guys" go right to your tissues. DHA and EPA are known as preformed omega-3 fats, which means that your body does not have to biochemically manipulate them before sending them to your brain cells. The "short guys" in plants, however, have to be converted into "tall guys" by enzymes in your liver. The name of one of these liver enzymes is appropriately called *elongase,* which, if it could talk, would say, "I convert the short guys into tall guys."

The problem is that not every person makes this conversion efficiently. This is why during the breastfeeding consultations in our medical practice we draw a fingerstick (three drops) of blood so that we can test the omega-3 level of breastfeeding mothers, just to be sure they have a sufficient level of DHA and EPA for themselves and their babies. If you're a vegan and concerned about your DHA and EPA levels, algae sources of omega-3s are a good choice.

READ AND LEARN MORE ABOUT IT

For an in-depth look into the reasons why omega-3s are so good for you and your baby, read *The Omega-3 Effect: Everything You Need to Know About the Supernutrient for Living Longer, Happier, and Healthier,* which Bill wrote with our son Jim. For the safest seafood sources and blood tests for omega-3s, see VitalChoice.com.

Nursing tip: *Prepare "fast foods."* Stock a bunch of make-ahead meals in your freezer so you can spend more time with your baby than you do in the kitchen. Babies often have their neediest periods (what we dub "happy hour") in the late afternoon, making it difficult to cook dinner.

INCREASE YOUR WATER INTAKE

While you are breastfeeding you should drink extra water, but you don't need to overdo it. Follow the commonsense "in and out" principle of hydration: if more fluid goes out, you must take more in. Since the average six-month-old consumes around one quart of breast milk daily, and 90 percent of that milk is water, it stands to reason that mother should drink four extra eight-ounce glasses of fluid daily. But don't become a compulsive water drinker. Drinking more water than you need won't produce more milk. In fact, by a strange biochemical quirk, forcing fluids into your body has been shown to diminish milk production. Here's how to get the right amount of water:

- Drink enough to quench your thirst plus a bit more, since thirst is not a completely reliable indicator of fluid needs.
- Tote a water bottle with you in your diaper bag.

Get in the habit of drinking an eight-ounce glass of water every time you breastfeed, plus one or two more each day. When baby drinks, mother drinks. If you get into the habit of drinking an eight-ounce glass of water every time your infant feeds (which is usually eight to ten times a day), you will meet your needs for fluid.

Because milk-making hormones help your body conserve water, failing to drink enough water will not affect the fluid content or volume of your milk. But not getting enough fluids can contribute to maternal constipation, fatigue, and impaired concentration. Watch your body for signs that you are not drinking enough fluids. If your mouth is wet, you are not constipated, and your urine is colorless to slightly yellow, you are probably drinking enough liquids. If your urine is consistently the color of apple juice, your kidneys are telling you to drink. If you feel dry, you probably are dry.

> **DRINK AT LEAST TEN EIGHT-OUNCE GLASSES OF WATER EACH DAY (FILTERED IS BEST)**

NUTRITIP:
Water versus juice

It's best for lactating mothers to drink mostly filtered water. If you want more variety, flavor the water with a squeeze of lemon or lime or a bit of your favorite juice. You can also drink herbal tea and add pieces of your favorite fruit or even cucumber slices to your water. Fruit juices, however, are not nutrient-dense foods. They pack a lot of calories into a small amount of volume and deliver minimal nutrition. Drinking too much juice can cause weight gain.

The Calcium Story

You may have heard that a breastfeeding woman can lose calcium from her bones while she's breastfeeding, and you may be worried about getting osteoporosis. In fact, reports that breastfeeding leaches calcium from a mother's bones tell only a half-truth. During lactation, the mother's body does take calcium from her bones and use it to make milk, regardless of the mother's own calcium intake. But what nature takes nature gives back. The calcium loss is only temporary. The good news is that after weaning, mother's body returns more calcium to her bones than lactation took out, resulting in a healthier bone density than she had prior to breastfeeding. In fact, the incidence of osteoporosis and bone fractures later in life is lower among women who have breastfed. Breastfeeding is designed to protect the health of the mother as well as the baby, and while you are breastfeeding, your body strives to conserve calcium. Certain hormones increase calcium absorption from your intestines and lessen the amount of calcium that is excreted by the kidneys. The calcium story is just one of the many health perks you enjoy when you breastfeed and allow your body to follow its natural reproductive cycle.

"LACTADE" SUPER SMOOTHIE

Depending on what you add to it, this recipe is a perfect balance of around 30 percent healthful fats, 25 percent protein, and 45–50 percent healthful carbohydrates, and it contains the calorie equivalent of two meals and two snacks.

8 ounces 100 percent green vegetable juice, such as BluePrint (available at Whole Foods)
8 ounces coconut milk or almond milk
1–2 cups plain organic full-fat Greek-style yogurt or kefir
1 cup fresh or frozen blueberries
1 fresh or frozen banana
½ avocado
1 cup cut-up mixed fresh or frozen fruit (such as strawberries, papaya, mango, and pineapple)
2 tablespoons ground flaxseed or 1 tablespoon flaxseed oil
1 teaspoon cinnamon
1 tablespoon coconut oil

Optional additions/substitutions

Figs for extra fiber and sweetness
1–2 tablespoons peanut butter for extra energy and satiety
Goat's milk (such as Meyenberg)
Organic fresh kale or spinach for extra folic acid
1 teaspoon Hawaiian spirulina for extra iron and B_{12}
Multinutrient protein powder (such as Complete by Juice Plus+)
1 serving soy lecithin
Grated fresh ginger

Combine all ingredients in a blender and blend on high speed until smooth. Serve immediately.

FOODS TO AVOID

Most breastfeeding mothers can eat whatever they want and find that the foods they eat don't bother their baby. Don't let strict food rules dampen your enjoyment of breastfeeding. In fact, eating a wide range of your favorite foods is one way to train your baby's developing tastes to appreciate the popular foods of your culture. The flavor of mother's milk reflects what she eats, so this can be a way for your baby to get used to the taste of your family's cuisine.

Sometimes a baby's fussiness or other problems can be traced to a food in the breastfeeding mother's diet. In the first six months, baby's intestinal lining is immature and thus more easily irritated by certain substances that piggyback into baby from mother's digestive system via her milk. Also, because of baby's intestinal immaturity (leaky gut), some substances that get into mother's milk from her diet can trigger unwanted responses, such as rashes and colicky behavior, in a hypersensitive baby. After six months, the intestinal lining becomes less leaky and more mature—through a process called closure—so that baby is less sensitive to certain things in mother's diet. (This may explain why diet-related "colic" usually subsides in most infants by six months.) While food sensitivities are highly individual, the foods listed below are ones most often reported to bother breastfeeding babies.

DAIRY PRODUCTS

Research has shown that the potentially allergenic protein beta-lactoglobulin, which is found in cow's milk, can travel through a mother's intestines into her milk. It's then absorbed through baby's immature intestines and enters baby's bloodstream in small amounts. Studies have shown that eliminating dairy products from a breastfeeding mother's diet can lessen colicky behavior in some babies, as many breastfeeding mothers have long suspected. Often the sensitivity to dairy products (and other foods) subsides after six months, when baby's intestinal lining becomes mature enough to screen out potential allergens. Remember, it's the cow's-milk protein in dairy products—as well as other proteins, such as gliadin, from the gluten in wheat—that are potentially allergenic, not lactose or other factors, and milk proteins can appear in processed foods under various names. (Check the ingredients list for whey, casein, and sodium caseinate.) If baby's colicky behavior is related to mother's diet, usually such behavior subsides within a few days after mother eliminates the suspect food. But since the protein in dairy products lingers in

mother's bloodstream longer than most other proteins do, it may take as long as ten days to two weeks for this protein to be completely eliminated from mother's and baby's systems. If you eliminate dairy products, you need to be sure you are getting enough calcium in your diet: 1,200–1,400 milligrams daily.

Nursing tip: *A little bit of the offending food may be all right.* Most food sensitivities have a threshold effect. While a lot of the offending food may bother the baby, smaller amounts may not. Drinking a small glass of milk may not produce symptoms in your baby, but drinking four glasses may mean a week of upset baby gut. Eating smaller amounts of a potentially offending food in multiple mini meals throughout the day may bother baby less than overdosing on that food at one meal. Dairy and wheat products as well as citrus fruits commonly show this threshold effect: too much bothers baby; a small amount doesn't.

NEW RESEARCH ON INFANT FOOD ALLERGIES

Once upon a time, especially if there is a family history of allergies to certain foods, such as peanuts, it was customary to advise the breastfeeding mother to avoid these foods in her diet.

New research, though still in its infancy, suggests otherwise. Scientists are discovering that feeding infants tiny amounts, called *micro exposures,* of peanuts actually lessens the chances of these infants becoming allergic to peanuts later on.

Coincidentally, while we were writing this section, we attended a scientific seminar on this subject. The presenting immunologist theorized that gradually exposing the

immune cells, which are being trained in baby's maturing gut lining, to recognize these foods as "good guys" and not fight them makes the immune system less likely to trigger allergic reactions. We think this could be why breastfeeding infants tend to have a lower incidence of food allergies when they get older. Could micro exposures to foods such as nuts, eggs, seafood, and soy in a breastfeeding mother's diet eventually lessen her baby's risk of allergies to these foods? Stay tuned for more research on this fascinating subject, which we will post on our website: AskDrSears.com/breastfeeding.

A MILK OF MANY COLORS

A mother's milk may reflect not only the flavors of her diet but also the colors of the food she eats. Diets high in green and yellow vegetables (containing lots of beta-carotene) can affect the color of your milk. Tinges of color from varied diets shouldn't come as a surprise—after all, your food becomes your baby's food. Some medications may also change the color of your milk. You may even notice that your milk is affected by artificially colored drinks (for example, those containing red or orange dyes, such as fruit punch). The small amounts involved probably won't affect your baby, but this stuff really shouldn't be getting into your mouth in the first place.

Gassy Foods

Do gassy foods in mother's diet cause gassy babies? Folk wisdom tells breastfeeding women to avoid cruciferous vegetables such as broccoli, cauliflower, cabbage, and brussels sprouts, along with onions and green peppers. It is likely that there are substances in these vegetables that do enter mother's bloodstream and eventually her milk, but don't eliminate these nutritious vegetables from your diet unless you are certain they bother you or your baby. Often you can avoid the intestinal effects by eating smaller amounts more frequently or by eating your vegetables cooked instead of raw (or the reverse, if that's what works for you and your baby). If baby is hypersensitive to a gassy food in mother's diet, baby will usually show symptoms within two to twenty-four hours.

SPICY FOODS

Unless baby is exquisitely sensitive, it's rarely necessary for a breastfeeding mother to stick to a bland diet. In fact, as we mentioned earlier, exposing your baby to a variety of flavors in your milk is one way of shaping young tastes and helping baby appreciate your family's favorite foods. One experiment showed that one to two hours after mothers ate garlic, their milk took on a garlicky flavor, but their babies actually nursed more enthusiastically and drank more milk when it was garlic flavored. While an occasional baby may protest the flavor of your milk the morning after a binge at your local ethnic restaurant, most babies tolerate changes in the taste of mother's milk quite well. Mild fussiness from your baby is probably just a reaction to the small change in the flavor of your milk rather than a true sensitivity. The flavor of your milk will return to normal within twenty-four hours of omitting the unwelcome spice and probably a lot sooner.

CAFFEINE-CONTAINING FOODS

There is good news for coffee-loving nursing moms: science is on your side. Studies on mothers consuming substantial amounts of caffeine-containing beverages showed that very little of mother's caffeine intake was transferred via her milk to her baby. And what little caffeine was present in the milk did not seem to affect either the heart rate or the sleep of the infants. One word of caution: since premature babies eliminate caffeine from their systems much more slowly than full-term babies do, it would be wise for a mother to limit her caffeine intake while breastfeeding her premature infant. Sometimes maternal observations are at odds with science, and some mothers find that their babies do seem to be caffeine sensitive. If you suspect your baby is bothered by caffeine, cut down on caffeine-containing coffee, tea, soft drinks, dark chocolate, and certain cold remedies.

FUSS FOODS

While food sensitivities vary tremendously from baby to baby, the following are the most common foods that have a reputation for bothering babies:

Broccoli, especially raw	Onions
Brussels sprouts	Peanuts and peanut butter
Cabbage, especially raw	Prenatal vitamins (prescription type, with iron salts)
Cauliflower, especially raw	Shellfish
Citrus fruits in excess	Soy products
Corn	Spicy foods
Dairy products	Tomato
Egg whites	Wheat gluten
Hot peppers	
Iron supplements	

HOW TO DETECT FOODS THAT CAUSE FUSSING

Mothers have been known to go to great lengths to pin the rap for their baby's fussiness on certain foods. They eliminate many nutritious foods from their diets and risk not getting enough of certain nutrients for themselves. But you don't need to go to dietary extremes to figure out if something in your diet is affecting your baby. Here is a simple four-step procedure for identifying foods you eat regularly that may be upsetting your baby. (You can use this same procedure to track down hidden food sensitivities in anyone—a baby who has started solids or even yourself.)

Step 1: Make a fuss-food chart. List the symptoms and behaviors that you believe might be related to problem foods, such as colicky episodes, bloating, severe constipation or diarrhea, painful night waking, fitful, restless sleep, or a red ring—the "target sign"—around baby's anus.

Step 2: Ask relatives about foods they have had problems with. Survey family members on both sides of the family about foods that have bothered them. Go beyond the most common culprits (dairy, wheat, egg whites, corn, nuts, soy, and cruciferous vegetables).

Step 3: Eliminate the food suspects. One by one—or all at once, if your baby is really miserable—eliminate the suspect foods from your diet for a week to ten days. Be as objective as you possibly can. Pick out the most obvious signs and symptoms and see if they disappear. It can take as long as ten days to two weeks to completely eliminate some foods from your system, so you may have to wait before you see results. (If you are eliminating a great number of foods from your diet, it would be wise to seek the advice of a nutritionist to ensure that you get the nutrients you need while on this restricted diet.)

SAMPLE FUSS-FOOD CHART		
Suspected Fuss Food	Troublesome Behaviors	Results After Elimination for One Week
Milk	Long (1–2 hours) crying jags in the evening	Less colicky Woke at night, but without screaming
Peanuts	Waking up four or more times at night crying	No apparent effect

Step 4: Challenge your results. When you think you have pinned down an offending food, try eating it again, starting with a small amount and gradually increasing how much you eat. If baby's symptoms reappear, scratch this food from your diet for at least a couple of months and then try reintroducing it when your baby is older. You may not have to eliminate a food completely from your diet. Your detective work may show you that it's possible to eat a small amount of this food or that your baby can tolerate it if you eat it only once or twice a week.

The good news is that as baby's intestines mature, the need for eliminating fuss foods from your diet will gradually diminish and you can slowly return to your prebreastfeeding cuisine.

QUESTIONS YOU MAY HAVE

Special situations require special nutrition to ensure that both mother and baby thrive.

VEGETARIAN DIET

I switched to a vegetarian diet shortly before I became pregnant, and I feel much healthier eating this way. Can I continue to avoid eating animal foods while I'm breastfeeding?

Yes. Being a vegetarian won't affect your ability to produce milk. However, because of new research,

we do have some reservations about vegetarian diets during breastfeeding. The term *vegetarian* means a person who sticks to a plant-based diet. A strict vegetarian, or vegan, avoids all foods of animal origin, including dairy products and eggs. Lacto-vegetarians include dairy products in their diet. Lacto-ovo-vegetarians eat dairy products and eggs. Pesco-vegetarians eat fish, dairy products, and eggs along with plant foods. Our nutritional research has led us to the conclusion that for most people, especially breastfeeding mothers, the *pesco-vegetarian diet* is the most healthful, largely because these moms still need to consume the "smart fat" omega-3s DHA and EPA (see page 86).

Nutrients at risk. We recommend that mothers who follow a strict vegan diet during lactation seek the advice of a professional who is knowledgeable about nutrition during lactation. Besides eating more omega-3 DHA, vegans should take special care to get enough of the following nutrients, most of which are found in the animal sources vegans avoid:

- *Vitamin B_{12}.* Vitamin B_{12} is necessary for peripheral nerve function. While animal foods are still the best source of vitamin B_{12}, a deficiency of this vitamin can be avoided by taking B_{12} supplements.
- *Zinc.* Zinc is necessary for healthy skin and a healthy immune system. A deficiency can be

prevented by eating lots of grains, wheat germ, chickpeas, lentils, tofu, artichokes, nuts, flaxseeds, and beans.

- *Riboflavin.* Also known as vitamin B_2, riboflavin is necessary for maintaining the health of cell membranes. A deficiency is often reflected in unhealthy skin and fatigue. Small amounts of riboflavin are found in fortified whole grains, avocados, and nuts. Vegetarians may prefer to depend on multivitamin supplements to get enough of this nutrient.

Calcium is seldom a problem in the milk of otherwise well-nourished vegan mothers, since there are many alternative plant sources of calcium, and moreover, dietary calcium is more efficiently stored by a lactating woman than nonlactating women.

GRAZING FOR TWO

While taking care of my new baby, I find it's hard to sit down to three square meals a day. I end up nibbling all day long. I feel like I'm not eating very well.

As long as you nibble on nutritious foods, you have nothing to worry about. Well-nourished breastfeeding mothers often wind up "eating like a baby," consuming six to eight mini meals in a day rather than three big meals. In fact, both little bodies and big bodies were designed for grazing throughout the day rather than for eating large, less frequent meals. You may want to continue the same grazing habits you enjoyed while pregnant, when your growing uterus made it hard to fill your tummy with a big meal. If you enjoy grazing, stick to nutrient-dense foods and skip the cookies and potato chips, especially if you have extra weight to shed. Nibbling a mere one hundred extra calories of junk food each day can add up to twelve pounds of extra fat in a year. Instead,

prepare a nibble tray with your favorite nutrient-dense foods from the top twenty-four foods listed earlier in this chapter. (In the early weeks, delegate the job of having these items on hand in the refrigerator ready for you to grab.) Place the tray at your nursing station and nibble while you nourish your baby.

NUTRITIONAL SUPPLEMENTS

Should I take supplements while breastfeeding?

Generally speaking, it's best to get your nutrients from foods rather than from supplements. Well-nourished mothers of full-term, healthy, thriving babies usually do not need vitamin or mineral supplements. Yet many breastfeeding mothers and their health-care providers feel that continuing to take either prenatal vitamins or other vitamin-and-mineral supplements provides nutritional "insurance" during lactation. Certainly this precaution would be wise if baby has extra nutritional needs or mother's nutrition is marginal. Be aware, though, that prescription prenatal vitamins containing iron have been thought to contribute to fussiness in some infants. For tips on how to choose science-based nutritional supplements, see AskDrSears.com/supplements.

DRINKING ALCOHOL

Is it safe to have an occasional drink while I'm breastfeeding?

Yes, it's safe, but only if you drink according to the guidelines we set out below. Once upon a time alcohol was touted as a way for nursing mothers to relax so that their milk would let down, and beer was believed to boost a mother's milk supply. However, new studies cast doubt on the wisdom and safety of drinking alcohol while breastfeeding. Alcohol is rapidly absorbed into the bloodstream of the mother. It is present in milk in the same concentration as in blood, and it reaches its peak concentration in breast milk within thirty to sixty minutes when consumed on an empty stomach and within sixty to ninety minutes when taken with food. As with all drugs, the side effects of alcohol are dose related—that is, it depends on how much you drink.

Studies have shown no negative effect on the milk-ejection reflex when mothers drink a small amount, such as a four-ounce glass of wine or a bottle of beer. Yet dosages exceeding .05 grams of alcohol per kilogram of body weight (approximately eight ounces of wine or two twelve-ounce bottles of beer for a sixty-kilogram, or 130-pound, woman) can suppress the milk-ejection reflex with a possible reduction in milk delivery to the infant. In experiments, alcohol has been shown to suppress prolactin and oxytocin and consequently milk supply. In one study, consistent regular drinking (approximately one or more drinks every day) was associated with slightly lower scores on motor-development tests in infants one year of age, although no effect on mental development was noticed. It's important to note that many studies on alcohol and breastfeeding are inconclusive, which might well lead many mothers to the conclusion "when in doubt, leave it out." At this writing, the research seems to support the belief that an occasional drink, such as one glass of wine or beer, will not harm either mother or baby. Higher amounts and drinking every day are suspect. Higher alcohol intakes will also render you less able to respond to your baby's cues and care for him. The American Academy of Pediatrics states: "Breastfeeding mothers should avoid the use of alcoholic beverages, because alcohol is concentrated in breast milk and its use can inhibit milk production. An occasional celebratory single, small alcoholic drink is acceptable, but breastfeeding should be avoided for 2 hours after the drink."

If you drink an occasional glass of wine (for example, during a much-needed dinner date with your mate), you can minimize the amount that gets into your baby. Breastfeed your baby before drinking, limit alcohol consumption to *one glass* of wine or beer, sip it slowly with food, and if possible wait two hours after drinking to breastfeed your baby.

That said, there's no need to "pump and dump" your milk after drinking a small alcoholic beverage. The alcohol concentration in your milk is roughly at equilibrium with the concentration in your blood, which means that any alcohol in your milk will be eliminated as your body metabolizes the alcohol in your blood. However, if you drink to the point of intoxication and become engorged, then you will need to pump for comfort until you're sober and dump this milk, as it will have alcohol in it.

SMOKING AND BREASTFEEDING

I'm addicted to cigarettes, but I want to breastfeed my baby. Is smoking harmful while breastfeeding?

Smoking and babies don't mix. Even though smoking is one of the most difficult habits to break, you owe it to your baby, yourself, and your family to quit—or at least drastically cut down on the number of cigarettes you smoke. The risks of just about everything you don't want to happen to your baby go up when you smoke.

Suppose you were about to take your baby into a room when you noticed a sign that read: WARNING: THIS ROOM CONTAINS APPROXIMATELY FOUR THOUSAND KINDS OF POISONOUS GASES, SOME OF WHICH HAVE BEEN LINKED TO CANCER AND LUNG DAMAGE AND ARE ESPECIALLY HARMFUL TO THE BREATHING PASSAGES OF YOUNG INFANTS. Naturally you wouldn't take your baby into that room. Yet that's exactly what your baby is exposed to when you or other family members smoke.

We're not going to apologize if the information that follows seems like we are going overboard in our indictment of smoking. In our experience, because of the nature of nicotine addiction, unless mothers truly understand the disastrous things that can happen when they smoke, they won't be sufficiently motivated to quit. Consider the following research about how babies are affected by smoking when they are in the womb and after they are born.

Smoking stunts growth. Studies have shown a correlation between a mother's smoking during pregnancy, especially heavy smoking (more than one pack a day), and the growth and brain development of her children. Children of mothers who smoked during pregnancy are more likely to have decreased Apgar scores at birth and be smaller (a condition called intrauterine growth retardation). In childhood they are shorter and have increased learning difficulties, increased hyperactivity, and increased behavioral problems.

Smoking endangers pregnancy outcomes. Smoking increases the risk of infertility as well as the following pregnancy complications: infertility, ectopic pregnancy, placenta previa (premature separation of the placenta), placental abnormalities (known as smoker's placenta), and prematurity. When mothers smoke during pregnancy, the chances of the newborn dying at birth increase by 20 percent—35 percent if mother smokes more than thirty-five cigarettes a day.

Smoking bothers baby's brain. Studies show retarded growth of baby's brain in the womb, resulting in decreased mental-performance scoring at one year, decreased academic performance in school, and reduced IQ. In addition, research in experimental animals has shown that nicotine harms the development of the breathing control center in the brain.

Smoking hinders baby's breathing. Cigarette smoke deprives the infant of oxygen, which could interfere with the development of the brain center that controls breathing. When the body is chronically deprived of oxygen, it tries to compensate by increasing the production of a chemical called 2,3-DPG, which facilitates oxygen transport. Researchers have found that this substance is higher in children exposed to smoke, indicating that these children are trying to compensate for chronic oxygen deprivation. Babies who are exposed to cigarette smoke have a much higher incidence of respiratory illnesses, including pneumonia, asthma, ear infections, bronchitis, sinus infections, and croup.

Smoking hurts little hearts. Besides being harmful to growing lungs, smoking may harm growing hearts. Levels of HDL, the "good cholesterol" that may provide protection from heart disease, were lower in children whose parents smoked. Toxins from cigarettes have also been implicated in problems with the automatic regulation of heart rates.

Smoking blocks little noses. Babies' nasal passages are exquisitely sensitive to smoke. When irritated, they produce mucus, causing stuffiness that makes it harder for babies to breathe. Babies are preferential nose breathers, meaning they insist on breathing through their noses and, unlike adults, do not easily switch to mouth breathing if their noses are blocked. The lower respiratory tract is lined with tiny filaments called cilia, which wave back and forth to clean mucus from the airway passages and help keep them open. Smoke paralyzes these cilia, leaving air passages clogged and susceptible to infection. Children whose parents smoke have two to three times more doctor visits related to respiratory infections.

Smoking interferes with breastfeeding. Studies have shown that breastfeeding mothers who smoke have a decreased milk-ejection reflex and decreased milk supply and tend to wean earlier. Studies of breastfeeding mothers who smoke also showed that the nicotine concentration in their breast milk was three times higher than in their blood, suggesting that babies don't only inhale tobacco poisons, they "drink" them as well. Cotinine, nicotine, and another nicotine by-product, thiocyanate, have been found in the blood of breastfed infants in levels proportional to the number of cigarettes smoked by their mothers.

Smoking interferes with natural mothering. Research has shown that mothers who smoke have lower levels of prolactin, the hormone that regulates milk production and is considered the biological basis of the term *mother's intuition.* Mothers with diminished prolactin may have a more difficult time caring for their babies. Couple this with the fact that babies of women who smoke tend to have a much higher incidence of "colic" (presumably because of the nicotine) and you have a situation in which baby has increased needs and mother is less able to meet them.

Smoking increases the risk of SIDS. Parental smoking is one of the big three risk factors for Sudden Infant Death Syndrome (along with tummy sleeping and not breastfeeding). Here are the deadly stats:

- Maternal smoking during pregnancy triples a baby's SIDS risk.
- When mothers smoke more than twenty cigarettes a day, the baby's risk of dying of SIDS is increased fivefold.
- If both father and mother smoke, the baby's risk doubles again. Having two parents who

smoke is twice as risky as when mother alone smokes.
- Even babies of mothers who don't smoke during pregnancy but whose husbands do have an increased risk of SIDS.

MINIMIZING YOUR BABY'S EXPOSURE TO CIGARETTE SMOKE

As you are weaning yourself from this harmful habit, try these tips to lessen your baby's exposure to cigarette smoke:

1. Never smoke in the same room with your baby, and never smoke in the car. This will lessen your baby's exposure to harmful chemicals (but baby will still inhale pollutants from your smoke-contaminated clothing).
2. If you must smoke, do it immediately after breastfeeding, so that your body has a chance to clear some of the nicotine from your blood by the next breastfeeding. The half-life of nicotine is ninety minutes, which means that an hour and a half after you smoke, half the nicotine will have been eliminated from your blood. So if you feed your baby three hours later, most, but not all, of the substance will have been cleared from your blood. Nicotine will still be present at the next feeding, though. Measurements of nicotine in breast milk have found levels higher in milk than in maternal blood. In fact, nicotine levels in breast milk are equivalent to the amounts needed to produce nicotine-related symptoms in an adult.
3. If you use nicotine gum or nicotine patches, the baby will still be exposed to nicotine, although it will appear in breast milk at lower levels than it would from

cigarette smoke. But baby will be spared exposure to all the other toxic substances found in cigarette smoke, including carbon monoxide and thiocyanate.

4. For information on how to quit smoking, contact the American Cancer Society (800-227-2345) or the American Lung Association (800-586-5872). *A Pregnant Woman's Guide to Quit Smoking* by Richard Windsor and Dianne Smith is a ten-day, twenty-step workbook offering practical ways to quit smoking. It's out of print now, but it may be available at libraries and online. Another resource is available online at Pregnets.org: *Smoking Cessation for Pregnant and Postpartum Women: A Toolkit for Health Care Providers.* You can ask your health-care provider for help using this resource.

TEEN NUTRITION FOR TWO

I'm a teen mom. Will I be able to get enough nutrition to breastfeed my baby?

Yes. If you can make a baby, you can make milk, but you should pay doubly close attention to good nutrition. Not only are you growing a baby, you are also continuing to grow yourself, so if your nutrition is marginal, your own growth may suffer, though your baby will probably be just fine. *Your baby needs a healthy, well-fed mother.* For your baby's sake, stay away from junk food (those with mega calories and mini nutrients) and settle down to a balanced diet that contains a variety of nutritious foods. Treat yourself to the top twenty-four foods listed on page 82. It's fine to snack and graze, but you need to be sure that the foods you eat deliver plenty of nutrients along with the flavor and fun.

STAYING FIT AND TRIM WHILE BREASTFEEDING

You don't have to be a cushiony, bosomy earth mother to breastfeed. In fact, breastfeeding can make it easier to lose those pounds left over from pregnancy. Making milk may require at most five hundred extra nutritious calories a day. The extra fat you stored during pregnancy was put there as nature's insurance policy, guaranteeing that you will have enough energy to make milk for your baby. When you breastfeed, your body draws on that fat, and those pounds eventually melt away without drastic dieting. How's this for a weight-loss perk? In one study, breastfeeding moms showed faster fat loss and larger reductions in hip circumference and a quicker return to their prepregnant weight than formula-feeding mothers. Another study showed that from four to six months postpartum, breastfeeding women lost more weight while consuming the same number of calories as women who formula fed (see page 15).

A safe and easily achievable postpartum weight loss (that is, fat loss) is one pound per month for a total of twelve pounds of excess body fat over the first year. That may not sound like much, but it actually is. Twelve pounds of fat is a pile the size of a basketball. With a crash diet, which we absolutely discourage, you might be able to lose more weight more quickly, but that weight loss would include water weight, which you are likely to regain. A slow and steady fat loss means it will be easier to keep the weight off. It also means you will lose fat, not muscle. If you want to lose more than one pound a month, or if you gained an excessive amount during your pregnancy, you can. We suggest that you plan on losing *no more than one pound a week,* or four pounds a month. You can achieve the one-pound-per-week goal by following this safe and simple formula: eat real foods and move more each day.

SAFE AND COMFORTABLE EXERCISING WHILE BREASTFEEDING

When your body belongs to both you and your baby, you have to take extra good care of it.

Get the milk out before your workout. Treat your baby, and yourself, to a long feed before beginning your exercise. This preexercise precaution not only settles baby but also makes mommy more comfortable. Some women find it uncomfortable exercising with full breasts.

Support your breasts. Wear a well-fitting cotton athletic support bra to reduce the jostling and nipple friction during vigorous exercise.

Prehydrate. Drink a couple of glasses of water before you exercise, sip water while you exercise, and drink some more when you're done. Unless you are exercising vigorously for more than an hour and almost to the point of exhaustion (which few breastfeeding mothers are able to do, want to do, or should do), water adequately hydrates your body and lessens muscle fatigue just as well as a sports drink—without the expense and nonnutritious additives.

Don't worry if baby rejects the breast after you exercise. In the '90s, researchers made headlines by suggesting that mother's milk "went bad" after exercise, causing baby to temporarily reject breastfeeding. Studies like this get a lot of press, even if the results don't make much sense. When you read any research in which science is at odds with common sense, suspect faulty science. The biochemical explanation proposed for this breast rejection was increased levels of lactic acid (the metabolic by-product of exercising muscles) in breast milk, giving it a bitter taste. A close look at this study shows that there are many reasons to doubt the researchers' conclusions, and in fact, the experience of many breastfeeding mothers over the years has not shown that breast rejection after exercise is a significant problem, especially when mothers stick to moderate exercise rather than working out to the point of exhaustion. If your baby seems fussy at the breast after your exercise session, wait a half hour or so and offer the breast again. Whatever was bothering him should be better by then. One other possible cause for fussiness could be salty-tasting skin or strong odors. Try rinsing or washing your breasts or even showering before nursing after a sweaty workout.

A L.E.A.N. APPROACH TO LIFE

What's good for mother is good for baby. When you feel fit and happy with your body, you're likely to feel better about yourself, your breastfeeding, and your parenting. At the same time, improving your lifestyle and your general attitude will make it easier to take care of your body and your baby. While there are many diets and fitness programs available, in our practice and in our family, we have found that there are a few simple keys to health and well-being. We call our approach the L.E.A.N. program, because it incorporates lifestyle, exercise, attitude, and nutrition. Being lean does not mean becoming skinny. It means having just the right amount of body fat for your body type, health, and well-being. In our view, being lean means more than just shedding fat. It means getting rid of habits that interfere with your health and concentrating on the things that are most important to you. Here's a brief introduction to the four components of the L.E.A.N. approach to healthful living.

L is for lifestyle. Take inventory of your overall lifestyle and trim away the things that interfere with breastfeeding and parenting your baby. Stay away from people who criticize your parenting (or at least stay away from the topic of parenting when you are talking with them). Avoid unnecessary energy-draining activities and overwhelming amounts of work in or outside the home. For example, if you have a job that drives you to junk-food binges and leaves you with no energy for your baby, you need to make some changes. Learn ways to relax: listening to music, practicing prayer or meditation, reading, enjoying quiet time alone or with your spouse. Laugh a lot. Enjoying a funny book or movie will help you feel better about life.

E is for exercise. Regular, brisk physical activity helps you control your weight and cope with stress. Exercise will help you make the changes called for in the other parts of the L.E.A.N. program. (See below for tips on getting enough exercise while caring for a baby.)

A is for attitude. Besides trimming the excess fat from your body, shed all the stuff in your mind that interferes with your mothering and your breastfeeding. You can't control situations, but you can control your reaction to them. If you're having problems with breastfeeding, don't dwell on them. Instead, get help solving them. Don't waste energy on life's little annoyances. Concentrate on the important things and find support for yourself in your endeavors. You are doing what no one else in the world can do as well as you: nurturing your baby with your milk.

N is for nutrition. Emphasize a right-fat, nutrient-dense diet containing lots of fresh fruits and vegetables and whole grains. Be careful about what you put in your body. Eating healthful food helps you stay healthy and cope better with stress.

Our L.E.A.N. program uses the principle of synergy. When you get all parts of the program working together, the whole is greater than the sum of its parts—sort of like 1 + 1 + 1 + 1 = 5, or maybe even 10! Once you try the L.E.A.N. program, it becomes self-motivating. You begin to feel so good that you want to do everything you can to perpetuate this feeling. Postpartum depression and mother burnout are two of the most common maladies that undermine breastfeeding and lead to premature weaning. The L.E.A.N. program can give you a physical and emotional boost that will help you avoid these problems while contributing to the health and well-being of both you and your baby.

LEARN MORE ABOUT L.E.A.N.

Check out the course for pregnant and nursing moms available at DrSearsWellnessInstitute.org.

Maintaining a Lean Diet

Here are some tips on what to eat that will help you get adequate nutrition, stay trim and healthy, and make enough milk for your baby. It's a review of everything we've said in this chapter.

Eat nutrient-dense foods. While you are breastfeeding, take the opportunity to do what you have probably thought you should do for a long time: get rid of junk food in your diet. Concentrate instead on those foods that pack the most nutrition into a relatively small number of calories. Avoid calorie-dense foods—those with a lot of calories and little nutritional value, including foods high in fat and/or sugar. Nutrient-dense foods are more likely to leave you feeling satisfied; junk foods leave you craving more. In one research study, people who were allowed to eat all they wanted consumed fewer calories when their choices were limited to nutrient-dense foods than when they included highly refined and processed foods.

Fill up with fiber. When you eat high-fiber foods, you feel full without consuming a lot of calories. High-fiber foods tend to be more nutrient-dense. Consider just the *a*'s and *b*'s of fiber foods: apples, artichokes, apricots, and avocados; bran, broccoli, beans, and berries. All these pack lots of nutrition into few calories while filling your tummy. Other nutrient-dense sources of fiber are lentils, sweet potatoes, prunes, pears, figs, spinach, grapefruit, and peas.

Little bites mean a lot. You may be surprised by how one indulgence a day, such as one chocolate chip cookie or five to ten potato chips, can add up to ten pounds of extra fat in a year. These little bites provide little nutrition and a lot of unneeded fat and calories. Be particularly wary of foods that taste yummy but contain an alarming amount of unhealthful fat, such as coffee cake, piecrust, hot dogs, doughnuts, and croissants. For some women, trimming just one of these indulgences out of their diets each day is all that is necessary to stay trim. As an alternative, make a trail mix of raw almonds, sunflower seeds, raisins, walnuts, dried papaya, and even a few chocolate chips. This is something healthful to nibble on with just a touch of decadence to satisfy your sweet tooth.

MAKING THE EFFORT TO EXERCISE

As we mentioned earlier, exercise is the safest way to lose fat while breastfeeding, but fitting exercise into your daily life is often the hardest part of the L.E.A.N. program for breastfeeding mothers, especially mothers who are blessed with a high-need baby. When you have a baby who is in your arms or at your breast most of the day, you tend to remain sedentary. Exercise may be the furthest thing from your mind, especially when you are coming off an "all-nighter," a fussy period, or twenty-four hours of marathon nursing during one of baby's growth spurts. If your family also includes a toddler or older children, it can seem even harder to find time to exercise. Yet you owe it to yourself, and to your baby, to get some exercise. Actually, the best remedy for a fussy baby or for a mother in burnout is to get out and get walking. Put baby in a sling or heavy-duty stroller and walk briskly for as long as two hours in the morning. Come home for lunch and rest and then go out again as needed. This will also help lift your mood and fight depression.

In our experience, postpartum weight-loss programs do not work without incorporating some kind of exercise program that gets mother moving briskly a minimum of thirty minutes four times a week. Exercise raises your basal metabolic rate (BMR) — sort of like turning up the idle speed on your car engine so it will burn more fuel. Your body burns fat while you're exercising and continues to burn fat for six to twelve hours after you exercise. Exercise also helps you regulate your appetite. Burning energy through exercising helps bring your cravings in line with what your body really needs.

Even more important to your well-being is the fact that exercise releases endorphins, the body's own mood-elevating hormones. The days when you least feel like exercising are the days when you most need to get out there and get moving. This is when you'll notice the endorphin effect the most. Endorphins relieve tension, soothe stress, calm you when you're anxious, and help pull you out of a depression. Exercise is the least expensive antidepressant, and the side effects are all good ones.

EXERCISE FOR TWO

"But I'm too tired, and I don't have time to exercise," you say with a sigh. It may seem hard to believe, but regular exercise can cure fatigue. Try it, and you'll soon notice the benefits. Also, remember this medical truism: "If you don't take time to exercise, reserve more time to spend in the doctor's office."

To help burn off unwanted postpartum weight, put your baby in a sling and take a brisk thirty- to sixty-minute walk. Bringing your baby along makes the walk possible, and it increases the intensity of your workout. As baby gains a pound or two a month, mommy will lose a pound or two. If you also have a toddler or preschooler, put her in a stroller and take a walk as a threesome.

A walk with baby in a carrier is a boon for fussy babies, especially during "happy hour," that late afternoon fussy period that is so common to babies (and can often be found in adults). Soothe your baby with a walk around the neighborhood or through the park. Babies often settle, and even nap, in the sling of a moving mother.

There are other ways to include your baby in your exercise program. Try these tips from experienced mothers:

- *Put on some music and dance.* Hold your baby in your arms or in a sling and move vigorously to the music for half an hour. You'll have fun, burn some calories, and blast away your tensions. This is good during the winter months, when you can't get outdoors regularly because of bad weather.
- *Play with your baby as you exercise.* If you're doing sit-ups on the floor, put your baby on your lower abdomen, resting against your bent knees, and say "Boo" every time you raise your head and shoulders. Lift and lower your baby with your arms to build upper-body strength. Hold your baby in a sling or backpack while you do low-impact aerobics. Watch your form if you're holding baby while you exercise so that you don't strain muscles by using them incorrectly.
- *Keep your baby entertained.* Some babies may be content to watch you while you work out as long as you continue to talk, smile, and entertain them.
- *Look for opportunities during the day to be active.* When you're caring for an infant, you have to be flexible. One day you might get your exercise by walking to the store with your baby in the sling. On a rainy day, find something to do inside your home, even if it's housework with baby in a sling or backpack.

When you want to exercise without your baby, or when you just need a break from mothering, hand baby off to your partner or another caregiver and go for a brisk walk on your own. You'll be calmer and happier when you return.

As an added hormonal perk, prolactin, the milk-making hormone, has been shown to be elevated for twenty to forty minutes following exercise. Exercise boosts immunity by increasing the production of antibodies and white blood cells, which fight disease. Weight-bearing exercise, such as walking, builds strong bones and helps to prevent postmenopausal osteoporosis because it conserves calcium—another perk for breastfeeding mothers. Building muscles with exercise increases your metabolic rate because it takes more calories to maintain muscle than fat.

5

Taking Medications While Breastfeeding

WHAT GOES INTO YOUR BODY can also go into your milk, so before you take any medication, you need to consider how it will affect your baby and whether it has any effect on lactation. A breastfeeding mother and her baby should be thought of as a single biological system, since baby is dependent on mother for nourishment. This chapter is a guide to using medications wisely and safely while breastfeeding.

SAFE MEDICINE TAKING WHILE BREASTFEEDING

First some general principles about taking medications while breastfeeding. There are three issues to consider: Do you need the drug? Will it affect your baby? Will it affect your ability to make milk? Answering these questions should give you an idea of the risks and the benefits you can expect when taking a particular medication.

QUIZ YOURSELF

How sick are you? Be honest. There are times when taking medicine is better for you and thus indirectly better for baby, even if baby is

exposed to a small amount of the medication in your milk.

Trying to tough it out for several days may actually decrease your milk supply, and you may not be a very good mother to your baby during this time. Taking medicine may lessen the severity and duration of your illness, and in some situations it's absolutely necessary. On the other hand, if you have a minor ailment, such as a cold, consider alternatives to taking medicine. While nearly all over-the-counter cold remedies are safe to take while breastfeeding, many are only marginally effective, and you can get more natural relief by treating your cold the old-fashioned way: steam, extra fluids, rest, and the tincture of time.

QUIZ YOUR HEALTH-CARE PROVIDER

For illnesses beyond "just a cold," be sure to inform your health-care provider not only that you are breastfeeding but also that this relationship is very important to you and your baby and you don't want to wean. Impress upon the prescribing provider that you are willing to explore alternative treatments and go to some extra effort if it means you can avoid even a temporary interruption of breastfeeding. Give the clear message that your goal is both to heal yourself and continue breastfeeding. Once your provider realizes how important breastfeeding is to you and your baby, he or she will be motivated to do some research and consider other ways to treat your illness. Since there are very few drugs that are not compatible with breastfeeding, you and your provider will probably be able to agree on a course of treatment that will not require weaning. However, if you can't agree because of a provider's lack of knowledge about a medication, seek a second opinion or consult the resources in this chapter. Better yet, give the prescribing provider the resources listed in this chapter. Wise physicians and other providers are open to learning from the most up-to-date information on the safety of medications while breastfeeding. Realistically, there are very few medical situations that would make it necessary for you to wean your baby prematurely. See the box below for some resources you can use.

An insider's tip for dealing with physicians and other providers: Many decisions about whether a medication is needed fall into a gray area—for example, will a lingering cold clear up without an antibiotic, or has it progressed to a

sinus or chest infection for which an antibiotic is needed? If you give the provider a clear message that you take a lot of personal responsibility for your health and are open to nondrug alternatives, he or she is likely to be less quick to prescribe medication. Let your provider know that you are asking for the benefit of his or her judgment, not necessarily for medicine. If, however, it is perceived that you expect to leave the office with a prescription, you are likely to get one. Talk to your baby's pediatrician or your family-practice provider about the medication. These professionals are usually more familiar with information about drugs in human milk than are specialists who see mainly adults or older children and rarely treat nursing mothers. You can also ask specialists to talk to your baby's health-care provider about medication questions.

Factors to Consider in Choosing a Medication

Here are some of the factors that may influence the choice of medications that can be prescribed while you are breastfeeding. Using the resources listed above, you can better discuss with the prescriber the safest choices while breastfeeding.

- While most drugs do pass into your milk, most of those appear in only minute amounts—usually around 1 percent or less of the amount you take.

- If there are several drugs that can be used to treat your illness effectively, the prescriber should choose the one that enters your breast milk in the lowest concentration. The route of administration also influences how fast the medication enters and clears from your blood and therefore your milk. For example, some medications come in both oral and inhalant forms; each has a different clearing time.

- It's better to use a short-acting medicine that is taken three or four times a day than to use a

---

RESOURCES FOR TAKING MEDICATIONS SAFELY WHILE BREASTFEEDING

- LactMed, the drugs and lactation database of the US National Institutes of Health
- Dr. Thomas W. Hale's *Medications & Mother's Milk,* online at MedsMilk.com
- American Academy of Pediatrics policy statement *The Transfer of Drugs and Other Chemicals into Human Milk*
- World Health Organization publication *Breastfeeding and Maternal Medication*

long-acting, once-a-day form of the medication. Although less convenient, short-acting medications clear from your blood and milk faster. They're also easier for babies to metabolize, so there is less risk that the drug will accumulate in the infant's system.

- Consider the age of your baby. More caution is called for when giving medication to a mother who is breastfeeding a premature or newborn infant ten times a day than to a mother who is breastfeeding a one-year-old four times a day. An infant who feeds more frequently naturally gets more of the medicine, and the smaller size of the younger infant means that the drug will be more concentrated in the baby's body. Also, the liver and the kidneys of older infants are better able to metabolize and eliminate the drug.

- If there are concerns about possible effects on your baby, can the baby be monitored during the time you are taking the drug? This might involve checking levels of the drug in your milk or in the baby's blood or watching carefully for changes in your baby's behavior.

- If a medicine that is not compatible with breastfeeding is prescribed but it's the right one for your illness, you may need to temporarily wean. Until the medication clears your system, you can keep up your milk supply through hand-expression or pumping and then reestablish breastfeeding once you have finished the medication.

- Some drugs do not harm the baby but may affect your milk volume by suppressing the milk-making hormones.

- The "when in doubt leave it out" policy is common among health-care providers, since it's impossible to keep up with all the research on the safety of taking drugs while breastfeeding. Many providers will recommend weaning when they are uncertain about the effects of a drug in human milk. Yet this approach assumes that formula is equal to breast milk. While many physicians and other providers as well as the general public make this assumption, it is not true. The risks of exposing a baby to a drug in breast milk should be weighed against the risks of exposing a baby to infant formula.

- If it is necessary for you to wean permanently because of a drug or a particular medical procedure, ask if you can safely delay the treatment until your baby is older or weaned. Drugs in breast milk present less of a problem to an older breastfed baby. However, if you're planning to nurse until your baby weans herself, the day when you will no longer be breastfeeding may be a lot further off than anticipated.

- Be particularly cautious about taking more than one drug while breastfeeding. While each drug taken separately may be listed in the safe category, together they may be unsafe. Be sure to tell the provider about any medications you are already taking before he or she prescribes another. A pharmacist is often the most reliable source of information on drug interactions.

Safety tip: If you have your baby sleeping in your bed with you—as many mothers do for easier night nursing—suspend this arrangement if you need to take a sedative or drowsy-formula cold remedy. These medicines can diminish your awareness of your baby (see page 192).

Understand how to take the medicine. Once the alternatives have been weighed and a decision has been made to take a medication that is in the best interests of both you and your baby, be sure you understand the dosage, the possible adverse effects on you (such as stomachache, headache, diarrhea), and any possible adverse effects to watch for in your baby. When you pick up the medicine at the pharmacy, check the label and be sure it agrees with what your provider told you.

Providers often overlook discussing possible adverse drug reactions: the pharmacist can help you with those, but keep in mind that pharmacists generally do not have good information about what is and is not compatible with breastfeeding. You may need to educate them as well.

Timing the dosage. In general, it is unnecessary to try to time feedings around a medication in order to minimize your baby's exposure to it. But there may be a few exceptions, such as a medication that should be used with caution or a once-a-day medication. If so, then be sure to ask for any information about the medicine that would help you time the dosage and the baby's feedings. Most drugs reach their maximum concentration in breast milk one to two hours after being taken. So usually taking medication right after you feed allows much of the medicine to be cleared from your milk before the next feeding. It's best to take once-a-day medications just before your baby's longest period of not feeding (usually right after putting your baby to sleep at night), unless the side effects of the medication could keep you awake. The timing of once-a-day medication has less effect on its peak concentration in breast milk than the timing of medication taken three or four times a day.

While timing your dosage may help minimize your baby's exposure to the drug in your milk, don't make yourself and your baby crazy trying to delay or schedule feedings. If you have a baby who nurses frequently throughout the day and night, you will probably both be calmer and better off if you take the medicine as directed and nurse your baby on cue.

Pump and dump. Some drugs, such as radioactive substances used in X-ray diagnostic procedures, require temporary weaning, or what we call interruption weaning. If you are advised to wait to nurse your baby until a potentially harmful drug is out of your system, first check your resources to confirm that interruption is necessary and, if so, for how long. If it is truly necessary, then pump your milk every three to four hours during the time you are not nursing and discard the milk. Meanwhile, use the safe milk you previously stored in the milk bank in your freezer.

BUILDING UP YOUR MILK BANK

Just as you put money in the bank to save for a rainy day, it is wise to save breast milk in your freezer in case you run into circumstances that would prevent you from breastfeeding for a day or two. Open a "milk account" in your freezer and stockpile a few days' supply of your white gold.

THE MOST COMMON QUESTIONS ASKED ABOUT THE MOST COMMON DRUGS

Even breastfeeding mothers get sick and need treatment. Mothers can safely take most medications while breastfeeding. You may also choose to use some time-tested remedies that lessen the need for prescription or over-the-counter medicines. And in the case of some chronic illnesses, you may even find that your symptoms are not as severe during the time you are nursing your baby.

You should always tell your health-care provider that you are breastfeeding if a medication is being prescribed. Some mothers are reluctant to mention that they are still nursing an older baby or a toddler. While the information that follows provides general guidelines for taking medications while breastfeeding, it does not take the place of a discussion about your particular situation. Many prescribers learn a lot from patients who are open about their desire to continue nursing while being treated for an illness.

ALLERGIES

My allergies and asthma really get me down. What medicines can I safely take while I'm breastfeeding?

When illnesses get you down, you'll have a hard time maintaining a good milk supply and taking care of your baby. It's good to do something about your symptoms rather than thinking you must suffer through them because you are breastfeeding. Breastfeeding is especially important when there are allergies in the family. The longer you breastfeed, the less likely your child is to inherit your allergies, and breastfeeding may also decrease your own allergy symptoms for a while. If stress triggers or aggravates your asthma and allergies, breastfeeding can stimulate your natural tranquilizing hormones, which may, in turn, reduce the severity of your allergies. Most of the prescription and over-the-counter medications commonly used to treat allergy symptoms are safe to take while breastfeeding. These include antihistamines, inhalant bronchodilators, decongestants, and cortisone sprays and tablets. Unless your doctor has a good reason for suggesting otherwise, it's better for nursing mothers to take inhaled or topical rather than oral medications. Any inhaled or topical medication is less likely to be absorbed into the mother's bloodstream and therefore is also less likely to be present in the milk. Be aware that although they rarely bother the baby, oral decongestants and sometimes antihistamines can lower milk supply. The supply should bounce back if you promptly stop the medication.

ANTIBIOTICS AND COLDS

I get lots of colds during the winter months. Sometimes they progress to bronchitis and I need antibiotics. What medicine can I safely take?

All the commonly used antibiotics as well as prescription and over-the-counter cold remedies (decongestants, antihistamines, and cough medicines) are safe to take while breastfeeding, *except codeine-containing medications.* You can use a cough syrup that contains dextromethorphan, or DM, if you are unable to sleep. Rather than once-a-day, long-acting medications, use short-acting medicines that are taken three to four times a day, and try to take them just after breastfeeding. Try single-ingredient medications (either decongestants or antihistamines) before trying combinations. Finally, don't forget nondrug cold remedies: a "steam clean" and a "nose hose." Twenty minutes of inhaling steam from a facial steamer loosens secretions in clogged breathing passages. Add one drop of eucalyptus oil and one drop of lavender oil for a better effect. Spritz your stuffy nose as needed throughout the day with over-the-counter saline nasal spray. Put honey in your herbal tea for a cough. These safe and simple remedies treat symptoms and can keep the secretions that accumulate during colds and allergies from collecting in sinuses and breathing passages and serving as media for bacteria growth, and thus they may prevent a cold progressing to sinusitis or bronchitis.

RX COMMON SENSE!

Concerning the safety of antibiotics while breastfeeding, we usually follow the rule that if it's safe to give the antibiotic directly to the infant, it's certainly safe for the mother to take it while breastfeeding.

ANTIDEPRESSANTS

My doctor wants me to take antidepressants and suggests that I wean my baby, but I don't want to give up on breastfeeding. Can I take antidepressants and still breastfeed?

Recommendations for antidepressants given to breastfeeding mothers need individual attention, so we refer you to the resources list at the beginning of this chapter. Discuss these resources with your prescriber to get the best information currently available.

ANALGESICS

Is it okay to take medication for fever and aches and pains while breastfeeding?

Yes. Nearly all pain- and fever-relieving medications are safe. Acetaminophen (Tylenol) is the safest medication for relieving pain and fever, since only a tiny amount enters the breast milk. Ibuprofen (Advil, Motrin) is also considered safe. Most narcotic analgesics are considered acceptable to take while breastfeeding, but they should be used with caution, especially once your milk changes from colostrum to mature milk. *One exception is codeine.* Because breathing difficulties and slow heart rates have been reported in breastfed infants whose mothers are taking codeine, it is now considered contraindicated. The reason other narcotics should be used with caution and only for short periods of time is that they may make babies sleepy and less eager to nurse. So monitor your baby closely and use them only when nonnarcotic analgesics are not controlling your pain. Also, sometimes taking just half a narcotic tablet in between doses of a nonnarcotic analgesic such as ibuprofen will be enough to control your pain. On the other hand, pain suppresses lactation, so if you need the full tablet, then take it right after a feeding and monitor your baby. It is always possible to work out an analgesic regimen that is both effective for mother and safe for baby.

CANDIDA AND OTHER VAGINAL INFECTIONS

I tend to get a lot of vaginal yeast infections. What can I safely take while breastfeeding?

Nystatin is one of the oldest and safest medications to use for the treatment of yeast

FACTS ABOUT TAKING MEDICINES WHILE BREASTFEEDING

The more you understand about how drugs can affect your milk and your baby, the more wisely and safely you can take medicines while breastfeeding. There are many characteristics that determine whether a drug enters your milk — and if it does, how much of it gets through. These are the factors that various drug safety lists consider:

- *How fast the drug clears from your system.* This is measured with a concept called half-life: how long it takes for half the drug to leave the bloodstream. A drug with a short half-life is preferable to a long-acting one.
- *The solubility of a drug.* A drug that is soluble in fat will linger in breast milk longer than a water-soluble drug will.
- *The molecular weight.* The larger the size of the molecule, the less likely it is to squeeze through the glandular membranes into the milk.
- *Absorption of the drug.* Some drugs, such as some laxatives, act locally on the intestines and are not absorbed into mother's bloodstream enough to affect baby.

Many other biochemical factors affect how much of a drug enters the breast milk. Using what is known about a drug, we can often predict whether significant amounts will appear in breast milk.

infections (candida). It is also the one used most frequently to treat oral thrush and diaper rash candida in baby. Since it is not well absorbed through the mucous membranes of the mouth and vagina, or through the intestines, very little of the medication used by the mother gets into the breast milk. Antifungal creams, such as Mycostatin and Gyne-Lotrimin, are also effective against yeast and may be preferable to an oral medication. Only a tiny bit of the active ingredient in these creams is absorbed into mother's system, so very little gets into her milk.

Diflucan (fluconazole) is safe to take while breastfeeding. If mother also has a yeast infection on her nipples, baby should be treated for thrush at the same time (see chapter 6).

DENTAL WORK AND LIGHT ANESTHESIA

I need to have some cavities filled. Is this safe to do while breastfeeding?

Yes. Since just a tiny bit of local anesthetic is used, only an insignificant amount could get into your milk, so it is completely safe to breastfeed following a local anesthetic for dental work. Also, dental X-rays pose no problem to the breastfeeding mother or her baby.

Breastfeeding is also usually considered safe following a light general anesthetic, which is the type used in dental offices when patients don't want to be awake and aware during dental work. Unfortunately, many dentists are still telling mothers to pump and dump for twenty-four hours after receiving any anesthetic! Refer to the resource list at the beginning of this chapter if your dentist says this to you. Since the inhalant (usually nitrous oxide) is cleared rapidly from your bloodstream, it is unlikely to enter your milk in significant quantities. Unless you are advised to the contrary, it is safe to breastfeed as soon as you

are able to. If there is some specific concern about a certain anesthetic passing into your milk, breastfeed your baby before the anesthetic is administered, followed by a three- to four-hour wait until the next feeding. Confer with your health-care provider and consult the resource list to determine how rapidly the particular medicine will clear your system.

HORMONAL CONTRACEPTIVES

Is it okay to use hormonal birth control while breastfeeding?

Based on the available evidence, we do not feel it is okay to use hormonal birth control at any time, including while breastfeeding. There are three kinds of risks: risk to the mother's health, risk to the baby's health, and risks to the life of a newly conceived baby, whether intended or not.

First, let us address one other concern about birth control hormones during breastfeeding: the effect on milk production. Some hormonal contraceptives contain both estrogen and progestin, and we know estrogen suppresses milk production. Estrogen-containing birth control should not be prescribed early postpartum. In most women, the progestin-only pill (called the mini pill) does not affect milk production, though individual women vary greatly in their response to hormones, and suppression of milk production does happen. Mothers of preemies and mothers exclusively pumping may be more at risk for loss of milk supply. But all mothers need to be warned to watch their milk supplies if they begin taking any birth control pill, especially if they are exclusively breastfeeding. Depo-Provera long-acting injections are often offered right after delivery; we do not recommend these because of concerns about milk supply. In addition, we suggest that mothers who are considering a long-acting progesterone method such as Depo-Provera, the Mirena IUD, or

Implanon first try the shorter-acting and easily reversible mini pill to see if it has any effect on their milk supply.

Now let us address the risks to the health of the mother and baby. We know that oral contraceptives damage the mother's intestinal flora (and probably the baby's, too), leaving her gut vulnerable to colonization from pathogenic strains such as *Candida albicans,* streptococci, and staphylococci. Gut imbalance negatively affects the ability to digest food and absorb nutrients. We also know that hormonal birth control depletes zinc in the body. We advise breastfeeding women (and all women) to get informed about what these chemicals do in their bodies and consider other ways to manage their fertility. Steroidal hormones affect the pituitary gland, the master gland of the body—a huge health concern. Hormonal contraception works by tricking your body into thinking, and acting like, it is pregnant all the time. A small amount of these steroids does enter the breast milk, and no one really knows what the long-term effects on sexual or reproductive development of the baby might be.

Combination pills are classified by the World Health Organization as a group 1 carcinogen (the most likely to cause cancer); studies show an increased risk for breast cancer going all the way back to the 1990s. Women have a right to be informed of this and other risks associated with combination pills, including blood clots, strokes, and heart attacks. And some hormonal contraceptives are riskier than others. For example, in 2013 the FDA advised the pharmaceuticals company manufacturing NuvaRing to warn users of the drug's serious risks for elevated blood clotting leading to pulmonary embolism, which can cause disability and death. The contraceptive patch and a few combination pills also use a newer type of progesterone that is riskier. The risk of adverse side effects can be as low as three in ten thousand for women using older progesterones and/or lower estrogens and up

to twelve in ten thousand for women using the newer progesterone drugs. The list of other known side effects of hormonal contraceptives is long: headaches, weight gain, swelling, constipation, nausea, spotting, breast tenderness, depression or mood swings, yeast infections, vision changes, contact lens problems, loss of libido, and more. By reading the package inserts for the various forms of hormonal contraceptives, you can do the research for yourself.

And now for the third risk, which is not well identified in the package insert. The package inserts will inform you that birth control hormones also thin the lining of the uterus, but what they won't tell you is that this makes it difficult or impossible for a newly conceived embryonic baby to implant in the uterus, and the baby thus dies. That's what is called the abortifacient potential of hormonal birth control, and some mothers find this risk unacceptable.

There are programs and apps that teach women to manage their fertility and overall health. Some of the better-known examples include the Billings ovulation method, the sympto-thermal method, and FEMM (fertility education and medical management). We have already mentioned the program of Natural Family Planning International (NFPI; see page 73). NFPI also teaches a cross-checking form of fertility awareness that its manual calls the complete approach.

Despite the risks, however, some mothers may have certain medical or personal reasons for choosing to use hormonal contraception. If this is the case for you, it is recommended that you delay the use of oral progesterone-only contraceptives until at least six weeks (preferably three months) postpartum for two reasons: your milk supply and breastfeeding pattern will be well established by that time, and your baby will be better able to metabolize any hormones that may appear in your milk. It is even safer if you can wait until six months postpartum. If you must use the combined estrogen and progestin pill, it's even more important to try to wait until six months postpartum, when other foods are introduced into baby's diet. A particular brand of hormonal contraceptive may affect one woman's milk supply and not another's, so prescriptions should be customized to your individual needs based on your body's reaction to the medication. If your milk supply is affected by hormonal contraceptives (or if you don't want to take them simply to find out whether they will be), consider other ways of avoiding pregnancy. And remember, ecological breastfeeding (see page 72) is nearly as effective as contraceptives, at least for the first six months, and it doesn't carry the risk of blood clots and other dangerous side effects. (See the discussion of lactational amenorrhea and natural family planning in chapter 3.)

HERBS TO INCREASE BREAST MILK

Are herbal teas safe to drink while I'm breastfeeding? I've heard that some can even increase my milk supply.

Remember, herbs are drugs. In fact, many commercial drugs were developed from herbs. Use the same wisdom and precautions when taking an herb as you would when taking an over-the-counter or prescription drug. In fact, use even more caution when taking an herb, because most herbs aren't subject to FDA regulations. Neither their safety nor their effectiveness has been confirmed. While the herbal teas that you find in your grocery store are not likely to have any medicinal effects, larger doses of other herbs should be used with caution.

Herbs called galactagogues are touted to increase milk production, but as of this writing, only a few small scientific studies find that they increase milk supply. This does not mean that galactagogues don't work or aren't safe; it just means they have been insufficiently studied. Some of the most popular galactagogues are fenugreek (*Trigonella foenum-graecum*), goat's rue (*Galega officinalis*), milk thistle (*Silybum marianum*), and blessed thistle (*Cnicus benedictus*). Other common herbal galactogogues are anise, fennel, hops, stinging nettles, and malunggay. Mother's Milk tea and More Milk Plus supplements are two popular brands that contain a mixture of herbs. Most of these herbs seem to be generally harmless, but we can't say for sure because they haven't been studied thoroughly enough. However, there are some helpful resources that will serve as a guide to recommended dosages, possible side effects, and precautions. Be especially cautious of possible harmful side effects when taking fennel, comfrey, sassafras, ginseng, and licorice, and be even more cautious if you take them in excessive amounts or in a mixture of herbs. Poor feeding and lethargy have been reported in a couple of infants whose mothers drank an herbal tea blend in high doses (two liters a day).

Is it possible that these herbs only have a placebo effect? Sure, it's possible. In fact, we believe that this is often the case (although some herbs may increase the milk supply through a pharmacological action). But the placebo effect is not necessarily a reason to write them off: any substance that a mother believes will increase her milk supply probably will. Also, consider the ritual effect. The mother takes time to prepare the tea just for herself, takes time to drink it, and therefore takes time to relax. Under these circumstances, she probably will make more milk. Remember, though — the only guaranteed way to make more milk is to nurse your baby more often.

For more information about galactagogues, see *The Complete German Commission E Monographs: Therapeutic Guide to Herbal Medicines,* edited by Mark Blumenthal et al., or visit NiceBreastfeeding.com and Drugs.com.

HERBS TO INCREASE BREAST MILK (GALACTAGOGUES)*				
Common Name	Fenugreek or methi	Goat's rue or French lilac	Milk thistle or silymarin	Blessed thistle or holy thistle
Scientific Name	*Trigonella foenum-graecum*	*Galega officinalis*	*Silybum marianum*	*Cnicus benedictus*
Dosage	Capsule (500–610 milligrams): 3–4 capsules 3 times per day Tea: 1 cup (240 cc) 3 times per day	Tincture: 1–2 milliliters 2–3 times per day	Infusion: 12–15 grams per day Extract (as silibinin): 200–400 milligrams per day	Capsule: 3 capsules 3 times per day; maximum 2 grams per day Tincture: 10–20 drops 2–3 times per day
Side Effects	Common: Maple syrup odor in sweat, milk, or urine Rare: Diarrhea or gassiness in mother or child	Rare: May lower potassium levels and interfere with absorption of iron and other minerals	Common: Diarrhea Rare: Other gastrointestinal symptoms such as bloating, gas, upset stomach, and nausea; headache and skin reactions	Rare: In high doses may cause nausea and vomiting; can increase stomach acid
Warnings	(1) Allergic reactions may occur, and if you have a history of reactions to foods in the pea family—e.g., peanuts, soybeans, chickpeas, or legumes—you are at higher risk (2) Use with caution if you have a history of peptic ulcers or reflux (3) In high doses, may lower blood sugar and interfere with blood thinners (4) May exacerbate asthma	(1) Allergic reactions may occur, and if you have a history of reactions to foods in the pea family—e.g., peanuts, soybeans, chickpeas, or legumes—you are at higher risk (2) Increases the risk of low blood sugar; use with caution if you are on medications for diabetes (3) Intoxication may occur if used with guanidine derivatives (muscle stimulants) (4) Stop if headache, jitteriness, or weakness occurs	(1) Allergic reactions may occur, and if you have a history of reactions to plants or foods in the asteraceae or compositae family—e.g., daisy, ragweed, marigold, artichoke, kiwi, or common thistle—you are at higher risk (2) Should not be used if you have a history of breast, uterine, or ovarian cancer (3) Use with caution if you have uterine fibroids or endometriosis (4) Can lower blood sugar; use with caution if you are diabetic (5) May interfere with medications broken down by the liver	(1) Allergic reactions may occur, and if you have a history of reactions to plants or foods in the asteraceae or compositae family—e.g., daisy, ragweed, marigold, artichoke, kiwi, or common thistle—you are at higher risk (2) Do not use if you have inflammatory intestinal problems such as Crohn's disease or colitis (3) If you have an intestinal infection, do not use until the infection is treated

HERBS TO INCREASE BREAST MILK (GALACTAGOGUES) (continued)				
Current Evidence	A few small limited studies show an increase in milk supply	One small strong study shows increased milk supply when used with a milk-thistle derivative	See goat's rue	Anecdotal evidence only

* *This list is not all-inclusive.*

RADIOLOGY STUDIES

I need to have X-rays done as part of a medical evaluation. Is this harmful while breastfeeding?

No. X-rays, even mammograms, are safe while you are nursing. The flash of radiation used to produce an X-ray has no effect on your milk. On the other hand, diagnostic tests that involve radioactive compounds called radionuclides, such as those used for bone scans and thyroid and kidney studies, usually require that you stop breastfeeding for a day or so. Some compounds are eliminated more quickly than others. Radiopaque substances are considered safe, and no interruption is necessary. Ask your health-care provider to use the substance that will be least disruptive to breastfeeding, and consult a physician who specializes in nuclear medicine to determine how long it will take to clear the radioactivity from your body. Feed your infant as soon as possible before the study, then pump for the duration of the study. You can save this pumped milk for later, as it loses its radioactivity over the course of a few days (but make sure to have it tested before using it). Meanwhile, feed your infant breast milk that you stored before you underwent the procedure. If your physician is in doubt about when it is safe to resume breastfeeding, or if you want to determine whether the milk you pumped is no longer radioactive, expressed milk can be scanned for detectable radioactive substances in a radiology lab.

6

Troubleshooting the Most Common Breastfeeding Problems

A NURSING INFANT needs a healthy mother. But, like any other organ of the body, breasts can get sick, sore, plugged, and infected. Fortunately, most mothers avoid these problems. We want to prepare you for the most common problems breastfeeding mothers encounter and tell you how to prevent them, treat them, and continue on to a successful breastfeeding relationship.

SORE NIPPLES

Breastfeeding should not hurt. Having said that, mothers commonly experience sixty seconds or less of slight soreness when baby initially latches on over the course of the first week. Signs that your discomfort is not the normal, "common" soreness include pain that lasts throughout the feeding, barely bearable pain, pain that persists beyond the first week, and pain that does not get better despite improving the latch-on. Nipple soreness, trauma, or cracking should also start to heal within twenty-four hours of fixing the latch-on. When it doesn't heal quickly, there could also be a medical problem in mother or baby causing nipple pain, such as vascular or

structural irregularities or infection, which require help from an experienced lactation consultant or health-care provider. Pain has a purpose. It's a signal that something's not right, and you need to make a change. When breastfeeding is painful rather than pleasurable, you need to take some corrective action.

IMPROVE THE LATCH-ON

The first and most important thing to do if you have sore nipples is to evaluate how baby is being positioned and how baby is latching on. Improving the way baby takes the breast will put the sucking pressure on your areola rather than on the sensitive nipple. A horizontal red stripe across the tip of your nipple or a temporary indentation at the base of your nipple is a sign of this. It indicates that baby is sucking or gumming your nipple instead of milking the areola. Review the latch-on instructions in chapter 2 and check the following points:

- Be sure that baby is latched on far enough back on the areola.

- Be certain that baby has both lips turned out. It's often hard for a mother to see if baby's lower lip is turned out when he is latched on, so ask an experienced breastfeeding mother or a professional lactation consultant to evaluate your baby's latch-on (and to guide you in the "open-wide" and the lower-lip flip techniques).

• Check baby's tongue while breastfeeding. If you gently pull down on baby's lower lip, you should be able to see the front of the tongue

extended over the lower gum and cupped between the lower lip and your breast.

• Try the nipple sandwich (see chapter 2) to get more of the breast into baby's mouth.

• When you position your baby for nursing, wrap her body around you and pull her very close into your breast (see chapter 2).

• Discontinue any bottle or pacifier use.

SORE BREASTS: STAGES OF SEVERITY

Factors	Normal breast fullness	Engorgement	Plugged duct	Mastitis	Infections of the ducts
Usual onset	Two to four days after birth	Within the first two weeks	Most noticeable after feedings	Most common around the third week postpartum; may occur at any time during lactation	Anytime after two weeks
Where	Both breasts	Both breasts	Localized area in one breast	One breast but can be both	One or both
How breasts feel	Generally swollen and uncomfortable; not hard but tight	Hard, swollen, sore, warm	Mildly tender lump beneath areola, reddened skin above	Very painful: hot, tender, swollen, red streaking	Sharp, shooting, and/or burning pain at random, either during feedings or after; no redness, but tender areas can be found with palpation; may have recurrent plugs and nipple soreness
Maternal fever	None	Less than 101°F	None	Higher than 101°F	None
How mother feels generally	Well	Well	Well; may see a white milk plug in a nipple opening	Achy, tired, chills, as if she has the flu	Well

		SORE BREASTS: STAGES OF SEVERITY (continued)			
Factors	**Normal breast fullness**	**Engorgement**	**Plugged duct**	**Mastitis**	**Infections of the ducts**
Treatment	Give frequent, unrestricted feedings; empty breasts	Give frequent, unrestricted feedings; empty breasts; alternate warm and cold compresses; rest	Give frequent, unrestricted feedings; apply moist, hot packs; massage plugged duct to loosen plug and encourage milk flow	Give frequent, unrestricted feedings; empty breasts; rest and relax; apply oil and gently massage the affected area from the back of the breast toward the nipple; physician may prescribe antibiotics	Frequent breastfeeding; milk needs to be cultured and mother treated with antibiotics, antifungals, or both for several weeks

You have to keep working on getting baby to latch on well, even if it means taking baby off the breast and starting over several times at the beginning of feedings. If you do this early on, you'll soon be rewarded with pain-free breastfeeding. If your nipples have gone beyond the sore stage to the painful, cracked, or bleeding stage, or are tender to the touch, see a lactation consultant and/or your health-care provider.

Lessening the Soreness

Improving your baby's latch-on will make breastfeeding more comfortable in the long run. Realize this soreness won't last forever—in a few days it should be much less severe. To make breastfeeding less painful right now, try these suggestions:

Use different breastfeeding positions. Start with laid-back nursing (see page 000), using skin-to-skin contact, and allow the infant to self-attach. Try to do this at least once a day until things are better. For other feedings, alternate between the cradle hold, the football hold, the reversed cradle hold, the laid-back position, and the side-lying position. Varying positions from one feeding to the next changes the distribution of pressure on the sore areas during sucking.

Feed baby first on the side that is less sore. Let him fill up on the less tender breast first, or if you need to empty the sore breast, switch him to the sore side after you have had a milk-ejection reflex. The pain from sore nipples is usually less intense after the milk is flowing.

Encourage more frequent and therefore shorter feeds. Feed baby before he is desperately hungry, so his sucking is less vigorous and he can cooperate better and calmly latch on. Watch more closely for the subtle early cues of hunger rather than waiting for rooting or whimpering. If the only cues your baby gives are these late cues, try a few days of waking baby yourself so you can start the feedings well before full-blown hunger hits.

Pad your nipple. As you're putting baby to the breast, use your thumb and index finger to slide the skin of the areola forward with gentle compression. This forms a wrinkle at the base of the nipple, which adds extra padding to protect the sore nipple.

Use your finger as a pacifier. Long periods of comfort sucking at the end of feedings may be hard to endure. If baby needs to be pacified and your nipples are wearing out, let him suck on your index finger instead of a pacifier (dads, use a well-scrubbed pinkie finger pad side up). This way, baby will avoid the nipple confusion and nipple preference that can result when he is given a pacifier or bottle while he is learning to suck from mother's breast. A pacifier has a narrow base, so baby doesn't have to open his lips as wide to take it into his mouth. When he applies what he has learned from the pacifier to the breast, the result can be poor latch-on and even sorer nipples. When baby sucks on an adult finger for comfort, the skin-to-skin contact is still there, and the finger can be placed farther back in baby's mouth than a pacifier, simulating sucking at the breast.

Avoid becoming engorged. Be sure that you are not limiting the length of breastfeedings to the extent that you become engorged, which itself can lead to poor latch-on and sore nipples.

Numb your nipples. If your nipples are exquisitely tender, try numbing them before breastfeeding by applying ice wrapped in a damp cloth.

CARING FOR SORE NIPPLES

You'll want to do everything you can to help your nipples feel better and heal quickly. Here are some time-tested tips for soothing tender nipple skin:

- Air-dry or pat dry your nipples with a soft cotton cloth after feedings. Be sure the surface of your nipple is free of wetness when not "in use." Leave your bra flaps down and your shirt open if practical until the nipple is no longer wet. Or go without a bra, especially at night. You can sleep on a towel to absorb any leaking

milk. Use fresh, dry breast pads after feedings, without plastic liners, to be sure no moisture stays in contact with your tender skin.

- Don't use quick-drying methods, such as a hair dryer, to dry your nipples. While some nipples tolerate this technique, it can cause delicate nipples to crack because it dries the skin itself, not just the surface of the skin.

- Try exposing your nipples to a few minutes of sunshine during the day (but only two or three minutes!).

- Use a modified lanolin ointment from which the allergic properties of lanolin, such as those mentioned on page 137, have been removed. Massage lanolin into your nipples after nursing. Don't use oils or creams that need to be washed off before nursing (Ouch!) because they're not safe for baby. Medical-grade modified lanolin is especially helpful in promoting healing of cracked nipples. This ointment works on the principle of *moist wound healing,* allowing the skin of the areola and nipple to retain its natural moisture. This prevents cracking and speeds healing. (See the discussion of nipple ointments in chapter 7.)

- Avoid using soap on your nipples. The little bumps on the areola around your nipples are glands that secrete a natural cleansing and lubricating oil. Soaps remove these natural oils, causing dryness and cracking.

- Be sure your bra is not so tight that it compresses your nipples or so rough that it irritates them. Your nipples may feel better if you go without a bra and wear a soft T-shirt instead.

- If your nipples are irritated by clothing, try wearing breast shells in your bra (see chapter 7). These will hold the bra fabric away from your sore nipples and allow nothing but air to touch them. You can obtain breast shells through a lactation consultant. She can also help you determine the cause of your sore nipples and help you solve the problem.

When Nothing Else Is Working

If your nipples are tender to the touch and the above measures don't bring improvement within twenty-four hours, or if your nipples show any other signs of infection, see your health-care provider. It's also time to see a lactation consultant. You need expert help in fixing the cause of the soreness. If your nipples need a rest, she may suggest the following:

Try a nipple shield. This is a soft, flexible nipple made of silicone that fits over your nipple and areola (see chapter 7). The baby sucks on the shield to get milk out of the breast. Nipple shields can ease the pain during vigorous sucking and can also provide a temporary solution to some latch-on difficulties. In some situations, nipple shields can be a lifesaver, getting mother through a few days of intolerable nipple pain. Unless otherwise recommended by your consultant, use only a medium-size, thin, soft silicone shield, not a bottle nipple. Small shields and bottle nipples can limit how much milk your baby gets and diminish your milk supply. Once baby is latched on, be sure his lips are turned out and positioned high on the part of the shield that covers the areola — not just on the nipple. Try to use the nipple shield for a few days only. Long-term use can cause some babies to develop problems with latch-on, and shields can lead to problems with your milk supply, since the breasts don't receive as much stimulation. To wean your baby from the shield, try using it only at the beginning of feedings. Once baby is latched on and nursing, quickly slip the shield off and get baby reattached directly to your breast. Eventually, baby will take the breast without the shield at the start of the feeding. Regard nipple shields as pacifiers: if

necessary, use them; but don't abuse them, and quickly lose them.

Rest the breast with a pump. Let baby suck on the nipple that is less sore while you pump the sore side for a day or so. But be careful. You can irritate nipples by pumping if you use too much suction or if the nipple rubs against the flange of the pump. Use a cup, feeding syringe, or a spoon to offer your baby the milk you've pumped. Feeding pumped milk with an artificial nipple will often make it more difficult to solve the latch-on problems that caused the sore nipples in the first place.

If after trying all the above measures your nipples remain exquisitely tender, or even just tender to a light touch, suspect a yeast infection called candida or a bacterial infection. Nipple soreness that occurs after weeks or months of comfortable breastfeeding is almost always caused by yeast (see page 131).

ENGORGEMENT

Two to four days after birth, you may awaken to find your breasts have grown two cup sizes overnight. It's those milk-making hormones at work! If anyone has been asking you, "Has your milk come in yet?" you can now answer with a definite yes! As one mother described it, "Four days after my baby was born, I awakened with two painful boulders on my chest."

This dramatic increase in breast size and fullness is called physiological engorgement. It is the result of a rapid increase in blood circulation and milk production caused by changing postpartum hormones. In fact, it's not biologically correct to speak of your milk "coming in." Your body began producing colostrum, the first milk, late in pregnancy and made more after birth. It's more accurate to say your milk supply suddenly increases rather than "comes in." The sudden fullness and tightness may take you by surprise, and your breasts can be rather uncomfortable during those early days, when they seem to fill up faster than your baby can empty them. Much of this is caused by tissue swelling from glandular activity—and it will subside. Once you and your baby settle into a comfortable balance of milk production, and baby learns to take in more milk so the demand equals the supply, the discomfort will pass. Your breasts won't be so enormous, but they will make milk steadily and efficiently. Physiological engorgement is usually more dramatic and uncomfortable in first-time mothers and lessens in intensity with subsequent births.

When Normal Breast Fullness Becomes Painful Engorgement

If your breasts are not emptied by an efficiently nursing baby, this early, normal breast fullness progresses into pathological (abnormal) engorgement, in which mother's breasts feel painfully hard and tender and she may run a slight fever. The swelling in the breast flattens the nipple, preventing baby from latching on correctly. When this happens, baby can suck on only a nubbin of nipple and can't get enough of the areolar tissue into her mouth to compress the milk ducts under the areola. Lactation hormones keep on producing milk, but baby can't get it out of the breast, so engorgement gets worse while baby remains hungry. As the hungry baby sucks harder but incorrectly, the nipple gets traumatized. Germs may enter through breaks in the skin, setting mother up for an infection called mastitis.

Preventing and Coping with Engorgement

Fortunately, you can keep normal physiological engorgement from becoming a problem. Since engorgement gets worse when the breasts fill up faster than they can be emptied, you can prevent this uncomfortable problem by emptying the breasts. Here are some suggestions for preventing and coping with breast engorgement:

- Room-in with your baby immediately after birth and encourage frequent and unrestricted breastfeeding day and night. Ignore advisers who suggest you limit the length of feedings to five or ten minutes to protect your nipples. Studies have shown that restricting the length of feedings can actually contribute to sore nipples and increased engorgement because baby does not adequately empty the breasts.

- Whenever possible, use skin-to-skin contact and allow baby to self-attach to encourage efficient latch-on in the first days after birth. With or without self-attachment, make sure that once latched on, the baby has a wide-open mouth and the lower lip is flipped out as described in chapter 2. It's easier for baby to latch on correctly on the first and second days, when your breasts are softer and before your milk supply increases. Use the self-attachment approach discussed in chapter 2 as much and as early as you can.

- Use the nipple-sandwich technique (see page 34). Be sure to continue holding the breast after latch-on, or it might "spring back."

- If you are still having trouble with latching on, use "reverse pressure softening," which can also help letdown and milk expression (see page 122).

- If you are becoming uncomfortably engorged before baby has mastered efficient latch-on, either use a hospital-grade electric breast pump to release some of the milk or manually express some milk just before feeding. This will soften your areola enough to enable baby to latch on efficiently and empty your breasts (see the illustrations on page 122).

- Be careful if your breasts are painfully engorged. Be gentle with manual expression and use low pressure settings when pumping. Short, frequent expression—i.e., between five and ten minutes every hour—may be most effective. Expressing too vigorously can worsen the edema, block milk removal, damage the underlying breast tissue, and set you up for mastitis.

- When you express milk, express only enough to make you feel comfortable. Expressing more than that may stimulate the production of additional milk. However, if the engorgement is the result of poor feeding, or if it occurs during the first few days of life, pump as much as possible to protect the supply.

- Apply cold compresses to your breasts between feedings to alleviate the pain and reduce swelling. Try wrapping Ziploc bags of crushed ice in a lightweight dish towel, or try bags of frozen vegetables.

- Take a warm shower just before expressing your milk or feeding your baby. Direct the shower spray from the top of your breast toward your nipple as you massage your breasts. The warm water helps trigger your milk-ejection reflex, which gets the milk flowing more quickly when you begin to pump or baby begins to feed. Other ways to apply warmth and moisture to your breasts include leaning over a basin of warm water (gravity will help you express milk in this position) or applying moist warm compresses to your breasts. *Caution:* While warmth from a hot towel or a hot shower will relieve the pain, heat can actually increase blood flow to the breasts and aggravate engorgement. Use heat only to stimulate your milk-ejection reflex immediately before feeding or expressing.

- You may have heard about using thoroughly washed cabbage leaves, chilled or heated, to treat engorgement. Even though controlled studies have shown no benefit of this treatment compared to the standard treatments listed above, many mothers report a benefit. It is certainly easier to wear cabbage leaves in your bra (crush them first with a rolling pin) than it is to manage ice packs. Drape one or two leaves over each breast for twenty to thirty minutes two or three times in twenty-four hours, but only until engorgement is relieved.

- Basically, do whatever you need to do to get your milk out of your breasts. If baby is unable to nurse well, you need to pump milk on a regular schedule to prevent problems with engorgement and to establish your milk production. Frequent emptying of the breasts in the early stages of lactation will help you have a good milk supply in the weeks and months to come.

- Above all, don't stop breastfeeding. *The breasts must be drained.* If baby won't nurse, use a pump or express the milk by hand. Unrelieved engorgement can lead to a breast infection.

- Increase the length of each feeding to be sure that your baby empties your breasts until they feel soft after the feeding.

- Use ibuprofen to relieve pain and as an anti-inflammatory.

- To prevent sore nipples when your breasts are engorged, pump or express a few drops of milk several times a day and gently massage this soothing natural emollient into your nipples.

- Avoid bras that are too tight or that compress the lower part of your breast against your body, which traps milk and sets you up for engorgement and mastitis. (For help in choosing a proper breastfeeding bra, see chapter 7.)

- Rest, rest, rest! There is something magical about the way rest relieves engorgement. Double the frequency and duration of your naps.

REVERSE PRESSURE SOFTENING*

When mother has been hooked up to a lot of IVs during labor and postpartum, normal physiologic engorgement becomes complicated by edema in the breast tissue and especially the areolar tissue, which distorts the nipple and makes latch-on difficult or even impossible. Reverse pressure softening (RPS) is a simple intervention that has proved very helpful in the first fourteen days postpartum. RPS uses gentle positive pressure to soften a one- to two-inch area of the areola surrounding the base of the nipple, temporarily moving some swelling slightly backward and upward into the breast. RPS may be applied by the health-care provider and/or taught to the mother or significant others. The goal is to soften the area around the areola long enough for the baby to get a good latch. Immediately before attempting to latch, apply firm pressure inward, using the suggested positioning in the figures below and alternating quadrants around the nipple, for a minute or two each time (or longer if the areola is hard and swollen). If this causes pain, apply less pressure for a longer time. This works well, especially when pumping seems to make engorgement worse, and it is a good way to avoid nipple trauma and make it easier for milk to flow. In addition, applying this pressure will often trigger letdown (MER).

* Adapted from "Reverse Pressure Softening" by K. Jean Cotterman, RNC-E, IBCLC, and from diagrams by Kyle Cotterman

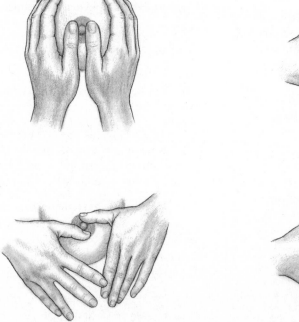
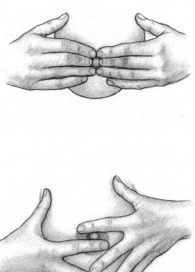

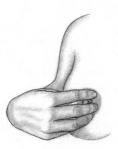

ENGORGEMENT AFTER THE EARLY WEEKS

If you have enjoyed weeks of trouble-free breastfeeding and then suddenly become engorged, take this as a signal that something is interfering with the balance between your milk supply and baby's demand: baby is going too long between feedings or isn't nursing well, or stress is affecting your nursing pattern or your milk-ejection reflex. Veteran breastfeeding mothers take engorgement as a cue to take a few days off from other responsibilities and reconnect with baby. They increase the frequency and duration of feedings and soon resettle into a comfortable breastfeeding pattern.

OVERSUPPLY AND OVERACTIVE LETDOWN

Some mothers make too much milk. This is both a blessing and a curse. It's a blessing because these moms have a much easier time during growth spurts, are less anxious about having enough milk, have an easier time storing milk for their return to work, and often donate their milk to milk banks. A breast milk bank is a service which collects, screens, processes, and dispenses by prescription human milk donated by nursing mothers who are not biologically related to the recipient infant. As of March 2014, there are eighteen milk banks in North America that are

members of the Human Milk Bank Association of North America. Too much milk can be a curse because it can be uncomfortable, increases the risk of plugged ducts and mastitis, and sometimes causes infant feeding problems. It is often associated with an overactive letdown and a foremilk-hindmilk imbalance. The overactive letdowns (also called a strong milk-ejection reflex) can cause baby to get gushes of milk that are more than he can comfortably handle. He gags, struggles, often refuses the breast, or may clamp down on the nipple to slow the flow. The foremilk-hindmilk imbalance causes these babies to get too much foremilk, which makes them become gassy or colicky and sometimes contributes to poor growth despite the mother's abundance of milk.

Several strategies are known to help mothers lower their milk supply, decrease the amount of foremilk ingested, and deliver the milk more steadily and comfortably to baby.

- Offer only one breast at each feeding. Use the other breast at the next feeding. This will bring your milk supply more in line with your baby's needs. If alternating breasts doesn't solve the problem, try using one breast for three hours— say, from noon to three o'clock—and then the other breast for the next three hours. If baby wants to nurse soon after a feeding, return him to the same breast.
- Try the following feeding positions:

  - Feed with baby sitting upright at nearly a ninety-degree angle rather than cradled across your chest.
  - Use the football hold, reclining back until baby is over the breast.
  - Try the laid-back position. Lie down on your back and let baby nurse while he is lying on top of your breast. Since the milk has to flow uphill, it won't come at him quite so fast.

- Don't delay the feeding. Watch for early hunger cues and feed baby before he is ravenous.
- Try manually expressing milk for a minute or so until the forceful part of the milk flow passes. Then put baby on the breast. Use a diaper to catch the milk so it doesn't spray across the room.
- Stop and burp baby several times during the feeding, especially if you notice her sputtering and gulping to keep up with the flow or if she has a lot of gas.

RESCUING YOUR NIPPLE

After baby clamps down and bites, she may not let go. Don't try to yank your nipple out of baby's mouth, because that will hurt more. Instead, work your index finger between baby's gums to pry the jaws apart. Then hook the end of your finger around the nipple to protect it as you withdraw it from baby's mouth. Your bony finger, rather than the tender breast tissue, will take the pressure of any further clamping down from baby.

In time, things improve. Mother's breast milk production will slow down, and her milk-making hormones will calm down. In addition, baby will grow, his ability to handle a faster flow will improve, and he will need more food per feeding. Nonetheless, if the aforementioned strategies are insufficient, then consult your health-care provider and/or lactation consultant for more strategies. In addition, certain herbs and medications, such as sage, pseudoephedrine, and combination birth control pills, have been used to lower supply—but only on a very short-term basis, until supply settles down.

PLUGGED MILK DUCTS

Sometimes a milk duct leading from the milk-making cells to the nipple gets plugged, resulting in a tender lump beneath the areola. There may also be a wedge-shaped area of redness extending from the lump back toward the wall of the chest. This is caused by something blocking milk removal from one area. Culprits can include a tight bra, a bad latch-on, skipping feedings, and bacteria or yeast. Unlike the pain of mastitis, the pain of a plugged duct generally comes and goes, and you will not feel ill. If left untreated, however, a plugged duct may become infected, resulting in mastitis, recurrent plugs, or a breast abscess. To unplug the duct and prevent subsequent infection, try these suggestions:

- Remember the golden rule of preventing engorgement and mastitis: **By any means, get the milk out!** Continue to breastfeed on the affected side. Use a breast pump or hand-expression if baby is unwilling to nurse.

- Drain the affected breast better by positioning baby so his chin points to the area of involvement. For example, if the lump is at the four-o'clock position on the areola "clock," use the football hold and position baby's chin at this point (see chapter 2).

- Apply moist-heat compresses for a few minutes before each feeding.

- Soak the affected breast in warm water or in the shower as described on page 121.

- Rest and nap nurse.

- Vary the baby's position at the breast so that all the milk ducts are drained. Be sure the baby is latched on well so that he can nurse efficiently. Try the football hold or side-lying position (see chapter 2). Before each feeding, massage the affected area by kneading your breast gently from the top down over the plugged duct toward the nipple.

- If you notice a small white head at the end of the milk duct on your nipple, that is the end of a plugged nipple opening. If this pore stays plugged, it could block milk drainage and lead to mastitis. Apply moist heat on this white blister and use a sterile needle to gently pop it. Then use an antibiotic ointment immediately after feedings, three or four times a day, for a day or two to prevent infection.

- Try a pressure massage on the area of your breast that is swollen and painful because of the plugged duct. This may help loosen the plug better than a typical circular massage on your breast, which would be more painful and less effective. To perform a pressure massage, you do not actually move your hand over the skin as you would during a normal massage, which could damage the breast tissue. You simply press increasingly firmly with the heel of your hand to move the plug in the duct down closer to the nipple. Start at the edge of the lumpy area closest to your chest wall. Apply pressure to that area with the heel of your hand to the point just before it becomes too painful. Hold the pressure at that point until the pain eases. Then increase the pressure again without moving your hand and hold it again until the pain eases. Continue to gradually increase pressure at that same site until you are pressing as hard as you can. Then pick up your hand, move it down about half an inch toward your nipple, and repeat the pressure massage in this area. Continue moving your hand half an inch and repeating the massage until you get all the way down to the nipple. This pressure massage may force the dried milk out from an opening in your nipple. It will look like a piece of spaghetti. Most of the time you don't see the plug come away. But even if the plug doesn't actually come

out, you will at least have dislodged it and moved it toward the nipple so that when baby goes to the breast and sucks, he will remove it with his suction. Always put baby to the breast on the plugged side first, at the beginning of the feeding, when his sucking will be the strongest.

- To prevent plugged ducts, feed baby in a variety of positions, with his nose pointing to various spots around the areola "clock," so that you empty all the milk ducts.

- Studies have shown that taking one tablespoon of granular lecithin per day, or a 1,200-milligram lecithin capsule three to four times a day, is helpful in preventing and treating plugged milk ducts. You can add the lecithin to your Lactade super smoothie when you make one (see page 89).

- Some mothers find that it helps to limit or avoid dairy products and other animal fats that may contribute to a tendency to get plugged ducts.

- Your health-care provider can order ultrasound treatments to relieve plugged milk ducts. If your provider is unfamiliar with this option, the prescription is: 1 MHz, 2 watts/cm^2, continuous for five to ten minutes to the affected area, once a day for up to two days.

- Once you have a plugged duct (or a breast infection), it is easier to get another one. It is important to figure out what caused it so you can lower the chances that it will happen again. Some typical causes are stress, baby missing feedings, baby sleeping through the night, a too-tight bra or an underwire bra, a baby-carrier strap that constricts part of your breast, and strenuous upper-body exercise or work, such as jumping rope or mowing the lawn.

- If plugs are multiple, recurrent, or associated with burning breast pain, suspect a low-grade fungal and/or bacterial infection (see page 133).

MASTITIS

Unrelieved engorgement often leads to an inflammation of the breast tissue called mastitis. Mastitis doesn't necessarily mean infection. The suffix *-itis,* as in arth*ritis,* means inflammation accompanied by swelling, tenderness, redness, and pain. It is often difficult for a mother (and health-care provider) to tell whether the inflammation is the result of engorgement or a plugged duct (neither of which needs antibiotics) or an actual infection (which usually, but not always, requires antibiotics). Another form of mastitis, ductal infections, is discussed on page 133.

SIGNS TO WATCH FOR

If you feel tired, run-down, achy, have chills, or think you have the flu, call your health-care provider. Mothers with mastitis will sometimes experience these flulike symptoms even before they get a fever or notice breast tenderness.

These are the other signs of mastitis:

- Part or all of the breast is intensely painful, hot, tender, red, and swollen. Some mothers can pinpoint a definite area of inflammation while others find the entire breast is tender.

- You have chills or feel feverish, and your temperature is 101°F or higher (but not always).

- You are feeling progressively more sick, your breasts are growing more tender, and your fever is more pronounced. (With simple engorgement, a plugged duct, or mastitis without infection, you gradually feel better instead of worse.)

- Recent events have set you up for mastitis: cracked or bleeding nipples, stress or getting run-down, missed feedings or longer intervals between feedings.

A BREASTFEEDING MOTHER WHO THINKS SHE HAS THE FLU PROBABLY HAS MASTITIS.

FOR MEDICAL PROFESSIONALS: HOW YOU CAN HELP

Because more mothers are now breastfeeding in a variety of circumstances, there are more mothers who require support from trusted professionals, such as hospital nursery nurses, pediatricians, family practitioners, and physician's assistants. Here's how you can help.

1. Believe in breastfeeding. Belief systems are contagious. The more you believe that mothers can and should breastfeed, the more mothers will believe it themselves. Breastfeeding has an important cerebral component: it requires an "I know I can" attitude. Your role as a professional is to advise, facilitate, and motivate in a way that develops a mother's confidence. Many mothers are victims of bad breastfeeding advice from bottle-feeding friends and relatives who give the message, "We weren't able to breastfeed, and you won't be able to, either." In the back of every new mother's mind is the worry, "Will I be one of those breastfeeding failures?" It's important for you to reassure a woman that even if she doesn't breastfeed or if she quits, *she can still be a success as a mother.* It is also your job to override negative advice and negative attitudes she picks up from others and

FOR MEDICAL PROFESSIONALS: HOW YOU CAN HELP (continued)

from the culture. Bill once had a mother of a newborn confide that she had previously decided not to breastfeed, but because Bill was so positive about breastfeeding and conveyed the message that naturally he assumed she would breastfeed, she decided to. She thanked him for his attitude. Our job as health-care providers is to convey to parents that breastfeeding is the norm; formula feeding isn't.

2. **Educate yourself.** The teacher needs to know the subject better than the student does. Read this book from cover to cover, especially chapter 2, "Getting Started." Helping a mother and baby get started with efficient latch-on is where you, as someone who sees lots of new mothers and babies, can really shine. Here are some educational resources you will find helpful:

- The Academy of Breastfeeding Medicine, at BFMed.org. Subscribe to their newsletter.
- The American Academy of Pediatrics breastfeeding promotion program; see their website, AAP.org.

When I told my nurse practitioner on my first prenatal visit that I would breastfeed my baby, she snapped, "Well, you better sign up for breastfeeding classes now. It's not as easy as people think."

3. **Employ a lactation consultant.** New parents now expect that medical practices caring for babies will either have a lactation consultant on staff or will have easy access to one. In fact, when expectant parents make their rounds to interview prospective health-care providers, many ask, "Do you have a lactation consultant in your office?" Large managed-care plans employ lactation consultants in their facilities (those that don't are *mismanaged*), and most insurance plans will cover the cost of breastfeeding consultation. (It's common knowledge that breastfeeding cuts medical costs.)

4. **Turn down free formula.** Beware of formula reps bearing gifts. Be discerning about posters, pamphlets, and educational materials from formula companies. Having the name of a formula manufacturer on the information you hand your patients about breastfeeding conveys the message that bottle feeding is the norm, as does having cans of formula around your office.

5. **Become a breastfeeding-friendly medical office.** In 1992 the Baby-Friendly Hospital Initiative (BFHI) was launched as a global program sponsored by the World Health Organization and the United Nations Children's Fund (UNICEF) to encourage and recognize maternity centers that create an environment that supports women and that implement policies to facilitate breastfeeding. Take the lead in bringing this program to the hospital where you work. BFHI has a poster entitled "Ten Steps to Successful Breastfeeding" (see box below) that is available for medical offices and when displayed will convey to parents your attitude about breastfeeding. Follow-up studies have shown that mothers are two to three times more likely to breastfeed at facilities that follow these steps than at those without the benefit of BFHI support. For information on how you can encourage your local hospital to become a member of the BFHI, and for office resources, contact Baby-Friendly USA at BabyFriendlyUSA.org.

FOR MEDICAL PROFESSIONALS: HOW YOU CAN HELP (continued)

6. Help the employed mother. Mothers who must return to work will consider continuing breastfeeding if given encouragement and support by their health-care providers. Be an advocate for the mother by negotiating with her insurance company to cover breastfeeding-related expenses such as breast pumps and whatever additional equipment is necessary for her to pump, transport, and store her milk. (See the sample letter on breast-pump rental in chapter 8.) If a mother desires to extend her maternity leave, help her out. Write a letter that describes the mother's need to be home with her baby as a medical necessity. The key to negotiating with insurance companies and employers is the phrase *medical necessity*. A letter stating that it is medically necessary that a baby receive mother's milk because of formula allergies is medically honest, especially when there is a history of allergies in the family. (We believe that all babies show at least microscopic intestinal allergies to formula.) Going the extra mile to help the breastfeeding mother conveys to her that you care enough to help her give her baby the best nutritional start.

7. What's in it for you? Breastfeeding not only benefits mothers and babies, it also benefits health-care providers. Breastfed babies are healthier, and they recover more quickly when they do get sick. This is especially true of gastrointestinal illnesses such as gastroenteritis, during which babies should continue to breastfeed to minimize dehydration and weight loss. Breastfeeding mothers are more intuitive. Because they know their children so well and have built a mutual trust, breastfeeding mothers are wiser disciplinarians. This benefit spares you time-consuming discipline questions. As an added perk, if your patients are covered under an HMO, you will reap a lot of financial benefits from fewer office visits for illnesses and phone calls for advice from breastfeeding families. Medical practices with a large HMO population have a financial incentive to be particularly breastfeeding friendly.

Mothers who realize that breastfeeding makes a difference will find a way to do it. The professional's job is to provide the information that convinces mothers that it makes a difference, then provide the support to help them achieve their goals. If you have a breastfeeding-friendly office, you can call yourself a truly successful health-care provider. When our sons Dr. Jim and Dr. Bob joined our pediatrics practice, we gave them our criteria for success: "Your success in life is directly proportional to how many lives you touch and make better." A breastfeeding-friendly medical office will truly improve the lives of the families you care for.

FOR *Mrs. Smith*

R

Because Mrs. Smith's baby is allergic to any milk other than her breast milk it is medically necessary to extend her maternity leave.

Refill ____ Times   Dr. *William Sears*

Sample medical-leave prescription

Preventing Mastitis

The best way to prevent mastitis is to prevent the situations that set you up for it. Relieve engorgement promptly (see above). Milk that doesn't flow gets thick and clogs the ducts, which is a setup for mastitis. Breastfeed frequently. Don't restrict the length of feedings. If you feel your breasts getting full, encourage your baby to nurse. You don't have to wait for baby to tell you he's hungry. Avoid sleeping on your stomach or so far over on your side that your breasts are compressed against the mattress. Take care of yourself and get plenty of rest (both mental and physical). Problems with recurrent mastitis can be the result of irregular breastfeeding patterns: missing feedings, giving bottles in place of breastfeedings, or skipping pumping sessions when separated from the baby. Recurrent mastitis may also mean that mother's immune system is generally run-down because of fatigue and stress. Mastitis is a sign that you need to take a closer look at your lifestyle and breastfeeding relationship and make some adjustments.

Treating Mastitis

Treating mastitis is much like treating engorgement (see above), only more intense:

- Rest, rest, rest. You must take a medical leave from all responsibilities other than breastfeeding and take your baby to bed with you and nurse. Rest relieves stress and replenishes your immune system.

- Alternate warm and cold compresses. Cold compresses relieve pain; warmth increases circulation, which mobilizes infection fighters in the inflamed area. Lean over a basin of warm water, stand in a warm shower, or soak in a warm bath. Moist heat, such as warm water or a warm, wet towel, is more effective than the dry heat of a heating pad. Many mothers find immersing their breasts in warm water less painful than the weight of a warm towel.

- While immersing your breasts in warm water, gently massage the area of tenderness. Or simply massage the area using an unscented massage oil. Massage from the back of the breast toward the nipple. This further increases circulation and mobilizes local immune factors.

- Breastfeed frequently on the affected side. If it hurts to nurse your baby, start the feeding on the breast that is not sore and quickly switch to the sore side after you notice your milk-ejection reflex. Breastfeeding is usually more comfortable when the milk is flowing. It's important to empty the inflamed breast. As in other parts of the body, fluid that is trapped in the breasts can get infected. Your baby can empty your breast more efficiently than a breast pump can. However, if your baby is not nursing well, you may have to pump or use hand-expression to get the milk out. This milk is safe to use.

- Vary the baby's position at the breast so that all the ducts are emptied.

- Take analgesics for fever and pain. Acetaminophen and/or ibuprofen (good for inflammation as well) are safe to take while breastfeeding. Unrelieved pain not only decreases your ability to produce and release milk but also suppresses your body's ability to fight infection.

- Drink lots of fluids, as you would if you had the flu. Fever and inflammation increase your need for fluids.

- Boost your immune system with good nutrition. (Try the recipe for the super smoothie on page 89).

- Avoid sleeping on your stomach or far over on your side, which can lead to engorgement and plugged ducts.
- Sleep without a bra. At other times, wear a loose-fitting bra that does not put pressure on the affected area.

When do you need antibiotic treatment? As we mentioned above, the inflammation of mastitis does not always mean that you have a bacterial infection. But it is often difficult to tell whether mastitis has become a breast infection. While it is always best to consult your health-care provider as soon as you suspect mastitis, you may not necessarily need an antibiotic in the following situations:

- You do not have a history of frequent episodes of mastitis.
- You don't feel *that* sick.
- You have not gotten progressively sicker over the last few hours.
- Your fever is not rising.
- The breast pain and tenderness are not increasing.
- You can easily correct whatever factors may have set you up for engorgement in the first place.

These are the signs that you do need antibiotic treatment:

- You have a history of frequent mastitis.
- Both breasts are affected.
- The pain is not controlled with analgesics.
- Your fever is rising.
- You are feeling increasingly ill as the hours go by or your symptoms are not improving after twenty-four hours.
- Your nipples are cracked or you see pus (cracks provide a likely entry point for bacteria to get into your breast tissue).
- You see pus or blood in your milk.

In our medical practice, we operate on the principle of *better to treat earlier than later.* In our medical experience (and research supports this), mothers who are given antibiotics too late in the course of mastitis are more likely to wean their babies from the breast, to have a more severe infection, and to have the infection recur.

Which antibiotics are best? The type of bacteria involved in mastitis is usually staphylococcus, and the two safest and most effective classes of antibiotics against this organism are cloxacillins and cephalosporins. Other frequently prescribed antibiotics are Augmentin, azithromycin, and sulfamethoxazole-trimethoprim. All these antibiotics are safe to take while breastfeeding. Even though you will feel better after a few days of taking them, be sure to complete the full course prescribed by your doctor (seven days or less is insufficient; you need at least ten and sometimes fourteen days), otherwise you run the risk of having the mastitis return. If you don't feel better after two or three days on an antibiotic, call your doctor, who may wish to prescribe a different medication.

Inflammation of the milk glands may increase the sodium content of your milk, giving it a salty taste. Most babies either don't notice or don't mind and go right on nursing. Some may object to the change and fuss or refuse to nurse from that side. Try starting the feeding on the unaffected side and finish on the salty side. As the inflammation subsides, your milk will soon return to its usual taste.

Don't quit nursing because you have mastitis. Weaning increases the risk of a breast infection turning into a breast abscess that requires surgical draining. It can also scar and damage breast tissue. Continuing to nurse your baby is the best treatment for engorgement, mastitis, and breast infections.

BREAST ABSCESS

Occasionally engorgement, mastitis, or a plugged duct can progress into a localized area of pus called a breast abscess, which is like a boil under the skin. Your health-care provider will suspect an abscess if the lump remains tender and does not go away with the treatment for plugged ducts and mastitis. A breast ultrasound may be necessary to locate an abscess deep in the breast. Often, surgical drainage and antibiotics are needed. In addition to the treatment recommended by your doctor, apply moist heat to the affected area and continue to nurse on the unaffected side. Depending on the location and the extent of the abscess, your health-care provider will advise you about whether it's possible to nurse on the infected breast. By all means keep the infected breast drained, either by baby or by pumping. If surgical drainage is necessary, ask your doctor to make the incision as far away from the areola as possible so that baby can continue to nurse immediately after the procedure.

CANDIDA (YEAST) NIPPLE INFECTIONS

Candida (also called yeast, monilia, and thrush) is a fungus that thrives in warm, dark, moist environments, such as the mucous membranes of the mouth and vagina, the diaper area, skin folds, bra pads, and persistently wet nipples. Suspect candida may be the cause of your sore nipples if any of the following is true:

- Your nipples are tender to the touch, sore, burning, itching, flaky, and/or pinker than normal.
- You experience shooting pains in your breasts during or just after feeding (especially during your milk-ejection reflex).
- The usual remedies for treating sore nipples aren't working.

BABY-FRIENDLY HOSPITAL INITIATIVE: TEN STEPS TO SUCCESSFUL BREASTFEEDING

1. Have a written breastfeeding policy that is routinely communicated to all health-care staff.
2. Train all health-care staff in skills necessary to implement the breastfeeding policy.
3. Inform all pregnant women about the benefits and management of breastfeeding.
4. Help mothers initiate breastfeeding soon after birth (within half an hour).
5. Show mothers how to breastfeed and maintain lactation even if they are separated from their babies.
6. Give newborn infants no food or drink other than breast milk unless *medically* indicated.
7. Practice rooming-in, allowing mothers and infants to remain together twenty-four hours a day.
8. Encourage breastfeeding on demand.
9. Give no dummies (also called artificial teats, pacifiers, and soothers) to breastfeeding infants.
10. Foster the establishment of breastfeeding support groups and refer mothers to them upon their discharge from the hospital or clinic.

- Baby has oral thrush (white, cottage cheese–like patches on the tongue and sides of the mouth) and/or a candida diaper rash.
- The sore nipples appear after a period of pain-free breastfeeding.
- You or your baby are taking or have just finished taking a course of antibiotics and your nipples suddenly become sore. Yeast infections are common following antibiotic treatment.

Preventing Candida

Here are some simple suggestions that can prevent yeast infection of the nipple or cure a mild case of it:

- Eat plain and unsweetened organic yogurt daily. Choose a brand that contains live and active cultures.
- Yeast organisms hate sunlight, so give your bra and breasts a sunbath. Expose your nipples to sunlight for several minutes several times a day. Lay out your bra in the sunlight.
- Air-dry your nipples after feeding.
- Avoid plastic-lined breast pads, which irritate the skin and trap leaked milk.
- Change nursing pads at each feeding.
- Wear 100 percent cotton bras and wash them and your breast pads daily in very hot water, using one cup of distilled white vinegar in the rinse cycle.
- Avoid using pacifiers, as they tend to carry yeast.
- Thoroughly wash breast shells, bottles, nipples, pacifiers, mouthable toys, and pump parts that come in contact with your breasts and boil them in water for five minutes daily. Towels and washcloths can harbor yeast, so use them only once before washing them.

Treating Candida

If the simple home remedies listed above don't bring relief, consult your health-care provider about the following treatments:

- Apply a small amount of an antifungal cream (such as Mycostatin, clotrimazole, or miconazole) to your nipples and baby's mouth after each feeding, since that is when the organisms are transferred. Use it until your symptoms have been gone for a few days.

- When you have a candida infection in your nipples, baby should be treated for thrush even if you can't see any white patches in her mouth. Your health-care provider will prescribe an oral antifungal suspension that should be painted on baby's tongue and the roof and sides of her mouth three or four times a day for a couple of weeks.

- Relief should come within one to two days. Continue the medication for three days after your symptoms are gone. If you feel no relief after two days, you may also have a bacterial infection or need oral medications, so be sure to see your health-care provider.

- Babies can also be given probiotics. Talk to your health-care provider.

- As a last resort, when topical treatments fail to work, oral fluconazole (Diflucan) can be prescribed for mother and/or child.

- If the candida is resistant to the standard treatments described above, in consultation with your health-care provider, apply a 1 percent solution of gentian violet to your nipples twice a day for three to seven days. Gentian violet is effective, though messy. Also apply a small amount once a day to baby's mouth, but be aware that overuse of gentian violet may irritate her sensitive oral mucous membranes. If you are concerned about purple stains on your baby's mouth, you can try applying Vaseline to baby's lips before using the gentian violet.

- If baby has a candida diaper rash, treat it with an over-the-counter antifungal cream.

- Be aware that freezing does not kill yeast, so if you freeze milk for later use while you are infected, use it sparingly.

- Be aware that your partner can harbor yeast and cause reinfection.

Many health-care providers worry that you need to wash the creams off your nipples prior to breastfeeding, but unless the cream is visible at the next feed, doing so is unnecessary. While nursing a baby on a candida-infected breast can be excruciating, it is necessary to keep the affected breast or breasts empty to prevent mastitis or a candida infection even deeper in the breast tissue. Pay particular attention to proper latch-on and easing your baby off at the end of the feeding, since infected nipples are more sensitive and prone to injury from improper sucking patterns. Pump and use expressed breast milk if necessary.

DUCTAL INFECTIONS

Ductal infections manifest themselves as burning breast pain that occurs randomly before, during, and/or after feedings. The breast can feel achy, and the pain can radiate to your back. It has also been described as sharp or shooting pain. The nipples may or may not be sore with this infection, and sometimes mothers will have recurrent plugged ducts. The condition often goes undiagnosed because there is no fever, redness, or flulike symptoms. Occasionally you can find some breast or areolar tenderness if you or your health-care provider does a careful breast exam. In rare cases, the milk can become bloody or pink. The cause of these low-grade infections include yeast, bacteria, or both. Many health-care providers are unaware of this type of infection, and it requires two to eight weeks of oral antibiotics, fluconazole (Diflucan), or both for adequate treatment.

If you need help educating your health-care providers about this condition so you can get adequate treatment, you can consult "Academy of Breastfeeding Medicine Clinical Protocol #4: Mastitis," at ncbi.nlm.nih.gov/pmc/articles/ PMC4048576/, and Christine Betzold's articles "An Update on the Recognition and Management of Lactational Breast Inflammation" and "Results of Microbial Testing Exploring the Etiology of Deep Breast Pain During Lactation" (both in the *Journal of Midwifery & Women's Heath*).

IV

BREASTFEEDING IN TODAY'S WORLD

Working and breastfeeding? We'll help you make it work. Need to combine breastfeeding and bottle feeding? We will help you. Because they know it makes a difference, an increasing number of mothers are finding ways to breastfeed despite the challenges of life in the twenty-first century. In this section, you will learn about shaping your lifestyle around your breastfeeding relationship. We'll tell you how to cope with your busy life as a new mother, and as you discover that breastfeeding is more than a nine-to-five job, we'll share ways to feed your baby at night while getting enough sleep yourself. We'll also tell you about the many products and gadgets available to help modern mothers enjoy breastfeeding. Some of these you need, some are nice to have, and some you can do without.

Modern life brings challenges to dads, too, as out of choice and necessity they learn to share the child care and to "father nurse." More than anything, breastfeeding mothers need the support and understanding of fathers.

In this section, we also let the experts—mothers—speak for themselves, as they share their tricks of the trade and their recipe for successful breastfeeding: education, professional help, commitment, support, and a pinch of humor.

7

A Consumer's Guide to Breastfeeding Products

IF YOU HAVE ANY DOUBT that there are a lot of breastfeeding mothers out there with money to spend, you need only look through catalogs for expectant and new parents. There are many products available that promise to make nursing easier. Which ones do you need? Which ones are nice to have? Which ones are a waste of money? How do you choose one type over another? Here's a guide to what's out there.

NIPPLE CREAMS AND OINTMENTS

Sore nipples are all too common, so any product that promises to prevent or soothe them will have a market. The important thing to remember is that in most cases, sore nipples are the result of inefficient latch-on or incorrect sucking, and the only way to cure the sore nipples is to fix what the baby is doing wrong at the breast. (See chapter 2.)

But while you are working on the breastfeeding problem, you might need to use something besides your breast milk on your nipples to help them heal. You can't use just anything on sore nipples, since this skin will be going into your baby's mouth. Look for products that contain edible food-grade ingredients that are specifically

marketed to breastfeeding mothers. They should also be hypoallergenic.

One recommendation is a product called Lansinoh, a highly purified, 100 percent natural form of lanolin with no allergens or additives. It's a sticky but very effective emollient that has been used for decades. A small amount softened between the fingers and patted on the nipple and areola will help the skin retain the internal moisture that speeds healing. It is especially effective on cracked nipples and prevents painful scabs from forming and then pulling off. A similar product is made by Medela. Other notable products are Motherlove Nipple Cream, Earth Mama Organic Nipple Butter, and Green Goo 100% All Natural Nursing Cream. You can also use any edible oil such as olive oil, but beware of using vitamin E oil, as it can be harmful to your baby.

Stretch marks on the breasts are common during and after pregnancy. There's not much you can do to prevent these; you're a victim of your own heredity, which gave you inelastic skin. If your breasts are dry or itchy during pregnancy or lactation, you can use your favorite lotion on them. Just avoid getting it on the nipple and areola, and avoid lotions with perfume. Babies don't like strong scents, and perfumes camouflage the natural scent of mother's body that baby is attracted to.

BREAST PADS

Breast pads help absorb milk that may leak between and during feedings. You wear them inside your bra to keep the bra dry and milk away from your clothing. Most mothers don't have problems with leaking after the first few weeks, so you probably won't need breast pads for long. But they're very useful at first.

You can buy pads that are disposable or cloth pads that you wash and use again. Look for pads that allow air to circulate to your nipples. While it might seem that plastic-lined pads will protect your clothes better, you should avoid them because they retain moisture, contributing to sore nipples and encouraging bacterial growth. You can make your own pads by tucking folded cotton handkerchiefs inside your bra or by cutting four-inch circles from cloth diapers. Change breast pads promptly when they get wet. If the pad dries and sticks to your nipple, moisten it first with warm water so that you don't remove any skin as you pull it away from your breast.

BREAST SHELLS

Used both to protect sore nipples and to shape flat or inverted nipples, breast shells are worn inside the bra during pregnancy and the early postpartum period. They have an outer shell that holds the bra cup away from the nipple and an inner ring that presses against the areola and allows the nipple to protrude through the opening in the center. Be sure to use the shell rings according to the manufacturer's instructions.

Breast shells can be helpful when nipples are so tender that they hurt when even soft bra fabric touches them. (But remember: nipples won't heal until you fix the cause of the soreness; see chapter 2.) However, breast shells are falling out of favor as a solution to flat or inverted nipples. Most lactation experts feel that teaching baby to latch on appropriately is the best solution to nipples that don't protrude.

LIVING WITH LEAKING

Yes, it's those hormones again. Women who leak milk have been shown to have higher than average prolactin levels. Mothers may even experience "long-distance leaking" when they're away from their babies at feeding time. Just the thought of your baby can cause a spurt of milk to leak, a reminder that breastfeeding is a brain activity as well as a bodily function. Leaking may occur at inopportune moments — during a board meeting or during lovemaking, for instance. Like spit-up on a father's tie, leaking milk is a telltale sign that you have a new baby.

This normal biological nuisance is most common during the first weeks of nursing. It improves with time, and most mothers stop leaking by three or four months postpartum, although some will still experience occasional leaking even after six months of breastfeeding. Here are some tricks of the trade for dealing with this side effect of nourishing your baby with human milk:

- Accept leaking as a natural part of breastfeeding. Breast milk may be wet, and it may be sticky when it dries, but it's not dirty. Expect leaking during lovemaking. Whatever arouses the mother arouses her milk.
- Since leaking occurs with a milk-ejection reflex, as soon as you feel one coming on, fold your arms over your chest and push gently inward for thirty seconds to suppress the squirts.
- Dress for the occasion. Prints camouflage wetness; solids make it obvious.
- Wear nursing pads when you're away from home. In a pinch, fold a tissue inside your bra, cut out a small portion of a disposable diaper, or use a handkerchief.

- Keep a cloth diaper under your breast to absorb the leaking milk during a feeding. Tuck one end of the diaper inside your bra to absorb leaks from the breast you are not using, and place the other end under baby's chin to catch his drips.
- Avoid becoming overfull with milk; feed regularly and/or pump if you're separated from your baby. If you have too much milk, taking steps to lower your supply will get the leaking under control faster. The first step is to use one breast for the entire feed instead of switching and feeding on both sides.

Breast shells press against the breast tissue while you wear them, so they may encourage leaking and even overstimulate your milk supply. If you have a reason to use them, don't use them all the time, and don't use them for days on end. Any milk that collects in the shell should be discarded, since germs can multiply in milk kept in the warm environment next to your skin.

NIPPLE SHIELDS

Nipple shields are made of thin, flexible silicone, and they cover a mother's nipple and areola while the baby is nursing. The baby sucks on the nipple shield rather than directly at the breast. Nipple shields are sometimes confused with the breast shells described above.

A nipple shield can be used to protect a sore nipple during feedings. It can also be used to help a baby who is having difficulty latching on to a flat or inverted nipple.

Nipple shields are very effective but should be used with help from a lactation specialist to prevent the following problems or complications. First, with a shield in place, the breast may not receive the same kind of stimulation that it does when a baby sucks directly on the breast. This leads to a reduction in milk supply. Second, baby learns to latch on to the nipple shield rather than on to the breast or starts to prefer feeding with the shield, which makes weaning from the shield a challenge. With correct guidance, both these problems can be prevented.

If working with a specialist is not an option, then you should know that when you're dealing with sore nipples or latch-on difficulties, it's better to avoid nipple shields and work directly on solving the problem. Generally, nipple shields should not be the first line of defense for dealing with sore nipples. Some lactation experts do find nipple shields useful in very specific situations in which the baby might find it impossible to latch on to the breast without the shield, such as a mother with very large nipples and a baby with an unusually small mouth and jaw structure.

If you do use a nipple shield, try to use it only in the first minutes of a feeding. Once baby is latched on and his sucking has pulled out a flat or inverted nipple, quickly remove the shield and get him to attach directly to your breast. If you can't get him to latch directly, you may need to pump after feeding to maintain your supply. It's best to have baby's weight monitored while you are using shields.

Back in the days when nipple shields were made of latex, mothers were told to trim a little bit off the nipple shield each day in order to wean the baby onto the breast. This can't be done with the newer silicone shields, since cutting them leaves a sharp edge.

NURSING PILLOWS

One of the nicest products for breastfeeding mothers is a nursing pillow—a firm semicircular support designed to cover your lap and raise your baby up to breast height. Some pillows also provide support for mom's lower back. Nursing pillows are great for mothers of twins, who never seem to have enough hands to get everyone properly positioned. These pillows may also be very helpful if you have a tiny preemie or a baby with low muscle tone who just seems to sink away into bed pillows or couch cushions. The My Brest Friend pillow works best for newborns, especially those of first-time moms. While some mothers enjoy the convenience of having one special pillow reserved for breastfeeding, others find that using a large towel that has been rolled up and taped is the most comfortable option.

One problem with some nursing pillows is that they encourage baby to lie *flat*. These pillows sometimes require a regular pillow underneath them to raise baby up to the level of the breast. To facilitate stomach emptying and keep milk out of the middle ear, babies should usually be fed propped up to at least a thirty-degree angle. This is easily achieved by angling the pillow and supporting it with another pillow underneath it on the side you are feeding on.

Nursing pillows, especially Boppy, may even have a life after breastfeeding. Certainly toddlers and preschoolers will be able to find inventive uses for a giant-size cushion. And similar pillows are marketed to people who do various kinds of needlework as support for their arms and their work as they sew.

NURSING FOOTSTOOLS

You can buy a nursing stool that is slanted at just the right angle to prop up your feet, raise your lap, and make your lower back more comfortable while you are breastfeeding your baby. You might decide this is a helpful addition to your nursing nook, a way to pamper yourself during the time you're giving so much to your baby. A footstool is a valuable tool for establishing proper position and latch-on. A box, toddler step stool, or milk crate might work just as well.

SPECIAL FEEDING DEVICES

There are various special food-delivery systems that are used for special babies, such as premature infants, infants with a cleft palate, or babies with

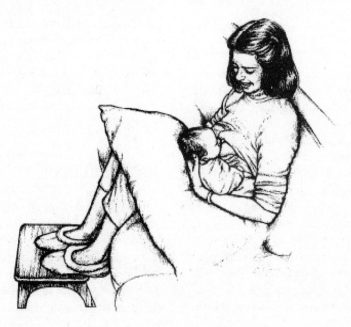

various neurological problems. These devices have special nipples or other ingenious ways of delivering milk. For example, a bottle known as the Haberman Feeder is used for infants with oral-facial abnormalities, such as a cleft lip, cleft palate, or receding jaw, and for babies who have developmentally delayed suck. This bottle has a long nipple and a valve that regulates the flow of milk. Lactation consultants and speech pathologists who have had special training in managing infants with anatomical or neurological challenges that affect feeding can recommend the best type of feeder for your baby.

IF YOU MUST SUPPLEMENT: ALTERNATIVES TO BOTTLES

Bottles are not the only option for feeding a baby at the breast. And since artificial nipples are likely to lead to nipple confusion and nipple preference, which makes breastfeeding problems more difficult to solve, bottles are not the best choice for giving supplements to young infants. What do you use instead? Consider these choices.

Cup feeding. If a medical situation temporarily delays breastfeeding, cup feeding is a safe and healthful alternative to bottle feeding. Cup-feeding infants are less likely to get nipple-confused and more likely to go on to successful breastfeeding than those who are fed by artificial nipples. Premature infants are especially prone to nipple confusion if bottles are introduced before the breast, and research has shown that not only are preemies able to drink from a cup, they also maintain a more stable blood-oxygen level during cup feeding than during bottle feeding. This helps them grow better. Some nurseries have used cup feeding in infants as preterm as thirty weeks. Babies get milk by using a lapping action rather than sipping, sort of like baby kittens do.

To give supplements to a baby, use a small cup (shot-glass size) that holds just one or two ounces of human milk or formula. Cups made of flexible plastic allow you to bend them into a spout shape. You can use a small plastic disposable cup or purchase cups made especially for infant feeding. These are available from many catalogs that sell breastfeeding supplies and from pump manufacturers. Plastic cups for supplementing breastfed babies may also be available from lactation consultants. Try these cup-feeding tips:

1. Fill the cup at least half full with the supplement.
2. Tuck a cloth diaper or hand towel under baby's chin to absorb drips or use an absorbent bib. You might want to swaddle baby in a receiving blanket to take his hands out of the action.
3. Fill several cups so you don't have to interrupt the rhythm of the feed to refill cups.
4. Hold baby on your lap in an upright, supported position.
5. Hold the cup to baby's lips and tilt it until the milk just reaches his lips.
6. Be patient. Allow baby to lap up the milk and swallow at his own pace. Don't pour the milk into baby's mouth; he may sputter and choke. Let baby set the pace and let him decide when he's finished.

Spoon feeding. You can also feed a baby supplements with a spoon. Support her

IF YOU MUST SUPPLEMENT: ALTERNATIVES TO BOTTLES (continued)

upright on your lap as you would for cup feeding and offer small spoonfuls of milk, placing the tip of the spoon on her lower lip. Allow her to take the milk and swallow at her own pace.

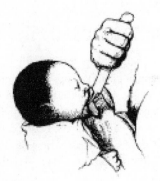

Syringe feeding

Medicine dropper or feeding syringe. Use a plastic medicine dropper to drip milk into baby's mouth while holding him upright on your lap. A feeding syringe is similar to a medicine dropper, but it holds more. You can also use a feeding syringe to supplement a baby at the breast. Insert the tip of the syringe into baby's mouth while he is latched on, and depress the plunger to reward the baby when he sucks.

Nursing supplementer (also known as an SNS, or supplemental nursing system). This device allows baby to receive supplements of formula or expressed human milk while sucking at the breast. A container for the milk (either a bag or a plastic bottle) hangs from a cord around mother's neck. Narrow silicone tubing runs from the container to the mother's nipple, and it is secured with tape.

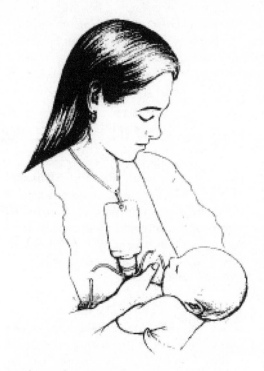

Supplemental nursing system

When the baby latches on to the breast, he takes the tubing in his mouth as well as the nipple and areola. When he sucks, he gets the supplement along with the milk from the mother's breast. The sucking helps stimulate the mother's milk supply, and the supplement rewards the baby for sucking properly, so he learns what to do at the breast.

A nursing supplementer is used for induced lactation by mothers who are nursing adopted babies as well as by mothers who are relactating (nursing their babies to reestablish a milk supply after a premature weaning). Nursing supplementers can also be used for preemies or babies with various kinds of

IF YOU MUST SUPPLEMENT: ALTERNATIVES TO BOTTLES (continued)

sucking problems. The baby, however, must be able and willing to latch on to the breast.

It can take a few days to become comfortable with using a supplementer, so it may not be the answer to a short-term need for supplements. However, supplementing baby at the breast eliminates the need to give baby an additional feeding after breastfeeding, which saves time and effort. And it keeps baby at the breast, eliminating the need for other feeding methods.

Talk to a lactation consultant before using a nursing supplementer. She can help you decide if this is the best choice in your situation and will also help you solve the breastfeeding problem that created the need for a supplementer.

Nursing tip: Give baby enough tubing to reach where your nipple will wind up. Because your nipple stretches during a feeding, extend the tip of the tubing half an inch beyond the tip of your nipple when you tape the tubing in place.

Finger feeding. Newborn babies will suck on an adult finger, and a nursing supplementer can be used with it to deliver milk. The supplementer's tubing is taped to the adult finger, and the finger is gently inserted (pad up) in the baby's mouth. When baby sucks, milk goes through the tubing and into baby's mouth. You can also use a feeding syringe for finger feeding. Gently insert the tip of the syringe into baby's mouth while he sucks on your finger. Depress the plunger to deliver milk. Finger feeding is the preferred method for supplementing when the baby is having trouble sucking correctly, and finger feeding can be used indefinitely

until the baby is finally able or willing to go to the breast.

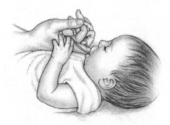

Finger feeding

How you deliver supplementary milk to your baby's tummy will depend on what sort of breastfeeding problem you are experiencing as well as on your own preferences. Cups, spoons, syringes, medicine droppers, and finger feeding are helpful while you are correcting a problem involving baby's inability to latch on. If baby can latch on to the breast but needs supplementing, we recommend an SNS. A lactation consultant can help you decide which method will work best for you and your baby and can help you locate and purchase special feeding equipment. She can also help you create a plan for gradually eliminating the need for supplements.

The best supplement to nursing at the breast is mother's own expressed milk. If your baby is not nursing well, you'll need to pump after breastfeedings in order to stimulate your milk supply. Milk that is expressed shortly after baby is fed at the breast has a high fat content and makes an ideal supplement.

If you must use formula supplements, consult your doctor about what to use and how much.

There are also a variety of soft cups and feeders that are useful for babies who have a temporarily weak suck, such as premature infants. These are preferable to bottle nipples, which can lead to nipple confusion and nipple preference.

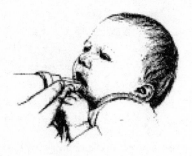

A special feeding device

SHOPPING FOR BRAS

You'll probably shop for new bras fairly early in your pregnancy. Breast changes begin in the first trimester, and most mothers outgrow their prepregnancy bras right along with their nonmaternity jeans. If you're buying new bras during pregnancy, go ahead and buy nursing bras. These may not fit immediately after birth, when your breasts are swollen as lactation begins. But they'll fit again at some point in your breastfeeding career.

Nursing bras are designed with cups that open. You can open the flap on the cup so that baby can nurse while the rest of the bra stays in place. You'll find nursing bras in the maternity section of department stores and in specialty shops. You can pay discount-store prices or a lot more for a higher-quality garment. Many catalogs for new mothers also sell nursing bras and provide instructions for using a tape measure to determine your size. You can buy nursing bras and nursing clothing on the Internet, too.

What to Look for When You Shop

At first buy only one of a particular style of bra to test it. When you find a bra you really like, purchase more of that type. Keep these factors in mind when you're looking for the right bra:

- Flaps should be easy to open with one hand. If you can refasten them with one hand, even better. Remember, your other arm will be holding a hungry baby. For discreet nursing in public, choose a bra with fasteners that you can open without looking at them.

- The bra should support the breast from beneath even when the cup is open. This makes feeding more comfortable and reclosing the bra less of a struggle.

- Avoid bras that open completely at the front for feeding. You'll have a hard time wrestling your breasts back into place when you're done nursing.

- Nursing bras should fit comfortably. Bras that are too tight can leave you vulnerable to plugged ducts and breast infections in the parts of the breast where straps or underwires block the flow of milk.

- Avoid underwires, especially in the early postpartum weeks. If you do choose an underwire bra, be very fussy about the fit. The breast's milk-producing tissue extends all the way back to your rib cage and up into your armpit. An underwire can obstruct the milk ducts in this area—besides poking and annoying you. (Underwire bras can also be miserable to wear during pregnancy. The wires will dig into your upward-expanding abdomen whenever you sit down.)

- Cups should be made of a breathable fabric, such as 100 percent cotton or one of the new synthetics that also allow the skin to breathe.

Many synthetics trap moisture next to the nipples and encourage bacterial or yeast growth and soreness. Don't buy a bra with a plastic lining.

- You'll need at least three bras: one to wear, one in the laundry, and one in the drawer. Owning a few more means you'll have to wash them less often.

Size

How do you know what size bra to buy? Breasts change dramatically postpartum. Here are some guidelines:

- Your breasts will enlarge considerably after birth, so perhaps purchase two or three inexpensive bras late in pregnancy that are one numerical size and one cup size bigger than what you're wearing. These will get you through your first several weeks postpartum.

- When your breast size settles down, usually after the second week, purchase additional bras that fit well.

- Most nursing bras have several rows of hooks at the back to allow for changes in breast size and rib-cage expansion during pregnancy. If you buy a bra that fits well when fastened on the second row of hooks, you'll have room to get a bit bigger and a bit smaller. Because the flaps are open on the sides, there's also some room for expansion in the cups of most nursing bras.

- If you purchase bras through a catalog, follow the retailer's instructions for measuring to obtain the correct size. You may not end up with the size bra you think you wear, but you'll probably end up with one that fits better than one purchased in a store.

- Large-breasted women need a bra with extra support.

There are many styles of nursing bras available, and many of them are quite attractive. Some mothers find they must be very careful about how their bras fit throughout the time they are breastfeeding. Others, especially those who are small breasted, become more casual about bras as time goes on. Some women simply go braless. Others may choose stretchy nonnursing bras that can be lifted above the breast and then pulled down again.

Do you absolutely need the support of a good bra while breastfeeding? Will it prevent sagging and stretching? Breast shape and firmness are influenced mainly by heredity, and even women who don't breastfeed will find that their breasts change after pregnancy. Some mothers feel that their breasts are smaller and droopier after weaning but become more firm as the months go by.

Most mothers are more comfortable wearing a bra, but much depends on what you are accustomed to. Go ahead and choose whatever works for you.

CHOOSING THE RIGHT BREAST PUMP

No woman ever fell in love with a breast pump. Pumps just don't look like babies, and they can't empty a breast as efficiently. But breast pumps are a fact of life for mothers working outside the home. For mothers whose babies are unable to nurse well at the breast, breast pumps make it possible for them to maintain their milk supply and work toward the day when they will be able to breastfeed their babies directly.

A Breast-Pump Primer

All breast pumps work on the same principle: suction is used to draw milk from the breast into a container. What differs is the power source behind the suction, how much suction the pump produces, how the suction-and-release cycle is controlled, and how many suction-and-release cycles the pump is able to produce each minute.

With hand pumps, mother provides the power and regulates the suction by mechanical means, usually by squeezing a handle. With electric pumps, the suction is generated by a motor. With some electric pumps, the mother uncovers and covers a small hole with her finger to regulate the strength of the suction and the suction-and-release cycles. With most electric pumps, the suction-and-release cycle is controlled by the pump, and the better models allow the mother to adjust the suction level and the speed.

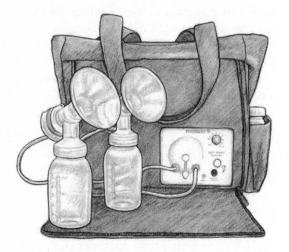

Portable electric breast pump

Generally speaking, pumps that allow for more cycles per minute are more effective. Cheaper electric pumps with small motors may be able to generate only five suction-and-release cycles per minute. The slower cycling rate is harder on your nipples, since they are subjected to longer periods of unrelieved suction. The better-quality electric pumps, the kind you rent, cycle up to sixty times per minute.

Some women can pump milk easily no matter what kind of pump they use, but most women get more milk if they use a better-grade pump. If you are pumping milk only to leave an occasional bottle for your baby or to store milk in your freezer for a rainy day, you don't need a top-of-the-line pump. If you are using a pump to establish or maintain your milk supply for a baby who cannot nurse at the breast or who has not yet learned how to nurse effectively, you should rent or buy one of the high-quality pumps. Using anything less is not worth the effort involved or the risk to your milk supply. If you are a working mother pumping while on the job, the kind of pump you use will depend on how long you are separated from your baby each day, where you will be pumping, how old your baby is, and other convenience factors. Don't try to skimp and make do with a less effective pump. The easier and more convenient it is to pump, the better you will feel about taking on the challenges of breastfeeding and working.

The pumps on the shelf at the local discount store or drugstore are not your only choices, and often they are not the best choices. Check with your childbirth educator, a lactation consultant, a local hospital that participates in the Baby-Friendly Hospital Initiative, or a breastfeeding support group for sources of better-quality breast pumps.

Picking the Right Pump for You

During pregnancy, seek the advice of a lactation consultant when selecting a pump. All the models and accessories available can get confusing. In addition, pumps have a breast shield (also called a flange or cone) that centers on your nipple; it is very important to make sure you obtain one that is not too small or big for your nipple. If your lactation consultant sells and rents only one brand of pump, you might also want to talk to another consultant, one who handles the competition's products. Most breast pumps are single-user items, except for the rental pumps, and for those you must purchase your own accessory kit. While many women now receive or request a pump as a baby-shower gift, you might want to wait and purchase one for yourself, especially if you aren't sure what your pumping needs will be postpartum.

The various breast pumps on the market fit into a few basic categories (see box). The more you depend on your pump to keep up your milk supply, the more important it is to use a high-quality pump. When you're considering whether to buy or rent and how much to spend, take these factors into account:

- What is your reason for pumping? Are you trying to establish and maintain a milk supply for a baby who can't yet nurse? If so, you need a better-quality pump than you do if you are pumping to keep milk in the freezer for an emergency.

- How old is your baby? Will you be pumping for many, many months? This may influence whether you rent or buy.

- Do you plan to have another baby, and will you use the pump again?

- Do you need the convenience and speed of double pumping (that is, pumping both breasts at the same time)?

- Compare the cost of the pump to the cost of the alternative: formula feeding. Even the most expensive pumps may come out looking economical by this standard.

- Battery-operated pumps go through batteries quickly. Pumps that come with an adapter for electrical outlets or the accessory socket in your car can give you the flexibility you need without having to depend on batteries for power every

time. Consider where you will be pumping the most, since not every place has an outlet.

- Do you need a pump that's lightweight and portable? Will you be carrying your pump back and forth to work every day, or will it stay in one place?

- Expect to pump each side for fifteen to twenty minutes (the average time it takes to breastfeed your newborn baby). A double-pumping system pumps both sides jointly and thus saves you time. It also increases the amount of milk you express. Moms who double pump also often have higher prolactin levels in the blood. It might seem that double pumping would require two hands, but enterprising mothers find a way to hold both breast flanges with one forearm, sometimes with the help of a desk or table. This leaves one hand free for answering the phone, turning pages, or eating your lunch. Breast pump companies sell a special bra for hands-free pumping. Other options include cutting a slit in an old bra for the flange to slip into, using two or three hair bands with a bra that has hooks, or, for some moms, loosening the nursing bra and slipping the flange inside.

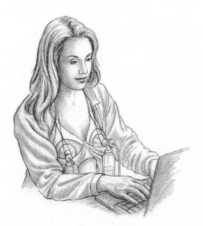

Homemade hands-free pumping solution

A GUIDE TO CHOOSING A BREAST PUMP

Type of Pump	How It Works	Cost*	Disadvantages
Hand pumps	Various mechanical means are used to create suction.	$20-$60 or less	Operating the pump becomes tiring. Generally, less effective than most other pumps. Not recommended to maintain or increase milk supply. Some require two hands and then mothers can only pump one side at a time.
Low-cost single electric or battery-operated pumps	A small motor creates suction. Can be used with batteries or an electrical outlet.	$40-$185 (may also need to purchase batteries)	Not recommended to maintain or increase milk supply. Can be noisy. Motor eventually wears out. The less expensive models are often much slower.
Portable double electric pumps	A motor creates the automatic suction-and-release cycles.	$130-$350	Not recommended to be used by more than one person. Sometimes the flange that comes with the kit is too big or too small. Most pumps come with a standard size flange that may not work for women with large or very small nipples. Suction power can be lost especially with long-term and frequent usage.
Hospital-grade double electric rental pump	A high-quality motor generates automatic suction-and-release cycles.	Rental rate $40-65/month or up to $3/day (plus purchase of accessory kit $50+). Rental rate goes down when rented several months. May require a deposit. Can be purchased for $400-3000.	Can be heavy! Requires an electrical outlet; some require a three-prong outlet. The standard flanges kits do not fit every mother and the suction strength may need to be checked.

Some insurance plans will cover the cost of a pump, especially for premature or ill infants.

A GUIDE TO CHOOSING A BREAST PUMP (continued)

Suggested Uses	Infant's Health	Length or Frequency of Separation	Comments
Prevention of engorgement and loss of milk supply for a normal healthy infant who is frequently breastfed. Treating engorgement or low milk supply if baby is effectively nursing. Occasional milk removal when separated usually no more than once a day or a few times a week. To express extra milk for storage.	Normal healthy infants who latch and effectively breastfeed on a regular basis. Use in infants with feeding problems ONLY when no other option is available.	Less than 20 hours per week; ONE 12-hour day or TWO non-consecutive 10-hour days.	Are light and easy to transport and no electricity is needed but some hand pumps can also be used with the same manufacturer's electric pumps. We don't recommend old-fashioned bulb pumps.
Same as for hand pumps but with the convenience of battery or electrical power.	Normal healthy infants as above. Use in infants with feeding problems ONLY when no other option is available.	Same as above.	Easier to use than a hand pump and cheaper than a double-electric pump but they are less effective. Works well for occasional separation or to store extra milk.
Same as above with the convenience of electrical power and pumping both sides together. Pumping regularly 2 or more times a day. To maintain milk supply for infants who are breastfeeding but need supplementation. Treats engorgement or low milk supply even when baby not effectively nursing.	Normal healthy infants who are directly breastfeeding but need some supplementation or when breastfeeding is temporarily interrupted for less than 72 hours. Use in infants who cannot directly breastfeed for 72 hours or more only if no other option available.	More than 20 hours per week or 2 or more 10+ hour consecutive days.	Designed for the convenience of working mothers. Less expensive if purchased without tote bags for storing the pump, the milk, and other accessories. Rechargeable battery packs and adapters for a car's cigarette lighter may be available. Get fitted or be sure that the flange is the right size for your nipple. If your nipples are rubbing or if the pump does not seem to empty your breast suspect an incorrect flange size followed by inadequate suction power or malfunction.
The gold standard for establishing and/or maintaining a milk supply for a baby who cannot directly nurse at the breast. May be used with short or long-term separations and/or for maternal convenience. Can be used for all of the above reasons as well.	Normal healthy infants and as above. Gold standard for infants who: are premature, have significant health problems, are unable to or infrequently directly breastfeed and/or need to be supplemented for most feedings.	More than 20 hours per week or 2 or more 10+ hour consecutive days.	The next best thing to a baby who can effectively breastfeed. Be sure to be fitted with the correct flange size and have the suction checked if there is poor milk removal, nipple pain, or a loss of supply.

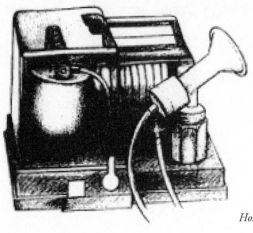 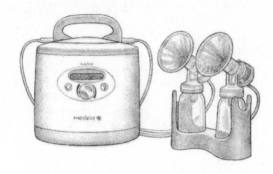

Hospital-grade breast pumps

Pumping Step by Step

All the pieces of your breast pump may look intimidating at first, but it's not hard to learn to use the device. Follow these basic instructions to pump milk for your baby. If you get your pump before the baby is born, put it together and take it apart prior to birth to familiarize yourself with all the components.

1. **Get ready.** Assemble the pump parts. If this is your first time using the pump, follow the instructions that came with it regarding cleaning and/or sterilizing before

Manual breast pumping

use. Sit in a comfortable chair next to a table that will hold the pump. Have a storage container handy for the milk (see below).

2. **Get set.** Take a few moments to breathe deeply. Close your eyes. Think about your baby at the breast. Or imagine yourself in a favorite calming setting. This step helps you relax so that your milk-ejection reflex will kick in.

3. **Go.** Center your nipple in the pump's flange (or flanges, if you're pumping both breasts at once). If the pump comes with several sizes of flange, choose the one that fits the best — not too big, but big enough to ensure that your nipple and areola do not rub against the plastic as you pump. Turn on the pump. If it has several suction settings, try the gentlest one first. You can increase the suction if necessary to get more milk. At first, you'll see only drops of milk appearing in the flange, but after your milk-ejection reflex is triggered, you'll see the milk spray out of your nipple. (Cool, huh?) If you have the type of pump that

requires you to control the cycling manually, hold for three to five seconds only; do not hold until it hurts! Pumping should not hurt; if it does, lower the suction, try a different flange size, and/or seek the help of a lactation consultant.

4. **When to stop.** Continue pumping until the milk is no longer flowing. (If your milk supply is low, pump each breast for fifteen to twenty minutes, even if the milk flow has ceased, because pumping also tells your body to make more milk.) If you're pumping one breast at a time, switch to the other side and pump until the milk stops flowing on that side, too. Then pump each breast again. If you're double pumping, you might want to pump a minute or two longer after the milk flow stops to see if you can trigger another MER and get more milk.

5. **Store it.** Pour the pumped milk into your selected storage container. Fasten the lid tightly, date the label, and refrigerate or freeze, depending on when you plan to use it (see below).

The Low-Tech Approach: Hand-Expression

Your hands are nature's original breast pump — and they are always handy! Expressing milk by hand works very well for many women. Even if manual expression is not your first choice for getting milk out of your breasts, it's a useful skill to have if you are caught somewhere with full breasts and no breast pump. Every mother should learn this skill. Mothers who do not need to express milk regularly may find that hand-expression is the only "pump" they need. Some women find that their breasts are more responsive to the skin-to-skin contact of hand-expression

than to plastic pump parts. Here's how to hand-express your milk:

1. Position your hand on your breast, with the thumb above and fingers underneath, about an inch to an inch and a half behind the nipple. If your breast were a clock, your thumb would be at twelve o'clock and your fingers at six o'clock. Don't cup your breast

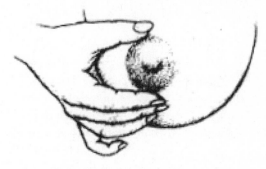

Hand-expression (front view)

in your hand. Instead, your thumb and fingers should be directly across the nipple from each other.

2. Press your thumb and fingers directly back into the breast tissue, toward the wall of your chest. Don't move them farther apart. Just press them back into the breast.

3. Roll your fingers and thumb forward to squeeze milk out of the milk ducts, which

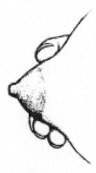

Hand-expression (side view)

17 TIPS FOR BETTER PUMPING

Stimulating Your Milk-Ejection Reflex

1. Whenever possible, pump as frequently as your baby nurses—usually every two to three hours. Follow a set routine for pumping: the place, the chair, the snack. Get your equipment ready, use your mental tricks to relax, and pump. This conditions your milk-ejection reflex.

2. Try a few minutes of breast massage before you pump. Start at the armpit and use the fingertips of your opposite hand to make small circles on the breast tissue in that one spot. Then move your hand slightly and do it again. Work your way around the breast and gradually down toward the areola in a spiral pattern. (This is similar to the breast exam that you and your doctor perform to check for lumps.) Finish the massage with a series of long strokes from the chest wall down to the nipple, again working your way around the entire breast. Then massage the other breast. If your milk flow slows down during a pumping session, a few minutes of breast massage may help get it going again.

3. "Prime the pump." Drink a couple of glasses of water right before pumping.

4. Get "pumped up" yourself. Visualize flowing mountain streams or rivers running toward the ocean as you pump. Or imagine yourself as a fountain of milk—whatever image helps your milk release and spray into the container.

5. Look at a picture of your baby while you pump. Or bring along one of your baby's blankets or a piece of clothing. Enjoy the baby smell on the fabric.

6. Right before you pump, call your baby's caregiver and find out what your baby is doing.

7. To minimize distractions while pumping, try using a portable stereo with headphones. You can enjoy your favorite music while you pump, or try one of the recordings that feature sounds from nature: the ocean, the rain forest—whatever appeals to you.

Problem Solving

8. If pumping is making your nipples sore, try a lower suction setting. Be sure that the nipple is not rubbing against the flange as you pump. If the flange is tight you can lubricate your nipple with a little olive oil. Some mothers with large nipples will need to special-order a larger flange if one is available for their brand of pump.

9. To soothe sore nipples after pumping and help them heal, use a small amount of nipple ointment (see page 137). Soften it between your fingers, then gently pat it onto the nipples.

Pumping More Milk

10. If you're worried about producing enough milk, pump more *frequently*. This is more effective at stimulating the milk supply than pumping for longer stretches at each session. If you're pumping to store milk, pump when you have the most milk, usually in the morning.

11. If you're not pumping as much milk as you once did, check your pump. Are you putting it together properly? Is a seal or some other part of it wearing out? Check with the manufacturer (there will be a phone number in the printed instructions). If you bought or rented your pump from a lactation consultant, she may be able to advise you about replacing any parts that are worn.

17 TIPS FOR BETTER PUMPING (continued)

Places that sell pumps often are able to test the pump's suctioning strength.

12. To get more milk for the bottles your baby drinks from while you're gone, try pumping on one breast while baby nurses at the other during an early morning or evening feeding. The baby will trigger the milk-ejection reflex, and you'll be able to collect milk from the other breast more easily.

13. For most women, double pumping yields more milk. Prolactin levels in the blood are also higher when you pump both breasts simultaneously. Good-quality electric pumps are the best and easiest way to double pump, but some manual breast pumps can be operated with one hand. If you get two of these, you can double pump manually.

14. If pumping is not going well, try another pump, preferably one that is a notch or two up the scale in quality from the one you are using. Rent a hospital-grade pump and try it for a week or two. You may be surprised at the difference! Cheap is not best when it comes to pumps.

Convenience

15. Wear two-piece outfits. It's easiest to pump (just as it's easiest to nurse discreetly) if you're wearing a loose top that can be pulled up from the bottom. Investing in several good-looking nursing blouses with camouflaged openings at the breasts can simplify both pumping and nursing.

16. Leaning forward while you pump—even leaning over a sink—will prevent milk from dripping on your clothes.

17. Pump hands-free. Hands-free kits are made commercially, but some moms find they can cut a slit in an old bra to hold the flange securely or use a nursing bra with hooks and some hair bands to attach the flanges. Still others can get away with just loosening their bra straps and securing the flange inside the cup. You may prefer to try leaning into the desk or table that's holding the pump, using the edge of the furniture and one arm to hold the pump flanges to your breasts. You'll have a free hand for turning pages in a magazine or eating your lunch. Or try using a footstool or thick book to raise your knees so that you can rest the collecting bottles on your lap as you lean forward. (For additional tips on pumping at your workplace, see chapter 8.)

---

collect under the areola behind the nipple. Don't slide the thumb or fingers along the skin—this will quickly make you sore.

4. Repeat this sequence (position, press, roll) until the milk flow ceases. Then move your hand so that the thumb and fingers are positioned at eleven and five o'clock and do it again. Use both hands to work your way around one breast, then switch to the other side until you have emptied all the milk ducts. As soon as you *see* milk squirting from your nipple, you know you are compressing the underlying milk ducts. (This position is also where baby's gums should be during efficient latch-on.)

The trick to hand-expression is discovering where to position your fingers. Experiment until

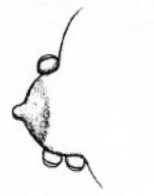

Hand-expression: press toward your chest

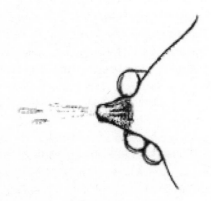

Hand-expression: roll and squeeze

you find the right spot. Having someone show you how is very helpful, too. Combining hand-expression with breast massage can be a very effective way to stimulate the milk-ejection reflex. Massage first, then express. Massage again, and repeat the hand-expressing routine.

When you hand-express, milk sprays out in all directions. If you're expressing just to make your breasts more comfortable, you can lean over a sink or express into a towel. If you want to save the milk, you'll need something in which to collect it. Some mothers manage to aim the nipple directly into a baby bottle. Or try a container with a wide mouth, such as a coffee mug. Medela makes a special funnel for hand-expression that collects

the milk and channels it down into a standard baby bottle.

STORING YOUR MILK

Human milk is not like a can of tuna. If it spoils, you can't just go to the cupboard and get more. A bottle of your milk is precious to both you and your baby. It represents commitment on your part and ideal nourishment for your baby.

You should handle your milk with care, but not with too much fuss. The same immunogenic properties in your milk that protect your baby also protect the milk from bacteria while it sits on the refrigerator shelf.

When you are pumping milk for a full-term, healthy baby, you do not need to worry about sterilizing storage containers or pump parts. Wash your storage containers in hot, soapy water, and wash your hands thoroughly with soap and water before you pump. Check the manufacturer's instructions for information on washing parts of the pump. (Mothers who are pumping milk for a sick or hospitalized baby will need to be more careful about milk handling and sterilization procedures. See chapter 11.)

Freezing does lower some of the immunogenic properties in human milk, so it's best if your baby is given fresh milk — milk that has been pumped or expressed and then refrigerated. Label each container with the date, so that you can use the oldest milk first and avoid wasting any.

The Container Debate

To store expressed milk, you can choose soft plastic (polyethylene) bags, polypropylene plastic bottles, and/or glass or steel containers. If you use plastic containers, be sure they are not made with bisphenol A (BPA), which can harm baby's endocrine system. The choice of container may lower the amount of antibodies, fat, some nutrients, and/or the white blood cells' ability to

STORAGE GUIDELINES FOR HUMAN MILK*

These guidelines are for mothers who are expressing milk for a full-term healthy baby. Use clean containers, and wash your hands with soap and water before expressing or pumping. When providing milk for a baby who is seriously ill and/or hospitalized, check with health-care providers for instructions.

Storage Location	Storage Temperature	Storage Duration
A cooler with reusable ice pack	60°F (15°C)	24 hours
Indoor counter, shelf, or cabinet	66–72°F (19–22°C)	6–8 hours
Indoor counter, shelf, or cabinet	76–85°F (25–29°C)	3–4 hours
Refrigerator**	Up to 39°F (4°C)	5–8 days
Open freezer compartment inside a refrigerator	Varies	2 weeks
Enclosed freezer above, below, or to the side of a refrigerator	Varies	3–4 months
Freestanding freezer that maintains a constant temperature	0°F (-17°C)	6 months optimal, 12 months acceptable

*Adapted from "Academy of Breastfeeding Medicine Clinical Protocol #8: Human Milk Storage," 2010
** Best to use within 48 hours to preserve nutrients

stay alive. However, no study has shown that these effects are problematic for baby. So just use the most convenient container unless you have an ill or premature infant; then you might want to use glass or plastic bottles, because plastic bags can lower antibodies by 60 percent (which is still 40 percent more than formula contains).

Sterilization is no longer considered necessary. Hot, soapy water or dishwasher cleaning makes reusing containers easy. But because convenience is usually the only concern, here are some factors to consider:

• Plastic bags take up less room in the freezer and in the ice chest you may be using to transport milk to and from your workplace and other locations.

• Plastic bags are one-use items, so there's no dishwashing involved. You'll save time and have one fewer chore to think about.

• The disposable plastic bags that are designed for use with infant feeding bottles are available anyplace that sells infant formula. However, they tend to tear and are not really designed for freezer storage. If you are storing your milk in these, use two bags to protect against breakage and freezer burn. Use twist ties to close the bags. (Sealing disposable nurser bags can get tricky; this is one of their disadvantages.)

• Plastic bags are associated with a higher incidence of sour-tasting or soapy-tasting (but not spoiled) milk. If baby refuses the milk, the soapy taste can be prevented by scalding the milk (heating it to 180°F [82°C]) prior to freezing. (Too much heat destroys enzymes.)

• Plastic bags made especially to hold human milk are available from breast-pump companies as well as most pharmacies and grocery stores that have a baby-care section. These bags are sturdier than formula-bottle bags, and some can be attached directly to their pumps. They have built-in closures that are much easier to use than twist ties. They are also designed to be used in the freezer, and many can be recycled. However, they cost more than formula-bottle bags.

- Plastic bags that fit into holders for feeding babies may be very convenient for your caregiver. Pouring milk out of a plastic bag into a bottle requires some care.

- Bags containing human milk should be placed inside another container in the refrigerator or freezer. This makes for better protection and easier handling. If you lay the bags down in a container in the freezer, you'll get flatter packages that will thaw more quickly. (But be sure they're sealed well, or you'll have a leaky mess.)

- Always leave some space at the top of the bag or bottle to allow for expansion. Like water, human milk expands when you freeze it. If there's no room for expansion in the bag, it will

break and you'll have to discard the milk. Squeeze out the air at the top of the bag and fasten it an inch above the milk. Leave about an inch of room for the milk to expand in the freezer in a hard container, too.

- Hard containers should have secure, one-piece tops.

How Much Milk to Store in Each Container

Store your milk in small amounts, about two ounces to each container, at least at first. (If you're pumping milk for a premature baby, you may want to store it in even smaller amounts.) Breastfed babies take smaller amounts of milk at each feeding than do formula-fed infants, and smaller amounts are quicker to thaw. After you've been back at work for a week or two, you may decide to put more milk in each bottle, based on your caregiver's report regarding how much your baby takes at each feeding. You can add more milk to already frozen milk, but cool the added milk in the refrigerator first. There should be less

SAVE OR DUMP?		
Type of Milk	**Save or Dump?**	**Why**
Milk remaining in the bottle that has been offered to baby	If fresh, refrigerate and use within 4 hours; if thawed, refrigerate and use within 1–2 hours; otherwise discard	Bacteria from baby's mouth will have entered the milk during the feeding, which could lead to bacterial contamination if it sits too long: one small unpublished study showed no increase in bacteria in leftover breast milk stored at 39–43°F (4–6°C) for 48 hours
Milk that has been thawed	Save in the refrigerator for up to 24 hours after thawing, then discard; do not refreeze	Milk that has been frozen has lost some of the immunogenic properties that inhibit bacterial growth in fresh refrigerated milk
Milk kept in the refrigerator for 8 days	Transfer to storage in the freezer	Bacterial growth is not a problem, but milk sometimes picks up odors or flavors from the refrigerator or container

added milk than already frozen milk to avoid having the frozen milk thaw and refreeze.

How Long to Keep the Milk

For recommended storage times, see the box above. Amazingly, research has found that human milk stored in the refrigerator for eight days actually has lower bacteria levels than freshly expressed milk.

Since human milk can be kept in the refrigerator for up to eight days, it may be possible to provide your baby with fresh, not frozen, milk most of the time. This ensures that your baby gets the maximum amount of nutrients and immunity boosters. Instruct your caregiver to use the oldest milk first and keep rotating the supply.

Previously frozen milk can be kept in the refrigerator for twenty-four hours after thawing. This means that you or your baby's caregiver can thaw milk for all your baby's feedings at one time, or you can thaw the milk in the refrigerator overnight. This can make it faster to prepare a bottle when your baby is hungry. Milk that has thawed should not be refrozen.

Transporting Your Milk

Research shows that bacteria do not grow readily in human milk and that it can be kept safely at room temperature for four to six hours (or more — see the box on page 155). You don't need to worry if you can't rush your milk to the refrigerator right after you express. But it still makes sense to refrigerate the milk as soon as possible and to keep it cool when taking it home or to the caregiver's location. If you have refrigerator space available at work, you can store your milk there until the workday is over. If not, you can use an insulated container with a reusable ice pack to keep it cool.

Pump manufacturers sell stylish carrying cases for electric pumps that also have compartments for keeping expressed milk cool. There might even be room for your lunch and snacks. You may not need such fancy equipment, but just the fact that it's available tells you that you're not alone in this pumping business.

Thawing and Heating Stored Milk

Heat can destroy human milk's enzymes, immunogenic properties, and other valuable components, so it requires gentle care before it is served to baby. Follow these guidelines:

- Defrost milk by holding the container under warm running water. Or, for a larger container, place it in a bowl of warm water on the kitchen counter. As the water cools, replace it with more warm water until the milk is thawed and warmed to body temperature.

- Do not heat expressed human milk on top of the stove. It's too easy to overheat it this way. Do not boil!

- Do not heat expressed human milk in a microwave oven. Even if the overall temperature of the milk stays below body temperature, there may be hot spots where the milk is overheated and some of its beneficial properties are destroyed. The uneven heating can be dangerous when the bottle is given to baby.

- Human milk, like any milk that is not processed or homogenized, tends to separate when stored. The cream rises to the top. Swirl the bottle gently to mix the layers.

- Human milk has a thin, bluish look to it, quite different from either homogenized cow's milk or the grayish color of infant formula. Your baby's caregiver may need reassuring that the color is normal.

- On rare occasions mothers report that their milk "spoils" (has a soapy smell) within hours and that baby rejects it even when it has been stored in a hard container. This is thought to be caused by higher levels of enzymes (especially lipase) in some mothers' milk. What happens is that the fat cells are being prematurely broken down by the lipase, causing the strong odor. In such cases scalding the milk (heating it to 180ºF [82ºC], or until you see tiny bubbles around the edge of the pan) seems to stop that process. Do this only if baby refuses the milk, since heat destroys valuable enzymes.

BREASTFEEDING WHEREVER YOU GO

There's no need to stay at home just because you're breastfeeding. Mothers nurse their babies anywhere and everywhere, and you, too, can learn to do this. Once you've experienced the freedom of being able to grab a few diapers and go, you may decide that when it comes to convenience, breast milk is the original fast food, a meal "to go" on a moment's notice.

Breastfeeding at home in the first weeks postpartum includes lots of skin-to-skin contact with baby and lots of "letting it all hang out." Nursing at the mall, the museum, or your mother-in-law's house is going to require a different approach. There's really nothing wrong with exposing a breast so that a baby can nurse, but in many social situations, most people are more comfortable when mothers nurse discreetly. Good manners suggest that you should take the feelings of others into account, but of course your first consideration should be your baby. When she's hungry or in need of comfort, she wants the breast!

Some simple strategizing can make breastfeeding away from home an easy and natural thing to do. Practicing at home helps, too. Ask your spouse or a friend for a critique of your discreet nursing style. A great place to practice and observe the style of experienced mothers is at a breastfeeding support group meeting. Here are some tips to help you feel more confident no

matter where you are when your baby starts giving cues that she wants to nurse.

What to Wear

Simple, accessible clothing is the key to nursing in public. Wear clothes that make it easy to nurse discreetly. Two-piece outfits with loose tops are

---

WARNING: DO NOT BREASTFEED IN A MOVING CAR

As tempting as it is to give your breast to your screaming baby to calm him in the car, especially since you are sitting right next to him and you both are securely buckled up, don't start this dangerous (and potentially illegal) practice. Moving your body so you can lean over your baby to nurse him, or for any other reason, causes your seat belt at the shoulder and hip to shift to an improper position. A collision in this situation will cause your chest to make hard contact with your baby's head. Leaning forward and over also loosens your shoulder strap enough to render it ineffective at preventing your head and upper torso from hitting hard surfaces. It goes without saying that you must never remove your baby from the car seat when the car is moving. If you think your baby is hungry and needs to be fed, have the driver get off the road and find a safe place to park, away from moving traffic. If baby is crying "just" because he hates being buckled in, and you are sitting next to him, try letting him suck on your index finger (as you do when giving your breast a break from being a pacifier). If you start this from the beginning, even on the car ride home from the hospital or birth center, he will get used to having this help in the months to come, when car rides will get easier on everyone.

the best. You can lift the shirt from the bottom so that baby can get at the breast. The rest of the fabric will drape around the baby's head to cover any exposed skin. If you're wearing a shirt or blouse that buttons, unbutton it from the bottom up rather than from the top down. Think of nursing in terms of snuggling your baby under your clothes rather than getting your breast out. Here are some additional clothing tips:

- A loose jacket or cardigan sweater can provide extra coverage for your middle.

- Drape a lightweight blanket or shawl over your shoulder and over baby as you nurse.

- An old T-shirt worn under a sweater or another shirt can provide extra coverage and protect your middle from icy drafts. Cut slits in the T-shirt at breast level. When you lift the outer shirt, the T-shirt stays in place.

- A baby sling is a real boon for discreet nursing. You can stroll through department stores or play with a toddler in the park while keeping baby latched on behind the fabric of the sling.

- Wear a large T-shirt over your swimsuit for discreet nursing at the beach. Or look for swimsuits made especially for breastfeeding women.

- If you yearn to wear dresses, look for special styles for nursing mothers, with hidden openings at the breast. These are available from catalogs and can sometimes be found in maternity shops. Or perhaps you can make your own.

- Nursing bras with cups that are easy to unfasten with one hand can make it easy to get your baby started at the breast, but refastening bra cups often requires two hands. You might have to wait to do this until you have a private moment—another reason to avoid clingy or sheer tops when you're out with baby.

- Prints and loose styles camouflage leaks and spit-up stains.

- Cotton is cool in the warm months and warm when it's cool.

BREASTFEEDING WHILE BABYWEARING

One day while attending an international conference on breastfeeding, we noticed several mothers from developing countries carrying their babies in attractive slings. In fact, many of their slings were made from the same fabric as their dresses. We noticed how these moms would casually nurse their babies while engaging in the activities of the busy conference. When we asked them why mothers in their cultures wear their babies, we got two very simple but profound answers: "It does good things for babies" and "It makes life easier for mother." Specifically, here are the good things babywearing does for breastfeeding babies and mothers.

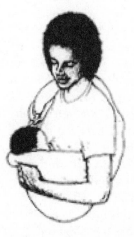

Sling nursing

BREASTFEEDING WHILE BABYWEARING (continued)

Babywearing facilitates breastfeeding.
Some babies breastfeed better on the move, especially those problem nursers who need movement to organize their systems. Tense babies and back archers especially breastfeed better in a sling because it keeps their bodies supported and relaxed. It's difficult for a baby to arch away from the breast in a baby sling. As baby's whole body relaxes, so do the muscles used in sucking. To try breastfeeding on the move, first position baby in the sling and get baby latched on. Then immediately begin walking at a slow, even pace, keeping your arm around baby to maintain secure latch-on. (This is not a "Look, ma, no hands" feat, but you do have one hand free.)

Holding regulates babies. Securely held infants show a heightened level of quiet alertness, the behavioral state in which infants best interact with and learn from their environments. A baby in the quiet, alert state will be more eager to breastfeed.

Carried babies cry less. Parents in our pediatrics practice commonly report, "As long as I hold her, she's content!" Parents of fussy babies who try babywearing relate that their babies seem to forget to fuss. A baby who fusses less is easier to feed.

Babywearing promotes a baby in balance.
Babywearing has a regulatory effect on the baby, primarily through the vestibulary system. Behind each ear there are three tiny organs that work as a kind of carpenter's level to control baby's sense of internal balance — one tracking side to-side motion, the other up-and-down motion, and the third back-

and-forth motion. Every time your baby moves, the fluid in these "levels" moves against tiny hairlike filaments that vibrate, which send messages to the brain to help balance her body.

Babywearing "reminds" baby of the motion and balance she enjoyed in the womb. The motion of mother's walk, which baby got so used to in the womb, is experienced again in the "outside womb" during babywearing. The calming effect makes baby easier to live with and easier to breastfeed.

Babywearing contains the infant. Wearing baby in a sling encourages baby to maintain longer latch-on. Using the sling to support baby in the football hold is particularly useful, since curling baby into this position generally relaxes baby's sucking muscles and encourages better latch-on.

Babywearing helps in toddler tending.
Babywearing is especially valuable when trying to juggle the needs of a new baby and the demands of an older toddler. As one mother in our practice told us, "Breastfeeding our new baby in the sling gives me an extra hand for playing with and enjoying our toddler. This has done wonders to lessen sibling rivalry and has allowed me to mother both children well."

Babywearing is good postpartum exercise.
What's good for baby is also good for mother. Wearing baby in a sling allows you mobility. You can take a relaxing walk — especially during "happy hour," that fussy period that many babies have toward the end of the day. Training your baby to become a "sling baby"

BREASTFEEDING WHILE BABYWEARING (continued)

allows you the mobility of going shopping, out to dinner, and incorporating baby into your daily activities. Also, being carried allows babies to interact with their environments. Babies learn a lot in the arms of a busy parent. And it's also good conditioning for you, strengthening your upper-body and back muscles as you gradually accommodate a baby who gets a little heavier every day.

Babywearing allows for discreet breastfeeding. Since sling babies are more content and cry less, you can more easily take them to places where having a baby with you might otherwise be socially awkward. When baby needs to nurse for food, comfort, or for settling, you simply nestle baby into the sling and use it as a cover-up. Martha has even breastfed several of our babies in a baby sling while being interviewed on national television. Babywearing while breastfeeding is not only one of the oldest ways of parenting, it is also quite contemporary.

Babywearing helps baby gain weight. In our breastfeeding counseling practice, we have found that babies who are carried more grow better. Mothers who have been encouraged to wear their babies in a sling for several hours a day report that their babies feed more frequently and in a more relaxed way and that their weight dramatically increases if they have previously been slow to gain. Proximity to mother encourages baby to feed more frequently, and the closeness enables mother to read and respond to baby's feeding cues better. Since baby is near the source of milk and comfort, she does not have to cry and waste energy summoning mother. Baby can then divert this energy from crying into growing.

BREASTS: NOT JUST FOR SELLING BEER

We can't let a discussion of nursing in public pass without commenting on one of life's ironies. In American culture breasts are exposed everywhere—in movies, in magazines, and especially in advertising. The woman who wears a cleavage-revealing swimsuit at the beach or public pool doesn't have to worry about social disapproval. But the new mother venturing out with her baby to a dimly lit restaurant with her husband shakes in her shoes when she discreetly nurses her baby with a shawl draped over both her breast and the baby's head. "What if someone says something?" she worries.

Fortunately, public opinion on breastfeeding is becoming more enlightened as the benefits become more widely recognized. While stories about women being asked not to nurse in public places occasionally make headlines, in the brouhaha that follows most commentators come down squarely on the side of the nursing mother. It's good public relations for businesses and public facilities to accommodate the needs of breastfeeding families. In recent years, many states have passed laws emphasizing that it's legal for mothers to nurse their babies anywhere,

---

BREASTS: NOT JUST FOR SELLING BEER (continued)

without fear of being cited for "indecent exposure." Of course, breastfeeding in public never has been against the law.

And keep in mind that thousands of mothers nurse their babies every day at the mall, the park, and the pool, and that thousands of other people either don't notice, don't care, or smile approvingly—which is what you should do when you notice a mother nursing her baby at the hamburger joint or the baseball game.

Nursing Without Being Noticed

One of the best ways to avoid drawing a lot of attention to yourself and your nursing baby is to be alert to your baby's hunger cues and feed her before she is howling. She'll latch on more easily, and you won't have lots of people scowling at you while you try to stop the noise. Expect that you will feed your baby while you're out at the mall or visiting friends. Don't nurse as a last resort, when all your attempts to distract your baby have failed.

Your breast could be exposed during the brief moment it takes for your little one to latch on. This is more of a problem with young babies than for experienced nursers. You can turn your back to the rest of the room while you get her started, or briefly go into another room and return once baby is latched on and blankets and clothing are discreetly arranged. Or drape a blanket over your breast, arm, and baby during latch-on. You can also pull up the fabric of a baby sling to cover your breast while baby is getting started.

If you're sitting on a bench or a chair without arms, use your diaper bag, a folded sweater or coat, or something else in your lap to bring baby up to breast level while you nurse. You'll enjoy your outing more if you don't go home with sore nipples or a cramp in your arm or back caused by poor positioning at the breast.

Remember, baby's head provides the crucial cover-up while she's at the breast. Keep an eye on your baby while she's nursing if she's the kind who likes to pop off and smile up at you from time to time. You'll want to flip your shirt down during these tender moments. If you have a baby who loves to push your sweater up to your collarbone, try holding that free baby hand in yours while nursing in public places. As your baby gets older, teach her good nursing manners. Climbing around on your lap while nursing may be okay at home, but you probably won't appreciate this behavior at the family reunion.

Sometimes people who are not accustomed to being around nursing babies simply don't know where to look while baby has his dinner. You can help them out with this awkward feeling by maintaining eye contact and chatting with this other person while your baby is latching on. That will help observers focus on your face and avoid looking at your breast, which will probably help them feel more comfortable. A brief positive comment about your breastfed baby will also help people who are new to the world of babies feel more at ease.

Where to Go When It's Time for Baby to Dine

Choose an out-of-the-way place to nurse your baby if possible, if it really matters to you. Here are some strategies for various locations:

- In a restaurant, ask to be seated in a booth at the side of the room rather than in the middle of everything. Sitting with your back to the room gives you more privacy.

BREASTFEEDING IN PUBLIC: DO WE REALLY NEED A LAW?

Unfortunately, yes: because having laws on the books that say mothers have the right to breastfeed in public is a way of protecting them from harassment and making everyone more aware of the benefits of breastfeeding. Women have always had the right to breastfeed in public, and courts have never regarded breastfeeding as "indecent exposure." Over the years, laws about public breastfeeding have been passed by many state legislatures, and eventually the federal government affirmed this by passing a law that says it is *legal* to breastfeed on federal property, even though it has never been *illegal* to breastfeed on federal property—in national parks, national museums, or the Capitol building itself.

Nursing in public is just one of several issues in which breastfeeding may be affected by the legal system. For more information about breastfeeding and custody decisions, visitation issues, and about getting an exemption from jury duty because of breastfeeding, contact La Leche League at LLLI.org.

• At the mall, look for a seating area with nooks or plants if you don't want to nurse in front of everyone who may be passing by. Or stop for a snack and nurse in a corner of the restaurant. Or choose a comfortable place to sit down where you can people-watch while you nurse.

• Nursing at a religious service is a real hurdle for some women. In many places of worship, you'll have more privacy and fewer comments from passersby if you nurse in a pew during the service rather than in a coatroom or even the women's restroom. If you nurse the baby before he starts to cry, most people won't even know what you're doing. (We know one woman who nursed a succession of babies while singing in the choir. Her only complaint came when the choir got new robes that made it much more difficult to find her breasts.)

• Many public places provide special areas where mothers can nurse their babies. Look for these, use them, and if you get a chance, write a note of appreciation. But don't feel that you have to hide in a special nursing mother's facility. It's often much more convenient just to breastfeed wherever you happen to be.

Taking the plunge. For some mothers, the biggest obstacle to nursing in public is their own mind-set: nursing in public may be fine for someone else, but it's just not me. You may not feel instantly comfortable nursing your baby anywhere and everywhere, but start small and give it a try. Babies need to nurse often, and mothers need to get out of the house. Breastfeeding shouldn't isolate mothers from the rest of the world. Maybe start by practicing in front of a mirror, then step it up by having a few girlfriends over. Focus on having fun and enjoying your new skills!

Many mothers find it easier to nurse around strangers than around certain friends or members of their extended families. What do you do if your father-in-law leaves the living room while you nurse? Or if your husband doesn't want you nursing your baby in front of his softball buddies? A lot depends on the relationships, but in many cases, it just takes time for people who are unfamiliar with breastfeeding to feel comfortable. Eventually people who care about you and your baby will take their cues from you. If you're comfortable nursing in front of the television during the World Series, they'll learn to be comfortable, too.

When you first venture out in public with your baby, take along a friend. A more experienced nursing mother can supply the confidence you need. So can a supportive husband. And smile proudly. You're doing the best for your baby.

8

20 Tips for Breastfeeding While Working

WOMEN HAVE ALWAYS WORKED and breastfed. The pioneer mother on the prairie had lots to do besides nurse her babies, and even modern mothers who are at home during the day struggle with the work of running busy households and often supplementing the family income while responding to the needs of their infants. Martha breastfed our first baby, Jim, while working part-time as a nurse. In 1967 Bill was a grossly underpaid intern, and we needed Martha's income to survive.

Today, continuing to breastfeed while working outside the home is much more common than it used to be. Working-and-nursing mothers can choose from a variety of pumps and products made just for them. In the United States, most pumping mothers are protected by a federal law that requires their employers to provide a clean, private place for milk expression as well as the time to do so. Some states have even more protections and allow more liberal maternity leaves than the usual six to eight weeks given to most US mothers. In some countries mothers are given as much as a year after birth to return to work. But no matter how old your baby is when you return to work, and no matter how many laws protect you, continuing to breastfeed after returning to work still presents plenty of

challenges. Here are twenty time-tested tips to help you continue to give your baby the best in nutrition after you return to your job.

YOUR WEEKS AT HOME

1. Make a commitment. Breastfeeding mothers want to give their babies the best possible nutrition, even if they can't be there to deliver it personally. Knowing how good human milk is for human babies is a powerful motivator. Mothers also continue breastfeeding after they return to work because they want to be more connected to their babies when they *are* with them. In fact, this connectedness stays with them during the hours when they are at work. They are, after all, breastfeeding working mothers. There is a physical and physiological identity that sets them apart as mothers who have made a commitment.

Juggling breastfeeding and working is not easy. There will be days when you wonder if it's all worth it. You'll develop a love-hate relationship with your pump. You'll leak at embarrassing moments, and you may be on the receiving end of less-than-supportive comments from ignorant coworkers. There will be days when you're ready to toss in the pump and reach for the formula. Yet once you make a commitment to continuing to breastfeed, you'll find a way to do it. If you believe that breastfeeding is important for your baby and for yourself, doing what it takes to continue this beautiful relationship will not seem difficult. And you'll enjoy all the practical benefits of nursing your baby full-time when you are together after work and on weekends.

To encourage new mothers to return to work, my wonderful employer provides a "mother's room," complete with a sink, refrigerator, cubbies for a pump, a nice comfortable chair, a phone, and a lock on the door. A strong pump was my key to success. I called it my double-barreled power pump. My milk supply did waver, but after a few weeks I was a pro. From six to eleven months, as my baby began to eat cereal and veggies and needed less milk, I reduced my pumpings to two per day. Then, as her solid-food consumption increased even more (eleven to twelve months), I pumped just once a day. Each day when I returned home, we nursed right away, which helped us reconnect. At one year, I ceased pumping altogether, and I am still nursing.

You may be worried that nursing and working will be a lot of bother. Friends may have told you about their own difficulties with pumping milk or arranging feeding schedules. Working and caring for a small baby *is* a juggling act, so you do need to think carefully about this choice and how you will manage it. If you're not sure that you want to continue breastfeeding after you return to your job, give it at least a thirty-day trial period. This way you'll have a chance to work out any problems and settle into a mutually rewarding experience for you and baby. Have confidence in yourself. You can do this!

2. Get connected. To build a solid relationship with your baby, you must banish the "what ifs." What if he won't take a bottle? What if he won't take a nap? What if she won't settle down without nursing? When I pump milk at home I can pump

only a little bit. What if I can't pump enough milk when I'm back at work?

Don't let these worries about the future intrude on your enjoyment of your first weeks with your baby. These are legitimate concerns, but at the same time, they are all problems that can be solved. It's good to plan ahead—but not too much. Look for the answers to these questions in

BENEFITS OF BREASTFEEDING WHILE WORKING

Choosing to breastfeed your baby means better nutrition and a special closeness, both compelling reasons for all mothers to breastfeed. Here are some other benefits enjoyed by mothers who continue breastfeeding after they return to work.

- Breastfed babies are healthier, so mother (and father) will miss fewer work days to stay home with a sick baby who is not welcome at day care.
- Breastfeeding saves money. A one-time pump purchase is cheaper than buying formula. Even renting a hospital-grade electric pump is cheaper than buying most formulas.
- Providing breast milk for feedings while you're gone protects your baby against allergies.
- Pumping, saving the milk, and even leaking while you're at work help you feel connected to your baby when you must be apart.
- Because only mother can breastfeed, a baby always knows whom he loves the most. Nannies, babysitters, and day-care workers are no substitute for a nursing mom.
- Mothers can look forward to a warm and cuddly reunion at the breast after hours of separation.

the pages ahead, but, as the saying goes, don't cross that bridge before you come to it.

Don't let your preoccupation with the day you need to return to work (W-Day) rob you of the joy of those weeks of being a full-time mother. We understand that you may be very worried about all the details of your return to the job, but you can't get properly attached to your baby if you're thinking constantly about the day you will need to leave her. Fears about how difficult it will be to leave your baby can get in the way of forming a deep attachment. Holding back on your feelings is bad for both of you. Nothing is more important to your success at combining working, parenting, and breastfeeding than building a strong attachment to your baby. You need this as much as your child does; it will be the foundation of your relationship in all the years to come. Your

baby needs to know that you, her mother, are the one special person she can always depend on. From your point of view, feeling connected to your child will help you keep your priorities in order when you're juggling job and family. So even if your maternity leave is only a few short weeks, use this time to allow yourself to be

---

BREASTFEEDING BENEFITS EMPLOYERS

Dear Employer:

You and your company will derive two major economic benefits by encouraging mothers to breastfeed and by giving them time and providing facilities where they can pump and store their breast milk when they are away from their babies. Mothers who breastfeed their infants take at least half as much sick leave because their breastfed infants suffer fewer illnesses. And by fostering a breastfeeding-friendly workplace, you will have happier, and therefore more productive, working mothers.

The American Academy of Pediatrics currently recommends that mothers breastfeed their babies for at least one year. For more information on creating a breastfeeding-friendly workplace, contact the Office on Women's Health at WomensHealth.gov or call 800-994-9662.

BEST FOR BABY, BEST FOR BOSS

Breastfeeding is not just good for mothers and babies. It's good for employers, too! It will be easier to get the support you need if you can show your employer that the company will benefit when you continue breastfeeding. Here's how:

- Mothers who enjoy the support of a breastfeeding-friendly workplace are likely to have more job satisfaction and show higher productivity (in milk making as well as in job performance).
- Breastfed babies are less likely to get sick, and their illnesses are milder than those of their formula-fed counterparts. Studies show that breastfeeding mothers have three to six times less absenteeism than mothers who formula-feed.
- Breastfed babies use fewer health-care dollars because they make fewer visits to the doctor and have fewer serious illnesses.
- Breastfeeding women are more relaxed and even-tempered, thanks to the hormonal effects of lactation.
- Breastfeeding women are less likely to become pregnant again soon. Women who continue breastfeeding probably won't be needing another maternity leave within twelve months.
- Supporting breastfeeding mothers helps companies hold on to valued employees.

MAKING THE MOST OF YOUR MATERNITY LEAVE

Maternity leave means just that: you leave out everything possible that drains your energy away from developing a relationship with your baby. There is both a cultural and a scientific basis for the traditional six weeks of maternity leave. Levels of prolactin, the milk-making hormone, are highest in the first six weeks postpartum. Many cultures have traditions that intuitively respect these six weeks of "maternity leave." Societies have learned that this is the minimum time necessary for mother to establish her milk supply and for her body to recover from childbirth. At the cellular level, lactation scientists now believe that it takes six weeks of frequent nursing to establish sufficient prolactin receptors, special sites on the milk-making cells of the breast that welcome prolactin as a trigger for milk production. The more prolactin receptors there are, the easier it is for the breasts to produce sufficient milk in the months ahead.

completely absorbed by your baby. Think of this time as a "babymoon"—like a honeymoon, with an emphasis on establishing a relationship with minimal intrusions. The stronger your attachment, the better you will be able to understand your baby. This will make caring for your baby much easier after you return to work.

If you're reading this during your pregnancy, you're probably thinking of all sorts of extra tasks you can accomplish while taking a few weeks or a few months away from your job. After all, with no work commitment, what will you do all day? (Mothers who quit their jobs to stay home full-time with their babies make these kind of lists, too.)

But here's a reality check: you're not going to get any of those things done. Wallpapering the bathroom is not a newborn-friendly activity. Nor is gourmet cooking. Expect to spend your time nursing your baby, holding your baby, enjoying your baby. This season of your life will never come again; treasure it while it's here. (You can organize those closets next year—or five years from now.) Mothering a newborn will absorb all your time. It should. These weeks after birth are when mothers fall in love with their babies. And as in any love affair, the two of you need time together to get to know each other.

Will focusing on just being a mother now make it more difficult to leave your baby later? It might. We've seen many mothers who had thought they would return to the workplace move heaven and earth to stay home longer so they would have more time with their babies. We've also seen the payoff for mothers who take the time to really get attached to their babies but who do return to their jobs. They work very hard at maintaining their close relationships with their children. They enjoy their babies more, and the benefits to the children are lifelong.

3. Get breastfeeding off to a good start. Doing everything you can to make breastfeeding work well in the early weeks is important to breastfeeding success after you return to work. You need to breastfeed early and often to encourage your breasts to produce lots of milk. Feeding your baby on cue will get your milk supply in line with your baby's needs. And your baby needs lots of practice at the breast, so that she has good sucking skills that will not be affected by artificial nipples later on. The more you can learn about breastfeeding at this stage, the more easily you will be able to solve any problems that might occur in the future.

Plan to take as much maternity leave as you can. Check with your human resources department to learn about what you are entitled to at the state and federal levels. If you don't have access to a human resources department, the National Conference of State Legislatures lists your entitlements at ncsl.org/research/labor-and-employment/state-family-and-medical-leave-laws.aspx. You can also use vacation time or, if financially possible, consider taking unpaid leave so you can stay home longer. (Sacrificing some income at this point in your life could turn out to be one of the best decisions you'll ever make—staying at home longer at first will lead to less sick leave and fewer health issues later on.) If there is a compelling reason why your baby must receive breast milk, or if your postpartum course is complicated by maternal health problems, you may be able to prolong your leave time by getting a letter from your doctor or by being placed on longer-term disability. The longer you can be with your baby, breastfeeding all the time, the easier it will be to continue when you are back on the job. Also, when you do return, consider working part-time, even if only for a month or two. This will simplify breastfeeding, provide an easier transition back to work, and aid in maintaining breastfeeding.

A SAMPLE LETTER

(on letterhead of requesting doctor)

Date:
To: Insurance provider
Insured: [find out whose name your insurer requires—yours or your baby's]
Subject: Rental [or purchase] of electric breast pump

As the physician caring for _____ [mother's or baby's name], I have found it to be medically necessary that _____ [baby's name] be fed mother's milk. Because of _____ [medical conditions such as prematurity, illness, inadequate weight gain, and so on], it is medically necessary that [name of mother] pump her milk with an electric breast pump so she can feed her baby her milk. Studies have proved that breast milk lowers the rate and duration of hospitalizations as well as the frequency of common illnesses of infancy and childhood. Studies have also shown that hospital-grade electric pumps with a double-pumping system provide the most milk. It is medically necessary that _____ [name of mother] either purchase or rent this pump, in addition to the materials necessary to transport and store her milk. I estimate that _____ [name of mother] will require the use of this pump for _____ [time— usually three to six months]. Please expedite the insurance coverage for this request. I will be happy to provide any additional information you require.

Sincerely,

[Name and signature of physician]

PLANNING YOUR RETURN

4. Explore your options. There are probably as many ways to combine breastfeeding and working as there are mothers, babies, and jobs. We'll give you a broad outline here, but it's up to you to fill in the details that work best for you and your baby (and your employer). Keep in mind that your plans will change as your baby grows and develops. For example, you may not have to provide quite as much pumped milk once your baby starts eating solid food. Often the best solutions to the challenges of combining nursing and employment are the creative ones. Consider these alternatives to spending the entire day away from your baby:

- *Take your baby to work.* This may not be possible on an industrial assembly line, but there are many workplaces that can accommodate the presence of an infant. We've known mothers who work in shops, in offices, in family businesses, and in other settings who have just packed up baby and brought her along when it's time to return to the job after a postpartum leave. Breastfed babies are very portable. Arrange a safe and comfortable place for naps, diaper changes, and floor play, and you'll be all set.

- *Try work and wear.* Wear your baby in a sling-type carrier to keep baby close to you while you assist customers, sort papers, work at the computer, or even attend meetings. You may have to work a longer day or accept less pay to make up for job time spent attending to your baby, but you'll save on the expense of child care and there will be less emotional wear and tear on mother and baby. Eventually, when your "sling baby" becomes a toddler explorer, you may have to make other arrangements, but by then baby will not be depending on you for as much of her nutritional needs. (For more on

babywearing while breastfeeding, see chapter 7.)

- *Take your work to your baby.* Working from home is becoming more common in these days of telecommuting. Perhaps you can arrange to complete some or all of your tasks at home. Even working at home one or two days a week and going into the office the rest of the time will give you more time to breastfeed your baby on cue. Some mothers who work from home concentrate on working during baby's naps, or they go to bed late or get up early. Some manage to work with baby close by or even on their laps, watching out for little fingers hitting the computer keyboard. Others find they need some in-home child care, but mother is still available for nursing as needed.

- *On-site day care.* Family-friendly employers are increasingly making child care available at the workplace. With this option, you can just go to another part of the building to breastfeed your baby on breaks or at lunchtime. Day-care workers can call you when baby is hungry, or you can let them know when you'll be in to visit and feed during the day.

- *Nearby day-care providers.* Many parents look for child care near their homes. But sometimes it's more practical to look for a babysitter near your workplace, which makes it possible to go to your baby and nurse one or more times during the day. You can also nurse the baby at the sitter's or at the day-care center before and after work. This will cut down on the amount of pumping you need to do while separated from your baby.

- *Visits from your baby.* Maybe it's possible for your baby to come and visit you while you're working, during your lunch break, or at other times during the day. Mothers who make this option work for them often have dad or grandma as chief child-care provider—

someone who's willing to go the extra mile (literally) for baby's health and happiness. Perhaps you could meet your caregiver and baby at a convenient lunch spot halfway between home and your workplace.

- *Part-time work.* Minimizing the time you spend away from your baby will make breastfeeding easier. Many mothers plan on working only part-time while their children are small—either shorter workdays or fewer shifts per week. Others ease back into a full-time schedule slowly when they and their babies are ready.

5. Be flexible. Babies have a way of derailing mothers from their preplanned career tracks. Try to remain flexible as you plan for your return to work and for the continuation of your breastfeeding. Your needs will change and so will your baby's. If something that worked well a few weeks ago is not working now, change it. Babies have different needs and preferences at different stages.

You may be surprised at the strength of your attachment to your baby. It may be more difficult to leave her than you thought it would be. You may also be far more stressed and tired out than you anticipated. Many couples reevaluate their lifestyles and their job commitments during the years when their children are young. Don't be afraid to explore possibilities you might not have thought of before you became pregnant—quitting your job, finding a job that is more family friendly, starting a home-based business, or even becoming a child-care provider who looks after other people's children so that you can spend time with your own.

6. Choose a breastfeeding-friendly caregiver. If you can, make your arrangements for a substitute caregiver while you're still pregnant, so that the search for a babysitter doesn't consume valuable time and energy that could be spent on your baby. Finding a caregiver whom you can trust to parent your baby in a sensitive way is vitally important to your baby's welfare and your peace of mind while you are working. You also want a caregiver who is supportive of breastfeeding. Be sure to tell your caregiver how much being able to continue breastfeeding means to you, and thank this person for helping to make this possible.

If your baby's caregiver is unfamiliar with breastfed babies and handling expressed human milk, you'll need to educate her. Share information about the benefits of breastfeeding and about how your baby is growing and thriving on your milk. Tell her how to thaw and warm your milk (written instructions will be helpful), and work out a system for preparing, labeling, and storing the baby's bottles. Make this as simple as possible so that the caregiver can devote her attention to the baby, not to the feeding procedure. To speed the delivery of your milk to your baby so that she doesn't have to wait for bottles when she is hungry, try these tips:

- Freeze milk in small amounts that thaw quickly if you have to leave frozen milk.
- Thaw the amount of milk needed for each day overnight in the refrigerator. Any milk left after twenty-four hours will have to be discarded (see storage guidelines on page 156), but if your baby's milk consumption is fairly predictable, you can do this without worrying about waste.
- Ask your caregiver to try giving your baby cold milk from the refrigerator. Some babies don't mind (though they prefer warm milk right from mom's breast).

Tell the caregiver that you want your baby held for all feedings and that your baby should be picked up whenever she cries or fusses. If the caregiver is having trouble getting your baby to accept a bottle during your first days back at work, share the list of suggestions in the box below with her. Tell her what to offer your baby when she wants to suck only for comfort (a pacifier or perhaps the caregiver's clean finger). Be supportive and sympathetic — a good relationship with this person is important. But first and foremost, remember that you are in charge here and that you are the one who is responsible for your baby's well-being.

7. Get to know your breast pump. At least two weeks before your planned return to the job, get that breast pump out of the case and figure out how to make it work. Read the directions carefully — they're your best source of information for how to put the pump together, how to get the best use out of it, and how to clean it. You may also find some helpful tips on maximizing the amount of milk you can pump. If you have bought or rented your pump from a lactation consultant, this person will be another source of support and guidance. (For more information on how to use a breast pump, see chapter 7.)

It's helpful if you can build up even a small stockpile of milk in the freezer before you go back to work. You'll feel more confident, and you'll be less likely to worry about pumping enough milk for your baby while you're gone. A good time to try pumping is early in the morning. Most mothers have an ample milk supply early in the day. Because your breasts make milk continuously, you'll still have milk for your baby's first morning feeding even if you pump several ounces before she awakens.

Nursing tip for beginners: Don't panic if you get only a small amount of milk the first several times you pump. Many a mother has gotten out her pump to start stockpiling milk for her return to work and managed to pump only half an ounce (or even less). When a few more attempts turn out the same way, she begins to feel very worried about her plans for working and breastfeeding. If this sounds like your experience, here's information to reassure you.

First, don't worry that your baby is not getting enough to eat. Your body does not respond to a pump the way it responds to your sweet, lovely baby, whom you love more than anything. Plus, your baby is much better at getting milk out of your breasts than the mechanical pump is.

Second, don't worry that you won't be able to pump enough milk when you're separated from your baby. When you squeeze pumping sessions in between nursings, there just may not be much milk in your breasts to pump. When you're at work and it's been two and a half or three hours since you've fed your baby, the milk will be there. And it will come out.

Third, with more practice, your milk-ejection reflex will become conditioned to the pump. Right now, your milk lets down after your baby sucks for a little while, or maybe in anticipation of your baby sucking. Your body will soon learn to react in a similar way to the pump and the routine that surrounds pumping.

8. Get baby used to the bottle — but not too soon. Someone is going to tell you, "Give your baby a bottle by two weeks of age so he'll get used to it. Otherwise, he may never take it." This is poor advice. It's best to avoid bottles, certainly during the first three weeks. Offering a bottle when your baby is learning the fine art of latch-on and you are building up your milk supply might interfere with both these processes. If the bottle is introduced too soon, some babies develop nipple preference. Other babies switch back and forth from breast to bottle without difficulty. Some quickly decide that it's easier to get milk from a bottle and have difficulty returning to the breast. Of course, you don't know that you have this kind of baby until after the bottle is introduced and baby is unwilling to take the breast. It's wiser not to take the risk, especially if your baby has had difficulty learning to take the breast. Give him some time to consolidate what he's learned about breastfeeding before you present him with a new challenge. A hungry baby will learn to take a bottle eventually, especially if your milk is in it. A couple of weeks before you return to work, begin offering baby the bottle as a toy and let him get familiar with it. Don't obsess about baby accepting the bottle, and don't force the issue. If baby takes the bottle, fine; if he doesn't, okay. Some babies refuse to take bottles from their mothers (they have sort of a "What's wrong with this picture?" reaction) but will take the bottle from another caregiver.

9. Check with your employer. If possible, talk with your human resources department about its policies as well as the state and federal laws that are in place to protect you. Under federal law in the United States, most women must be given a time and a place to pump their milk. The pumping area must be private and located somewhere other than a bathroom, and the amount of time allotted for pumping must be "reasonable" and consistently provided for the duration of the baby's first year of life. More information can be found at the United States Breastfeeding Committee website—USBreastfeeding.org.

If you are not covered by federal or state law, and your employer doesn't already have a pumping room, you'll need to talk—well in advance—with your employer and/or supervisor about your plans to pump at work. You don't want to be desperately looking around for a place to pump on your first day back, when your breasts are full and you've just realized that the women's lounge has no outlet for plugging in your electric pump. Depending on your employer's policies or lack thereof, you will need to consider when you will pump, where you will store milk, and whether other special arrangements can be made, such as being able to visit your baby or nurse during your lunch hour. If you know other women in your workplace who have pumped milk for their babies, talk to them about the problems they encountered and how they solved them. In putting together your plan, consider the following:

GETTING BABY TO ACCEPT A BOTTLE

It should come as no surprise that babies can be very opinionated about where their milk is coming from. A bottle and a rubber nipple are not the same as a breast, even if the bottle is offered by someone cradling the baby in secure, loving arms. Nevertheless, babies can and do learn to drink from a bottle when mother is not around. It may take some patience on the part of caregivers, but this is not an issue to obsess about throughout your maternity leave. Nor should you feel you must offer your baby bottles before four weeks of age—to "get him used to them." Undoing nipple preference and confusion (see chapter 2) in a young baby is more difficult than getting a slightly older baby to take a bottle, and problems with nipple confusion can lead to the end of breastfeeding.

Here are some tricks and tips for helping breastfed babies learn to accept milk from a bottle. If one approach doesn't work, try another.

- Introduce the bottle about two weeks before you return to work. If you introduce bottles earlier, don't make them a daily event. Baby doesn't need a bottle every day to maintain his skills; two per week should give him enough practice.
- Breastfed babies may not accept bottles from their mothers. (Why settle for something artificial to suck on when the real thing is only a few layers of fabric away?) Some discerning babies will balk if mother is even in the same room. So it may be best if dad or a substitute caregiver is the one to

GETTING BABY TO ACCEPT A BOTTLE (continued)

introduce the bottle. Fathers are often the logical choice to offer a baby her first bottles, but if your baby does not accept bottles readily from dad, avoid frustration and call in an experienced bottle feeder. This might be a grandmother, a substitute caregiver, or a friend with bottle-feeding experience. After baby has learned to take a bottle, dad can take over these occasional feedings.

- It may take some experimentation to discover your baby's bottle-feeding preferences, and the person offering the substitute feeding will have to be patient. Bottle feeding may prove to be a challenge that caregiver and baby will have to work on together. It shouldn't become a battle of wills. Experiment with different positions for bottle feeding. Some babies appreciate a bottle-feeding experience that is made to seem almost like breastfeeding: a familiar setting, the cradle hold, skin contact, lots of social interaction. Others see bottle feeding as a completely different activity. They may, at first, prefer to be held upright on the caregiver's lap, even facing outward rather than looking at her.

- Try walking around while offering the bottle. Using a baby sling can make this easier.

- Don't wait until baby is desperately hungry or in need of comfort sucking. For babies, as for adults, new experiences are easier to handle when they are well rested and not feeling anxious. A good time to practice is between feedings.

- Try nipples that resemble as much as possible the shape of your own areola and nipple. Use a nipple that has a wide, deep base that gradually tapers down to the tip of the nipple, much like the shape your breast takes in your baby's mouth. Avoid nipples that offer only a half-inch nubbin to latch on to or those with a short base. Orthodontic nipples are best, but be sure to buy the deep-base versions,

such as those made by Nuk and Avent. To judge how fast the milk flows, turn a full bottle upside down and watch the milk drip. One drop per second is easy for most babies to handle. A faster flow may overwhelm a baby who is used to the breast. A slower nipple will give baby more suck time.

- If baby is unhappy with one type of nipple, try another. No matter what the packaging claims, no rubber nipple is "just like mother."

- Warm the nipple under running water before offering it to the baby. Or cool it in the refrigerator if the baby is teething.

- Instead of inserting the artificial nipple into the baby's mouth, put it near his lips and encourage him to open wide and take the nipple on his own, as he does the breast, with a wide-open mouth. Be sure he latches on to the wide base and not just the tip of the nipple. If he starts using lazy latch-on techniques learned while bottle feeding when he nurses at your breast, you'll be sore.

- Don't bottle prop. Not only is leaving baby unattended during a feeding dangerous—what if baby chokes and needs attention?—but sucking from a bottle while lying down also allows milk to enter the middle ear through the eustachian tube and triggers ear infections (especially if baby is drinking formula). Remember, feeding time is a social interaction. *Nursing* implies both comforting and nourishing, whether by bottle or breast. Always put a person at both ends of the bottle.

Bottles are not the only alternative to breastfeeding. Babies can also be cup fed, finger fed with a nursing supplementer, or they can take milk from a spoon or medicine dropper. Babies who have begun to eat solid foods may get much of their nourishment from nonmilk sources while mother is away.

- When will you pump? You will need to pump about as often as your baby nurses, every two to three hours. If you work an eight-hour day, this means pumping at midmorning, at lunchtime, and at midafternoon. If you pump both breasts at the same time, allow fifteen or twenty minutes—thirty minutes if you pump each breast separately. You may have to arrive earlier and stay later at work to make up for time spent pumping.

- Where will you pump? Many women will find that their employers already have a special lactation lounge in place. For those that don't, federal law requires that the area provided must have a sink and cannot be located in the restroom. If you are not protected by law, you may be able to convince your employer of the need for a lactation program (see opposite), which might include a room set aside for pumping, hospital-grade pumps, and refrigerator space for milk storage, along with information and support for breastfeeding mothers. Other options include borrowing an office, using an empty room, pumping at your desk, or even using a closet. (Hang a DO NOT DISTURB sign on the door.) Pumping in your car is an option, and if all else fails, a stall in the women's restroom, while certainly not the best choice for pumping, is a workable option.

- Ideally the place you pump will have a comfortable chair, a sink, and a table. If you are using an electric pump, then it is nice to have an electrical outlet as well. If the room doesn't have one, then you will need a battery or, if pumping in your car, an adapter. Unless you have more than one kit and you can wash everything at home, you will need a sink to rinse off the parts of the pump that come in contact with your milk as well as a table for your equipment, your lunch, or any paperwork you might want to look at while you're pumping. If a sink is not available, special wipes can be purchased to clean your equipment.

- Where will you store the milk? A refrigerator where you can store expressed milk is handiest, but you can substitute ice packs and a cooler. Storing your milk in the employee refrigerator is considered acceptable. Be sure to label it with your name and date.

Present your plan to your employer and ask for support and problem-solving help where you need it. Even though it's wise to begin with a plan, be flexible enough to make the necessary on-the-job changes. Because you know that breastfeeding makes a difference, you will find a way. Here are a couple of creative stories from committed breastfeeding mothers:

I'm a letter carrier, and in the final weeks of my pregnancy I sent out a flyer to many of the homes on my route to see if any of these homes could offer child care for my baby. I was ecstatic to find just the right home midway through my route where I could stop and breastfeed my baby.

SETTING UP A CORPORATE LACTATION PROGRAM

To make your workplace more breastfeeding-friendly, Medela offers a packet of resources and free advice on setting up a lactation program in your company. Specifically, Medela can help you design lactation lounges, select which breast pumps are best, demonstrate how the employer can subsidize the cost of breast pumps, and show what other employers are doing to make their workplace more friendly to breastfeeding employees. Lactation programs have become more and more popular; more than 80 percent of the corporations listed in *Working Mother* magazine's "100 Best Companies for Working Women" (October 1998) offer this program to their employees. (For more information on this program, call Medela at 800-435-8316.)

I'm a security guard in a mall. I made arrangements with an understanding proprietor at the maternity shop to leave my electric pump at her shop. During my rounds, I would go into the back room of the shop and pump a couple of times a day. At the end of the day, I would pick up the stored milk from the shop's refrigerator. I figured that certainly a maternity shop would be sympathetic to my needs.

10. Ease into the new routine. Consider returning to your job on a Wednesday or a Thursday. You'll be less exhausted when the weekend arrives. Then you'll have two days to rest up before the workday routine begins again.

Many women arrange to work only three or four days a week while their children are small. With the kind of time that mothers put in caring for babies and children after hours, they certainly don't have to apologize for not working a full forty-hour week.

MAKING YOUR WORKING LIFE EASIER

11. Streamline your morning getaway. A baby adds a new wrinkle to the getting-ready-for-work routine. There's more stuff to manage and more potential interruptions. Here are some tips to help get you to the job on time:

- Set your alarm early so that you can nurse your baby before you get out of bed. Then you can shower and dress with fewer interruptions.

- Get things ready the night before: pack the baby's bag, have bottles of milk ready in the refrigerator, make your lunch, pick your clothing, and make sure your breast pump is clean and ready to go.

- Take the baby to the caregiver's in his pajamas.

- Make getting to bed at a reasonable hour a priority.

- Get a wash-and-go haircut to save time getting ready.

- If you're not back into your prepregnancy wardrobe, invest in a few basic pieces that coordinate with each other and flatter your new mommy figure. Don't start your day feeling fat with nothing to wear.

- Plan to nurse the baby one more time at the caregiver's before going to work. Your breasts will be empty and you'll feel more relaxed when you finally arrive on the job.

Because of my job schedule and unpredictable traffic, I didn't always arrive home at the same time every day. I would call my caregiver as I was leaving work. If I got stuck in traffic, I would call again and ask her to give my baby just enough milk to tide her over until I got home.

12. Enjoy a happy departure and a happy reunion. Breastfeed your baby at home or at the caregiver's before leaving for work and as soon as you return. This maximizes your baby's feedings at the breast and minimizes the amount of pumping you'll have to do. Plan ahead for the first return-from-work reunion. Ask your caregiver not to feed your baby a bottle within an hour of your anticipated arrival. Arriving with full breasts only to find your baby sound asleep with a full tummy does not make for a happy mother-baby reunion. If baby is hungry or you're going to be late, instruct your caregiver to feed him just enough to hold him over until you arrive. When you get home from work, take some time to reconnect with your baby. Settle down to breastfeed rather than plunging into household chores. Mute the phone, change into comfortable clothes, turn on relaxing music, and nestle down with your baby in your favorite nursing corner and get reconnected.

Nursing my baby as soon as I get home from work is not only great for her but it also helps me unwind after a tense day at work and fighting the rush-hour traffic. Partway through the breastfeeding, I get so relaxed I'm almost comatose.

BABIES WHO SPEAK UP FOR THEMSELVES

Many caregivers believe that breastfed babies are more work than their formula-fed day-care buddies. Some of this attitude has to do with the perception that human milk requires special care compared to bottles of infant formula; some of it may even stem from squeamishness about unfamiliar body fluids. Simplifying the preparation of feedings as much as possible may help to correct this misconception. So will some basic education about the advantages of breastfeeding.

But these caregivers may be on to something. Breastfed babies are used to being held while they are fed, and in general, they tend to be in mother's arms more than babies who are formula fed. Their mothers, who are very much in tune with their babies, may be more insistent that caregivers not prop bottles and that they pick up their little charges when they cry or fuss. Breastfed babies may also be less willing to accept pacifiers, especially if mother avoided offering one in the first weeks of baby's life.

Babies who are accustomed to feeling right will go on expecting the conditions that help maintain their equilibrium. This is good, even if it does make more work for adults. Perhaps you can help your caregiver see these behaviors in a positive light: your baby is smart enough to know what she needs and to ask for it.

Whatever you do, don't back down from expecting that your baby's needs will be met. It can be hard to stand firm, especially if you are a first-time mother, if your caregiver has had many years of child-care experience, and if the word *spoiled* is in the air. Remember, you can't spoil a tiny baby. Responding to infant cries teaches babies to trust, and this is a vitally important emotional skill.

You are the expert on your baby, and others are obligated to respect your judgment. If your baby's caregiver refuses to honor your wishes, it's time to look for another caregiver. On the other hand, be sure to let your baby's caregiver know how much her high level of caring for your baby means to you. Find ways to compensate her for going above and beyond, either monetarily or by other means that say how much you value her role in your baby's life. After all, it's important that she and your baby have a close bond and that all three of you trust one another. You'll have peace of mind and your baby will have the emotional security she needs to thrive.

---

13. Simplify pumping. Tucked into a discreet but stylish case, breast pumps are carried to work by thousands of women. At the end of the day, these mothers carry home pumped breast milk for their babies to drink during the next workday. We'd prefer to see more emphasis on keeping mothers and babies close when women must work so that babies could nurse directly at the breast and mothers could avoid having to pump. But in the conventional working world, pumps are a fact of life for nursing mothers, and anything that you can do to make pumping easier is worth trying. Here are some ideas that can make pumping less of a hassle:

- Find a pump that works well for you, since you'll be spending lots of time with this mechanical milker. Read the information on choosing a pump in chapter 7. If you don't like the first pump you try, invest in another one.

- With a good-quality electric pump, you can pump both breasts at the same time, clean up, and be finished in fifteen to twenty minutes. This alone may justify the price of a higher-quality pump. Hand-expressing milk or using a less efficient pump usually takes longer — around thirty minutes.

- Choose your work wardrobe with a nursing baby in mind. Select prints and loose-fitting blouses that camouflage leaking that may occur as you daydream about your baby during boring meetings. Two-piece outfits give you easier access for pumping and for breastfeeding your baby before you leave for work.

- Many pump parts or hand pumps can be washed in the dishwasher at home along with dinner dishes.

- If there are days when you don't have enough time for a full session, it's better to pump for five to ten minutes than not at all. Be careful. Skipping milk-expression sessions regularly will cause your milk supply to dwindle.

- If your workday tends to be unpredictable, you may have to discipline yourself to make time to express milk at regular intervals. You may also have to ask for the support of your employer and coworkers to make this possible. Don't think of your pumping schedule as an imposition on your freedom. Think of it as an opportunity to become better organized.

- If you're planning to pump in your office, rearrange the furniture to give yourself a bit more privacy in case someone barges through the door. A stack of books and papers strategically placed on a corner of the desk may save you and any unexpected visitors some embarrassment.

- If another woman at your workplace is also pumping milk for her baby, arrange to take your breaks or eat lunch together while you pump. This can be helpful if you miss the camaraderie of lunch with colleagues.

- Get some support from other women who are working and nursing. This might be friends from your childbirth class or a breastfeeding support group. (Call the leader ahead of time and ask if there are working mothers in the group.)

- Keep in mind that you'll be expressing milk for a relatively short time—not the rest of your working life or even the rest of your breastfeeding life.

- Don't cry over spilled milk. As you're getting used to a routine of collecting and storing milk, be prepared to drop a bag or two. While it's hard to see your "white gold" go splat on the floor, accidents happen even to the most careful mothers.

14. Gain the support of your coworkers. Your colleagues at work may make comments about your frequent breaks, your pump, the milk stored in the refrigerator, or the time you spend with your baby. This can make some mothers feel uncomfortable, or it can lead to resentment and problems between coworkers. Here are some suggestions for heading off comments and enlisting the support of the people you work with:

- Use humor. Laugh off any teasing that comes your way.

- Try being very discreet if this is what your workplace demands. Some people will never even wonder about what you're keeping in the lunch bag on the refrigerator shelf.

- Cite a medical reason for continuing to breastfeed, such as "My baby is allergic to formula." (Strictly speaking, this isn't a lie, since we believe most babies have at least microscopic allergies to formulas.) By claiming a medical reason, you aren't putting a guilt trip on the coworkers who chose not to continue breastfeeding.

- Share information about the benefits of breastfeeding, especially the ones that are important to you. ("My husband has terrible allergies, but breastfeeding will lessen the risk for our baby," or "Six months old and no ear infections yet!") If you've missed work because

GRANDFATHER'S ROLE IN BREASTFEEDING

If you are a new grandfather, you may think that you have absolutely no role to play in the breastfeeding relationship. However, even though your role may be indirect and distant, it's still a very valuable one. First, encourage grandmother to support and affirm the choices made by your grandchild's parents. When you were parents, you and your wife practiced a certain parenting style, one that was based on the prevailing practices and advice of the time as well as on your own ideas. You had your shot. This baby is the responsibility of your son or daughter and his or her spouse. Even if you disagree with the parenting choices they make, this does not mean that they are wrong and you were right, or vice versa. You did the best you could when you were new parents given the circumstances and advice that you had at the time.

Grandparents can also be helpful when they detect sources of stress in the lives of new parents and do what they can to remedy these without taking over. On the simplest level, this means bringing dinner when you come to visit your grandchild. There are other times when grandparents can help in bigger ways. For example, here is a story from our pediatrics practice:

One of our stockbroker friends—we'll call him John—used to call frequently with investment tips, most of which we declined. John's daughter had a new baby, and when she came into the office for her baby's one-month checkup, we noticed that she seemed worried and sad. She told us she needed to go back to work within a few weeks, and she dreaded this separation from her baby. It didn't feel right to her; she didn't want to return to her job, but her husband was a student and they needed her paycheck. She felt she had no alternative. Compounding her worries was the fact that she was blessed with a high-need child, a frequent breastfeeder who was often inconsolable when cared for by anyone but her. She emphatically said that she wanted to stay home with her baby, at least for the first year. We could see that economic pressures were at odds with her mothering instinct. Bill excused himself, stepped into the other room, and called her father. "John, have I got an investment tip for you!" Bill said.

John couldn't believe his ears. "You're calling me with investment tips?"

"Bet you've got an annuity and college fund already opened for your grandson," Bill said.

"You bet your life," he responded.

"How would you like to make another investment, the best one you can make in the physical, emotional, and academic future of your grandson, one that will guarantee returns?" Bill continued with his sales pitch. "This is probably the first no-risk investment you'll ever have a chance to make, but you have to act now or you'll lose this window of opportunity."

"Yes, quick, tell me what it is," replied John.

Bill went on to explain the dilemma John's daughter was in—that she really couldn't afford to stay home with her baby but wanted to. To sweeten the offer, he described the many advantages of breastfeeding, especially the benefits of a full-time mother to a high-need child. He explained the difference between just growing and thriving.

"Where do I sign?" John instantly replied. For the first year of his grandchild's life, John subsidized the family, whether in the form of a gift or a loan we're not sure, but he went on later to thank Bill and agreed that this truly proved to be the best long-term investment he'd ever made.

of the flu, point out that your baby had only a mild case — or no problems at all — because of the antibodies in your milk.

- Talk about how breastfeeding at home and pumping at work help you feel connected to your baby.

- Acknowledge and thank people for the times when they've covered for you while you've been pumping or feeding your baby. Return the favor when they need your help.

- Listen with sympathetic interest when coworkers share their breastfeeding stories with you — especially when breastfeeding didn't work out in their families. Acknowledge that they did the best they could under the circumstances.

- Wow them with facts and figures about breastfeeding, or just tell them that you're continuing to breastfeed because your pediatrician — not to mention the entire American Academy of Pediatrics — recommends it.

KEEPING UP YOUR MILK SUPPLY

15. Work in as many breastfeedings as you can. Depending on the work hours, most employed mothers can get in at least four breastfeedings: one early morning feeding before work, one when they get home, an evening feeding, and a before-bed feeding. (And of course most babies need to nurse once or twice at night.) If you are fortunate enough to have on-site day care, you may be able to breastfeed your baby during lunch and breaks, cutting down on or eliminating the need to express milk and give bottles.

16. Breastfeed full-time whenever you're not at work. In order to maintain and build up your milk supply, you need to have days when you breastfeed frequently, to make up for the times when you and baby are separated. Adopt the policy that baby is given a bottle only while you are at work or away from baby but is exclusively breastfed when in your care. This will build up a good milk supply and keep the two of you connected. Don't give bottles when you can breastfeed. Pumping does not stimulate the breasts to produce milk as well as a nursing baby does. You need to breastfeed your baby often during the time you are together in order to keep up your milk supply and ensure that your baby stays interested in the breast. Now is not the time to leave your baby with a sitter every Friday night to go out to a movie and dinner with friends. Pick a nice quiet movie and baby can go along or even join your dinner outing. Many mothers who work the usual Monday-through-Friday, nine-to-five work week find the amount they are able to pump dwindles toward the end of the week. After nursing frequently all weekend, their breasts feel much fuller on Monday and they're able to pump more milk and may even need to express more often to avoid uncomfortable engorgement. (Save this milk for later in the week, when your milk supply may be running low.) After a few weeks of juggling breastfeeding and working schedules, you will be amazed at how your body and your breasts adjust to making just the right amount of milk for your baby. Once baby starts taking some solid foods, around six months, some of the pressure to produce lessens.

17. Enjoy nighttime nursing. Many breastfed babies who are away from their mothers during the day nurse more frequently at night. They make up for what they're missing during the day by breastfeeding often during the evening and by waking up at night more to nurse. After mother returns to work, some babies reverse their daily patterns by sleeping more and feeding less during the day and then clustering their feedings during the night.

This is actually a good thing, and mothers who succeed at combining breastfeeding and working recognize this and even welcome it. They bring their babies into their bed so that they can nurse at night without waking up completely, and they appreciate this extra opportunity for closeness. (Working fathers like it, too.) In fact, many mothers report that they sleep better with their babies next to them, even if that means baby nurses through the night. Breastfeeding helps mothers unwind, relax, and sleep better, just as it helps babies feel calm and comforted. Also, a long feeding in bed in the early morning just before it's time to get up will help baby sleep or at least be content while you get ready for work. (See chapter 9.)

18. You can combine breastfeeding and formula feeding. Breastfeeding is not an all-or-nothing deal. While many mothers who combine nursing and working do supply all their baby's milk feedings for many months, others use formula as a backup when they are unable to pump enough milk. In other cases, baby nurses at the breast when mother is available and gets formula when she is not. If this second situation sounds like the direction in which you're headed, give some thought to how you will combine breastfeeding and formula feeding. Otherwise, you may discover one day long before you had planned on weaning that your baby has lost interest in the breast and you don't have much milk anyway.

Even if you are not expressing and saving milk for your baby while you are at work, you still may need to do some pumping to prevent plugged ducts and mastitis and to keep up your milk supply. Some mothers can go for four to six hours without nursing or expressing, but many can't. If you are away from your baby for seven or eight hours or longer, you will need to pump once or twice even if you don't save the milk. (We can't imagine any mother pumping and dumping that "white gold" routinely, but it would be better than not pumping and winding up with breasts so full of milk that they send the brain the message to stop milk production.)

If you're cutting back on pumping at work, nurse your baby frequently while the two of you are together and avoid long separations other than those related to your job. This includes nursing at night. Give baby lots of skin-to-skin contact and lots of time with you to keep her interested in the breast and to build your prolactin levels. If your baby seems to be losing interest in the breast, you may need to encourage her to nurse more frequently and do some expressing while the two of you are apart so that there is plenty of milk in the breast when baby wants to nurse. If your milk supply seems to be falling off, try a galactagogue (milk-encouraging herb; see chapter 5).

As babies near their first birthdays and eat a wider variety of foods, even mothers who have pumped regularly may stop expressing milk at work. They continue to nurse their babies into toddlerhood, and their little ones seek the comfort of the breast whenever mother is around.

LOWERING YOUR STRESS LEVEL

19. Take care of yourself. Faced with the demands of a job and a baby, you may find you can accomplish little else beyond doing your job and taking care of your little one. This is a completely realistic expectation. The one thing you should not neglect is taking care of yourself. Fortunately, breastfeeding can help you do this.

When you get home from work, head for the bedroom and nurse while you rest lying down. If you and baby can take a short nap, the whole family will have a more pleasant evening. Have a quick and nutritious snack, so that there's no pressure to start dinner right away, and enjoy being with your baby once more. If you have an older child, include him or her in this reunion.

You'll need to simplify your life at home as much as possible so that you can devote your attention to your baby and the rest of your family rather than to laundry, shopping, cleaning, cooking, and organizing. By keeping it simple your mate can more happily do his share. If you can afford it, pay someone to do many of these tasks for you. Some things—like washing windows or ironing clothes—you can simply ignore for a few years. While you're working around the house, carry baby in a sling so that you can enjoy some time together while you prepare supper or sort laundry.

20. Share the child care and the chores. If mom makes all the milk and some of the money, it's only fair for dad to share in the child care and housework. Breastfeeding while working is a family enterprise. Explain to your partner the benefits of continued breastfeeding. School-age children should also share in the housework. This is good modeling for when they become working parents. In fact, you model a double message: the importance of breastfeeding and the benefits of working together as a family. When you're breastfeeding and working, you simply can't "have it all." You will not have enough energy to make milk, make money, make dinner, and make love every night. Delegate all the household chores that could be done by someone other than you. Discuss these responsibilities with your partner and with older children in a family council. Try to shave or share as many of the energy drainers as you can. (See chapter 10 for more on a father's role in breastfeeding.)

9

Nighttime Breastfeeding

NEW PARENTS SOON DISCOVER that the only babies who sleep through the night belong to other people. *Nightlife* takes on a whole new meaning when one night you're awake feeding baby at 1:00 a.m., 3:00 a.m., 4:45 a.m., and again when the sun rises at 6:30 a.m. The key to surviving and thriving during the many months of night feedings is to develop a style of nighttime parenting that allows you to get enough sleep while baby gets enough milk.

WHY BABIES WAKE UP

To understand why infants wake up frequently during the night, it's necessary to appreciate certain basic principles of infant sleep.

There are two basic stages of sleep: light and deep. The younger the infant, the higher the percentage of light sleep. Throughout the night, babies cycle from light sleep to deep sleep and back again into light sleep, and as they pass from one stage to another, there is a vulnerable period in which they're likely to awaken. This happens approximately every sixty minutes. As babies get older, the percentage of deep sleep increases, sleep cycles lengthen, and night waking becomes a less frequent occurrence. We now know that newborns need about twenty minutes to cycle into deep sleep,

while an older infant only needs ten. So if you wait twenty minutes before putting your newborn down, your baby is more likely to stay asleep.

Babies don't sleep as soundly as adults, but the high percentage of light sleep in the early months, especially in the first six months, has survival and developmental benefits for baby. Light sleep itself stimulates baby's brain. Light sleep is also known as REM (rapid eye movement) sleep, an indication that dreaming is going on. Frequent waking gives babies more opportunities to nurse at night, when mother's prolactin levels are on the upswing and there is plenty of milk.

Infant sleep habits are determined more by their individual temperaments than by parents' nighttime parenting skills. It's not your fault your baby wakes up so much. We have to be honest and tell you that breastfed babies do awaken more frequently than formula-fed infants. Because breast milk is digested more quickly and completely than formula, breastfeeding infants need to feed more frequently — day and night.

SURVIVING AND THRIVING WITH NIGHTTIME BREASTFEEDING

During the first year you will spend a lot of time feeding your baby at night, so you might as well

THE GOAL OF NIGHTTIME PARENTING

You can't force your baby into a state of sleep. Your role as a parent is to create a sleep-inducing environment that allows sleep to overtake your baby naturally. We believe that the ultimate goal of nighttime parenting is *to help your baby develop a healthy attitude about sleep, so that your child grows up regarding sleep as a pleasant state to enter with no fears of either falling asleep or getting back to sleep*. To accomplish this goal, you will put a lot of effort into parenting your child to sleep and parenting her back to sleep when she awakens in the middle of the night. Eventually, your care and comfort will become part of her inner resources, and she will be able to do this for herself.

This goal is very different from training baby to sleep through the night as soon as possible by denying him parental comfort—in other words, letting him cry. This can lead a child to develop an uneasy attitude toward sleep. Worse, she learns that she can't depend on her parents to meet her nighttime needs. Meanwhile, mom and dad become less sensitive to their child's signals.

With the cry-it-out method, what's the lesson baby learns? "They aren't going to come, so I may as well give up," or "It doesn't matter how I feel." Less persistent babies give up quickly. Since they can't trust us to be there, they "cope" and learn a big lesson: you have to look after number one, because no one else will.

Think of nighttime parenting as a long-term investment. The middle-of-the-night time you put in now will save you sleep in the years ahead. Your children will sleep well when they are older, and the good relationship you have built with them will keep you from lying awake at night worrying about them when they are teenagers and young adults.

enjoy it. You have two nighttime goals: to get sufficient rest yourself and to meet the nutritional and emotional needs of your infant.

Develop a Realistic Mind-Set About Nighttime Nursing

Begin your parenting career without preset ideas about how your baby is going to sleep at night. This will make it easier to reconcile yourself to the realities of nighttime parenting. You may have a mellow baby who breastfeeds predictably by day and sleeps four- to six-hour stretches at night (for sleep researchers, sleeping a five-hour stretch qualifies as "sleeping through the night" in an infant under six months of age). Or you may be blessed with a high-need baby, one who will settle for nothing less than frequent nourishment and comforting day and night. Both types of babies are normal. Also, realize that when babies wake up frequently to nurse, they are only asking for what they need to thrive. *Thriving* means more than getting bigger; it means developing to the fullest potential—physically, emotionally, and intellectually. Nearly all babies know intuitively how much nursing they need for nourishment and for comfort. Remember that, at this young age, babies' wants are the same as their needs. So when your baby wakes up to nurse at night, respect his judgment. He really needs this feeding. In fact, as we'll later see, a common medical cause for an infant failing to thrive is not getting sufficient feedings at night.

Of course, part of what your baby needs at night is contact with you, and you may even learn to appreciate these nighttime feedings. Here's an

BE OPEN TO TRYING VARIOUS SLEEPING ARRANGEMENTS

There is no right or wrong place for baby to sleep. Whatever sleeping arrangement meets the nighttime needs of family members is the right one. Be open to trying various alternatives until you find what works for your family. Sleeping arrangements may vary at different stages of your infant's development. Some infants settle better when they sleep snuggled right next to mommy all through the night, while others seem to sleep better in a bassinet or crib in the parents' bedroom. Still others sleep well in various combinations of co-sleeping and solo sleeping. Most breastfeeding infants sleep best snuggled right next to mom. Where a baby sleeps is for mom, dad, and baby to decide. Do what seems right for you, keeping in mind safety issues (see page 192).

Some ultrasensitive infants are so stimulated by mother's close presence that they need a bit of distance from mom in order to settle. In this case, you can use a bassinet or cradle next to your bed or try the sidecar arrangement: place baby's crib right alongside your bed. For safety's sake, be sure to leave the side rail partly up so there is no crevice between the crib and adult mattress. This way baby is within arm's reach for nursing, but mother and baby are not so close that they keep each other awake. In 2016, the American Academy of Pediatrics recommended: "Infants should sleep in the same bedroom as their parents, but on a separate sleep surface such as a crib or a bassinet, and never on a couch, arm chair or soft surface."

The safest sleeping arrangement, which we have recommended for the past twenty years, is to use the Arm's Reach Co-Sleeper bedside bassinet. This criblike bed attaches safely and securely to the parents' bed and allows you and baby to have your own separate sleeping surfaces while enabling you to be within "arm's reach" of your baby for easier comforting and breastfeeding. Visit the product website at ArmsReach.com.

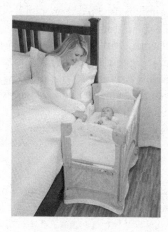

excerpt from the journal Martha kept while she was nursing our sixth baby, Matthew:

I look forward to night feedings. These are special times. No interruptions, just Matthew and me. We are both so relaxed and can truly enjoy one another. I cherish these special times because I know they will pass all too soon.

TIPS FOR EASIER NIGHTTIME BREASTFEEDING

Remember, a happy mother and a well-fed baby are the goals of both daytime and nighttime nursing. Here are some tricks of nighttime nursing that have worked for us with our eight babies and that mothers in our practice have shared with us.

SLEEPING THROUGH THE NIGHT — NOT RECOMMENDED FOR BABIES

"Is your baby sleeping through the night?" is a question you're guaranteed to hear a hundred times from friends and relatives who have been led to believe that a full night's sleep is every parent's most fervent desire. The question may also come across as a judgment about your parenting: only bad parents have babies who don't sleep through the night. Both experience and experiments have shown that breastfeeding babies usually wake up more frequently than formula-fed babies. Whether this is desirable or undesirable depends upon the parents' mind-set about nighttime parenting, but the facts suggest that breastfed babies wake more frequently for good reasons.

Breast milk is digested more rapidly than formula, so breastfed babies get hungry sooner. One of the main milk-making hormones, prolactin, is highest in the middle-of-the-night hours (usually between 1:00 and 5:00 a.m.). Could it be that a mother's body chemistry is designed for night feedings? It certainly seems that babies are designed for frequent waking. In one study, researchers compared the sleep-wake patterns in infants whose moms employed various nighttime parenting styles. Group 1 mothers breastfed on cue during the day and night and slept with their babies. Group 2 mothers breastfed their babies but tended to wean earlier and sleep separately. Mothers in the third group neither breastfed nor slept with their babies. Babies who breastfed and shared sleep with their mothers woke up more frequently and slept shorter stretches of time. Those who breastfed but did not sleep with their mothers slept longer, and the babies who neither breastfed nor slept with their mothers slept the longest. Which group of babies represents the norm is debatable, but cross-cultural studies of human behavior lead us to believe that nighttime breastfeeding, along with sleep sharing, is the norm. The focus, at least in the early months of breastfeeding, should not be on getting baby to sleep through the night but rather on learning to cope with his normal nighttime infant behavior.

Tank up baby with frequent feedings during the day. As babies get bigger, they get busier during the day and forget to eat. So they make up for missed feedings at night. This happens especially after six months of age. In this situation mother may be the one who "demands" that baby breastfeed at least every three hours during the day so that he does not need to nurse as much at night.

Refill tiny tummies before you retire. Wake baby for a feeding just before you go to bed. If baby nurses to sleep at 9:00 p.m. and you go to bed at 10:30 p.m., you may be wakened at 11:00 or 11:30 p.m., when you've barely had a chance to doze off. It's better to wake baby and fill his tummy right

before you go to sleep so that the two of you can enjoy a longer period of sleep at the same time.

Offer both breasts at a feeding. Since you're going to have to feed your baby in the middle of the night, you might as well do a thorough job of it and offer both breasts. Baby won't be hungry again quite so soon. There are two techniques for switching sides when nursing in the lying-down position. One is the *across-the-chest roll:* after your baby finishes nursing on the first breast, cradle him against your chest as you roll to the other side. Get settled, then latch baby on to your other breast. If rolling your baby across your body is more wiggling around than you want to do in the middle of the night, instead turn your upper shoulder toward baby as you adjust the level of that upper breast so your baby can latch on.

Change baby before a feeding. If baby's diaper is wet or dirty, change him before a feeding so he stays asleep after the feeding. This doesn't work for those "in and out" babies who seem to have a bowel movement every time milk goes in at the upper end.

Releasing the "all-night sucker." Some babies love to sleep with the nipple held in their mouths. After they have finished filling their tummies with milk, they continue to suck for a few minutes, then like to stay attached while they sleep. While some mothers can sleep with baby attached throughout the night or at nap time (they're just thankful that baby is sleeping), some mothers can't relax with baby still connected. An important comment here: sleeping with the nipple in the mouth once teeth have erupted is one breastfeeding behavior that leads to caries in cultures that have low caries rates. To avoid waking your baby as you disengage the nipple, gradually ease him off the nipple by inserting your index finger in the side of your baby's mouth to pry his jaws open gently. As the jaws release, slowly (or quickly—whichever works) draw the nipple out of his mouth, protecting it with your finger in case baby clamps down suddenly. Some babies will startle awake when they sense the loss of pressure inside the mouth. In that case, as you gently (or quickly) draw the nipple out, be ready to press with your index finger upward on his lower lip or chin as soon as your nipple is clear, and hold that pressure long enough for baby to adjust. Then slowly ease your finger pressure off. (Holding your breath seems to help, too!) If baby seems to wake, try patting his tummy gently. You may have to let him suck for a while and then try again.

Burping the night feeder. Many breastfeeding babies nurse less anxiously at night. They swallow less air and don't need to be burped. Even if you do need to help your baby bring up a bubble after nursing in the side-lying position, there's no need for you to get out of bed or even sit up. Drape baby over your side when side-lying and pat his back until he burps. See the illustration on page 77.

Prop your baby up at around a thirty-degree angle if he has GER. While most babies can night nurse while sleeping flat in the side-lying position, some suffer from gastroesophageal reflux, or GER, and wake up with colicky abdominal pain during or right after the feeding. In feeding GER babies, gravity is your best friend. Instead of nursing in the side-lying position with baby lying flat, elevate baby at about a thirty-degree angle on a firm foam wedge.

THE BENEFITS OF SLEEPING CLOSE TO YOUR BABY

"Is it all right to sleep close to our baby?" new mothers often ask. Of course it is. After all, you don't expect baby to be independent of you during the day, so why would you expect it at night? Most parents throughout the world sleep close to their babies. In fact, many mothers in Western cultures also sleep close to their babies at some time or other. (They just don't tell their doctors or their relatives.)

Our first three children slept in cribs, as did all our friends' babies. Because they slept fine, nursed once, then slept until morning (unless they were sick), we had no reason to consider any other arrangement. Then came our fourth baby, Hayden, whose birth changed our lives. Hayden was a high-need baby who craved frequent nursing and constant holding. She was one of those in-arms, at-breast, and (eventually) in-our-bed babies. For the first six months, she slept in a cradle right next to our bed, waking only once or twice to be fed. If she woke more than that,

SLEEP TRAINING — NOT FOR BREASTFEEDING MOTHERS

Ever since parenting books found their way into bedrooms, authors have touted magical systems promising to get babies to sleep through the night and follow a more convenient schedule. But while babies have a lot of wonderful attributes, convenience is not one of them. Beware of using someone else's training method to get your baby to sleep or get your baby on a predictable schedule. Most of these methods are variations of the tired old theme of letting baby cry it out. Before trying anyone else's method, see if it makes sense intuitively. Does this advice fit your baby's temperament? Does it feel right to you? Does it sound sensible?

With most of these baby-training regimens you run the risk of becoming desensitized to the cues of your infant, especially when it comes to letting baby cry it out. Instead of helping you to figure out what baby's signals mean, these training methods encourage you to ignore them. Neither you nor your baby learns anything good from this. Other risks include a drop in milk supply, mastitis, and resumption of menses and fertility. These risks are highest when the infant is under six months of age.

If your current daytime or nighttime routine is not working for you, think about what changes you can make in yourself and your lifestyle that will make it easier for you to meet your baby's needs. This is a better approach than immediately trying to change your baby. After all, you can control your own reactions to a situation. You can't control how your baby reacts. Be discerning about advice that promises a sleep-through-the-night, more convenient baby, because these programs involve the risk of creating distance between you and your baby and undermining the mutual trust between parent and child. On the surface, baby training sounds liberating for parents, but it's a short-term gain for a long-term loss. You lose the opportunity to know your baby better and become more of an expert on your baby. Baby loses an opportunity to build trust in his caregiving environment. You cease to value your own biological cues and your judgment and instead follow the message of someone who has no biological attachment to or investment in your infant.

Clicking into the cry-it-out method also keeps you from continuing to search for medical or physical causes of night waking, such as GER and food sensitivities. Night feedings are normal; frequent painful night waking is not.

Stay flexible. No single approach will work with all babies all the time or even all the time with any given baby. Don't persist with a failing experiment. If the "sleep program" isn't working for your family, drop it.

Follow your heart rather than some stranger's sleep-training advice, and you and your baby will eventually work out the right nighttime parenting solution for your family.

Martha could often lull her quickly back to sleep by swinging her cradle. When she outgrew the cradle, we put a crib in our room over against the wall, and that's when the frequent night waking started. She was up every hour, and so was Martha, nursing or patting her back to sleep. After a week, Martha was utterly exhausted. She realized our high-need baby was telling us she needed to stay closer to Martha. Finally, one night Martha said to Bill, "I don't care what the books say. I've got to get some sleep." That was a memorable night. She took Hayden into our bed, and we all slept, grateful for the closeness. Initially skeptical, Bill was quickly convinced. It was so easy! When Hayden began to wake up, Martha simply nursed her back to sleep. Usually Martha would not even awaken fully or remember how much she had nursed Hayden during the night. Martha slept so much better, and so did Hayden. Hayden broadened our view of nighttime parenting.

Sleeping next to Hayden opened not only our hearts but also our minds, leading us to research the physical and emotional benefits of parents sharing sleep with babies. And, as you may have guessed, we slept close to our next four babies and began presenting this wonderful style of nighttime parenting as an option to new parents, first in our pediatrics practice and then through Bill's first book, *Creative Parenting*. We expanded this message in Bill's next book, *Nighttime Parenting*, and then in several of our Sears Parenting Library books. Like all parenting styles, it may not work for all families. But when you truly understand the many benefits of sharing sleep, you may want to try this arrangement in your family.

Mother And Baby Go To Sleep Better

Because of the mutual benefits of *nursing down* (a term we use for breastfeeding off to sleep), babies usually fade out immediately after breastfeeding, as if they have been given a shot of sleeping medication. In fact, this may be what actually happens, since breast milk contains a sleep-inducing protein. Also, the act of breastfeeding raises the level of the hormone prolactin in mother's bloodstream, where it has a tranquilizing effect on her. When the breastfeeding pair drifts off to sleep, the mommy has put the baby to sleep and the baby has put the mommy to sleep. This is especially helpful for mothers who have busy schedules during the day and have difficulty winding down at night. Nighttime breastfeeding is a beautiful biological example of how mothers and babies benefit from doing what comes naturally.

Martha missed having this mothering-to-sleep tool with our last baby, Lauren, who came to us

by adoption. Lauren breastfed for ten months with the help of a nursing supplementer (see chapter 11), but this aid for breastfeeding never quite worked for getting Lauren off to sleep. Martha had to fall back on the long list of other ways to "nurse" a baby off to sleep (see chapter 10), and none of them was as satisfying or as easy.

When Martha was breastfeeding our babies, she noticed that just before they woke up for a feeding, her sleep would seem to lighten and she would become more aware of the baby. She could anticipate the baby's need to nurse and get him latched on just as he began to squirm and reach for the nipple. Getting him to suck immediately kept him from fully waking up, and they could both drift back to sleep right after feeding.

It was so obvious that our newborn would sleep better next to me. In my womb, he'd grown accustomed to the presence of my familiar breathing movements, my heartbeat, and my warmth.

Sleeping with our baby has brought us closer together as mother and daughter. Spending the night together, holding her, and breastfeeding her when she wakes up has made me feel more confident about mothering her during the day. Besides, as my husband says, "What better way to start the day than to wake up to see both your mate and your child lying next to you?"

Breastfeeding Is Easier

Breastfeeding mothers and infants often shift from light sleep into deep sleep and back again at the same time. This is why we prefer the term *sharing sleep* rather than *the family bed* or *bed sharing*, since babies and mothers do actually share sleep cycles. When baby begins to wake up during one of these transition periods, mother simply reaches out and soothes baby with her touch or breastfeeds him, and both drift back to sleep with neither member of the nursing pair having completely awakened.

Contrast sleeping with your baby with the crib-in-the-nursery scene. The separate sleeper wakes up alone, in his crib. He is out of touch. Separation anxiety sets in, and he cries. His cries escalate until he wakes up mother, who is not even in the same room. Mother is often startled out of a deep sleep by the cries of her baby on the monitor (being wakened from a deep sleep leads to the most problems concerning sleep deprivation) and goes to baby in the nursery. By the time mother reaches baby, he is wide awake and angry. Mother is wide awake and maybe just a little resentful. The night nursing that follows becomes a reluctant duty rather than a pleasant response. It takes longer to resettle a crying and angry baby than it does an infant who is half asleep right next to you. Finally, mother resettles baby in the crib, but now she is wide awake and may have trouble getting back to sleep easily herself.

We have three children, and I like my sleep at night. So we adopted a sleeping arrangement I call the lazy mom option, a way I could meet my baby's nighttime needs and get back to sleep. By having our baby sleep in bed with us, I could get to him quicker and nurse him before he became revved up and launched into a full-blown cry. He resettled faster, and so did I. When he became an older baby (and a squirmer), we placed a mattress on the floor beside our bed. I would nurse him to sleep on this mattress, and when he awakened during the night I would simply crawl down, nurse him, and then crawl back into bed.

Babies Grow Better

One of the oldest treatments for the baby who is gaining weight slowly is the medical advice "Take your baby to bed and nurse." Some mothers tell us that they often experience a stronger milk-ejection reflex at night, probably because they are more relaxed. A stronger milk-ejection reflex gives the night-nursing baby milk higher in fat and higher in the calories needed for growth. And some researchers believe that the closeness to mother and the skin-to-skin contact may actually stimulate growth hormones in the infant.

Benefits for Dads

Fathers often find that sleeping close to their babies helps make up for how much they miss when they are gone all day at work. Babies who sleep with mom and dad radiate a beautiful sense of trust in their parents and in their caregiving environment.

Bill remembers waking up in the morning and gazing at the contented face of our nine-month-old "sleeping beauty," Erin (our fifth baby, in our bed from day one). He could tell when she was ascending from her level of deep sleep to light sleep. As she passed through the vulnerable period for waking, she often reached out for her mother or me. When she touched one of us, an "I'm okay" expression would radiate from her face, her eyes would remain closed, and she would not wake up. However, if she reached out and one of us was not within touching distance, she often woke.

QUESTIONS YOU MAY HAVE

NAP NURSING

Our ten-month-old refuses to take a morning nap and usually doesn't get more than a half-hour nap during the day. I know he needs a nap, and I do, too. Help!

Babies and parents both need naps. While you can't force your baby to sleep, you can create conditions that allow sleep to overtake your infant. At around one year, baby may be ready to give up the morning nap, but you should still try to see that he gets two naps each day.

To encourage your reluctant napper to establish a predictable nap schedule, set aside a consistent time in the morning and in the afternoon to lie down with him. As nap time approaches, play soft music, nestle together in a rocking chair, or keep baby in the baby sling to settle him down. Then lie down on a bed and nurse him off to sleep. Once baby is in a deep sleep, you can ease him into the crib or just make certain he can't fall off the bed before you slip away—if you're not asleep yourself. (See the box on safe sleep sharing, on the next page, for tips on making your bed safe for your baby.)

You probably look forward to your baby's nap time so you can "finally get something done." Resist this temptation to tire yourself out while baby is resting. Naps are as important for you as they are for your infant, and napping alongside your baby is a good way to ensure that baby stays asleep and that both of you are well rested.

WAKES UP TOO SOON

Our two-month-old nurses to sleep but wakes up as soon as I try to lay her down in her crib. Then I have to nurse her some more. This takes forever, and I'm getting frustrated.

Your baby may be waking up so quickly because she is not fully asleep when you put her down (see "Why Babies Wake Up" on page 183). Breastfeed her for a long time, preferably on both breasts, then continue to hold her until she is in a deep sleep. It takes at least twenty minutes (usually longer) for an infant to go through the initial state of light sleep into the state of deep sleep. Your baby's body language will tell you when she has made the transition from light to deep sleep. In the state of light sleep, her muscles are tight, her fists are clenched, her eyelids flutter, and you'll see

a few muscle twitches, especially in the face, called sleep grins. She may stay latched on and suck during this light sleep stage. Continue to breastfeed her until deep sleep takes over. Her face will be motionless, her breathing more irregular, her eyelids will be still, and you'll see what we call the limp-limb sign: arms dangling loosely at her sides, hands open, and muscles relaxed. Once baby is in the state of deep sleep, you can ease her into her crib. If she awakens as you put her down, lie down with her for a while on your bed and continue to nurse in the side-lying position. Extending the time in your arms or at your breast will also allow you to take advantage of a second spurt of tranquilizing hormones. Appreciate these leisurely nights and nap times while they last, as the time your baby is in your arms and at your breast will pass all too quickly. Use this quiet nursing time to read, talk with your husband, watch a good video, or just dream.

FEAR OF SPOILING

I've been told that if my baby always goes to sleep at my breast, he won't learn to go to sleep on his own or get himself back to sleep without breastfeeding. Is this true? Am I spoiling him?

Forget spoiling, at least in the early months. Babies, like food, spoil only when they are left alone and ignored, not when someone responds freely to their needs. What you've been told about not letting your baby go to sleep at the breast is based on the principle of *sleep associations,* meaning that if you always use the breast to get your baby to sleep, your baby will associate going to sleep with breastfeeding and won't be able to go to sleep any other way or settle himself back to sleep in the middle of the night without nursing. This is true. The controversy arises over what you should do about this situation. We believe that for children to develop a healthy sleep attitude—that is, to grow up regarding sleep as a pleasant state to

SAFE SLEEP SHARING WHILE BREASTFEEDING

Around the world, the most common nighttime parenting practice, by far, is mother sleeping close to baby. The same subconscious awareness of boundaries that keeps you from rolling off the bed will keep you from rolling over onto your baby. In some instances, however, infants have been harmed because of unwise and unsafe conditions. Observe these safety precautions.

- *No smoking!* If even one parent is a smoker, bed sharing is dangerous—smoking is a very significant risk factor for SIDS. Don't allow any smokers near your baby, even when they are not smoking, since chemicals from tobacco on their breath or on their clothing are harmful to baby's breathing.
- Place baby next to mother rather than between mother and father. While mothers are physically and mentally aware of baby's presence while sleeping, fathers do not have that same sensitivity, so it is possible they could roll over or throw out an arm onto baby.
- Place baby to sleep on her back, the safest sleeping position and the one that gives baby easier access to the breast.
- Use a king-size bed with a firm mattress and a secure guardrail with no gap baby could slip into. Or, if you have a smaller bed, attach a crib securely alongside, flush with your mattress, with the crib rail partly up; or place the mattress on the floor away from other furniture. Avoid a headboard and a footboard, where baby can get entrapped in the space between the mattress and the board.
- Don't sleep with your baby if you are under the influence of alcohol, drugs, sleeping pills, or other tranquilizing medications (including nighttime cold medicines and seizure-disorder medicines) that diminish your sensitivity to your baby's presence.
- Use caution in falling asleep with your baby if you are obese or extremely large breasted.

- Avoid falling asleep with your baby in a recliner or on especially soft surfaces such as a couch, beanbag, wavy water bed (those without internal baffles), or any surface on which baby could get wedged in a crevice between the soft surface and mother's breast. Keep baby's face clear of pillows, blankets, and stuffed animals, and check that there are no ribbons or other objects that could choke an infant. Never put a baby to sleep on top of a pillow or soft, cushy bedding material, such as a comforter.
- Don't wear lingerie with string ties longer than seven inches, and avoid dangling jewelry.
- Extremely long hair should be tied up. Avoid anything in which baby can get entangled. Check for objects in the bed.
- Babies one year of age and younger should not sleep with other children.
- Avoid overdressing and heavy blankets, which could cause overheating, and never cover baby's head.
- Consider using an Arm's Reach Co-Sleeper bedside bassinet.

I was very worried about my level of awareness when I was asleep. So I usually cradled my baby in my arm or at least had her touching me somewhere. That seemed to heighten my awareness—or at least made me feel safer.

Sleep researcher Dr. James McKenna, professor of biological anthropology and director of the Mother-Baby Behavioral Sleep Laboratory at the University of Notre Dame, has done extensive studies on the benefits of sleeping close to your baby. For further reading, consult Dr. McKenna's *Sleeping with Your Baby* (2007) and enter the terms "Dr. James McKenna, safe co-sleeping guidelines" in your browser's search window.

enter—babies must be parented to sleep rather than left to cry themselves to sleep. (There are some "laid-back" babies who can soothe themselves to sleep, but even they would benefit from extra holding.) When babies fall asleep in a parent's loving arms, they develop pleasant sleep associations, and as they get older, these good feelings will allow them to drop off to sleep easily on their own. Other advisers use the sleep association principle as a basis for suggesting that babies be left to fall asleep on their own so that they don't need a parent's presence at bedtime. If tired babies went calmly off to sleep when isolated in a crib, this idea might have some merit. But the reality is that tired babies fuss and cry and often can't relax on their own. What they then develop is a fear of sleep as well as a distrust of parents who aren't heeding their appeals for help.

Parented to sleep doesn't always have to mean breastfed to sleep. Sometimes mom can walk or rock baby to sleep after she has nursed enough to fill baby's tummy. Other times dad can be the one who eases baby off into dreamland. (See the father-nursing tools in chapter 10.) Having a variety of ways to put your baby to sleep—as well as other available caregivers besides mother who can do it—will come in handy. Someone else can take over occasionally to give mother a break and make it possible for her to have a night out, confident that baby won't wind up crying himself to sleep.

WAKES UP TO NURSE

A month ago, our seven-month-old was sleeping through the night. Now she wakes up several times to nurse. What's going on?

Frequent night waking in the older baby is often caused by teething. If your baby is teething, give her acetaminophen at bedtime and then again in four hours if needed. Another cause is either mom or baby being busy during the day. A breastfeeding mother who has recently returned to work, who has been away from her baby much of the day, or who has been preoccupied during the day will often be reminded of her baby's need for her by a middle-of-the-night breastfeeding. Babies around six or seven months of age also enjoy rapidly developing visual and motor skills. They concentrate on playing a lot during the day, to the extent that they forget to feed. Then at night they make up for those missed feedings by waking to nurse. We call these babies "all-night suckers."

Some babies simply prefer night feedings. Can you blame them? Nighttime is quiet time. Baby has mom all to himself, and he milks this quiet time, so to speak, for all he can get.

To get baby back into a routine with more feedings during the day and fewer at night, temporarily shelve as many outside responsibilities as you can and offer to nurse your baby every two or three hours during the day. Between feedings, hold and play with your baby more and simply have a lot of touch time. A baby whose needs are met during the day is less likely to be demanding at night. If you are working outside the home, try this approach during the evening and on weekends. Don't let other activities distract you from paying attention to your baby.

In the first few months of his life, Martha attended to Peter (their third baby) and his need for night feedings rather mechanically. He cried, she got up and charged down the hall, picked him up, sat in the rocker, and nursed him back to sleep. (What is amazing is that she never once thought of taking him to bed during the night!) When he got to the point where he woke up only once a night, she looked forward to this nighttime togetherness. She was no longer exhausted and she could begin to appreciate what she was doing: being with her baby while the whole household was asleep, no interruptions or distractions—just the two of them. She learned not to rush him so she could get back to sleep. She would take him from his crib and go into the family room, turn on some quiet music, and spend an hour in this special place she had carved out of her busy life. It was so special to be alone with her baby that she often continued to sit and hold him long after he was asleep. This was an important bonding time, and she still treasures the memory of those moments.

DISCOURAGING NIGHT NURSING

We have found that a family bed works best for our family. But my one-year-old son, who spends most of the night with us, is on and off the breast all night long. As a result, I don't sleep well, and I get out of bed in the morning feeling tired and resentful. I'd like to continue co-sleeping, but how do I get my son to stop nursing all night so that I can get some rest?

Look at your present dilemma from your baby's viewpoint. He sleeps next to his favorite person in the whole world, and his favorite five-star restaurant, Mom's All-Night Diner, is open only inches away from his eager mouth. He seeks out the breast whenever he stirs in his sleep, and there it is! Why not latch on for a few delicious sips before sinking back into sleep? Babies don't realize that mothers need sleep.

It is normal for a one-year-old to wake up once or twice a night to nurse. Some wake more often, and this may be fine. Some mothers can tolerate this and still sleep well themselves. Others can take it for a while but then begin to feel restless as baby gets older, past his first birthday, and night nursing goes on and on.

If going to bed feels more like work than rest, you need to make a change. A general principle of parenting that we believe in is this: *If you resent it, change it.* You may need to change your style of nighttime parenting so that both baby's needs and your needs get met. Active toddlers need happy, rested mothers.

Of course, there are many physical causes of night waking at various stages—teething, growth spurts, illnesses, and less obvious conditions, such as GER and food or environmental sensitivities. You may want to investigate these possibilities (although some of the time, there isn't a physical cause for night waking), since approaches to nighttime parenting won't work if there is a physical problem. Here are ways to convince your little nocturnal gourmet that nighttime is mostly for sleeping rather than nursing:

- *Tank him up with more feedings during the day.* Many toddlers get so busy during the day that they forget to nurse, and they try to make up for the food and the closeness they miss during the day by nursing at night.

- *Wake him up for an extended nursing and a thorough burping before you go to sleep.* This may help him to settle down for a good long sleep, so that he won't wake you for a longer stretch of time. If he does wake again to nurse in an hour or two, you'll know that he can't possibly be hungry again and that it's appropriate to try other ways of "nursing" him back to sleep.

- *Get him used to falling asleep in ways other than nursing.* Try the technique we call wearing down. First, wear your baby in a sling-type carrier as bedtime nears. After baby has been fed but is not yet asleep, walk around the house or around the block with him still in the sling. Once baby is in a deep sleep, ease him down onto your bed and extricate yourself from the sling. This is a good way for dad to take over part of the bedtime routine. Eventually your baby will associate father's arms with falling asleep, and he'll be willing to accept comfort from dad in the middle of the night as an alternative to nursing. Other ways to ease your baby into sleep without nursing him include patting or rubbing his back, rubbing his feet, singing and rocking, or even dancing in the dark to some tunes you like or lullabies you croon.

- *Increase the physical distance between the two of you at night.* Try the sidecar arrangement (see page 185). Or, once he's past the age of eighteen months or so, try having your baby go to sleep on a mattress on the floor next to your bed. Sometimes a bit of distance will dampen a baby's desire to night nurse. He may waken once or twice to nurse, but once he is back in his sidecar or you have crawled back into bed from his mattress on the floor, he may sleep more soundly and wake up less often.

- *Ask dad to take a more active part at night.* Sometimes the give-and-take of the mother-baby relationship gets out of balance: babies take too much and mothers give too much, to the extent that mothers give out. If you persist with a nighttime parenting style that you resent, you are likely to carry this resentment into your daytime relationship with your baby. You'll also be too tired to enjoy your little one. Part of maturing as a parent is learning when to say yes and when to say no. If you're becoming so exhausted that it's time to say no to all-night nursing, it may be time for dad to take over.

  It's best to wait until your baby is around eighteen months old before you take this approach because by then most babies are developmentally mature enough to handle this level of frustration. Between now and then, work on the list of things we've already given you to try. If baby is waking consistently more than two or three times a night and seems physically irritated by this situation, look closely at physical causes again. Also, be sure your own expectations about your child's

sleeping pattern have not been influenced by others telling you how your baby *should* be behaving. Remember, you can trust your baby to know what he needs.

Nursing does not always have to mean breastfeeding, especially at night. While only you can offer nighttime breastfeeding, father can "nurse" at night in other ways. If you are a single mother, consider asking your mother or someone else whom the baby knows well to come in for several nights to help baby over this hump. One of the ways we survived when we had a toddler who wanted to nurse frequently during the night was for Martha to go off "night call" temporarily. Bill would wear Stephen down in a baby sling so he got used to Bill's way of putting him to sleep. When Stephen woke up, Bill would again provide the comfort he needed by rocking and holding him in a neck-nestle position, using the "warm fuzzy" and singing a lullaby (see the nighttime fathering tips in chapter 10). Babies may protest having father instead of mother, but remember, crying and fussing in the arms of a loving parent is not the same as crying it out. Dads, realize that you have to remain calm and patient during these nighttime fathering challenges. You owe it to both mother and baby not to become rattled or angry if your baby resists the comfort you offer.

Try this weaning-to-father arrangement on a weekend or another time when dad can look forward to two or three nights when he doesn't have to go to work the next day. You will probably have to sell him on this technique, but we have tried it, and it does work. Be sure to use these night-weaning tactics only when baby is old enough (around eighteen months) and your gut feeling tells you that your baby is nursing at night out of habit and not out of need. And for night weaning to be successful, be sure you increase the time you spend playing with and holding your baby during the day.

- *Try sleeping elsewhere.* If your baby persists in wanting to nurse all night, relocate Mom's All-Night Diner to another room and let baby sleep next to dad, but only for a few nights. He may wake less often when the breast is not so available, and when he does wake, he will learn to accept comfort from dad.

If your best efforts to get your baby to cut back on nighttime nursing are getting you nowhere, back off for a while. If your one-year-old becomes very upset when you ask him not to nurse at night, or if he becomes more clingy during the daytime, his nighttime nursing may still be a real need, not just a habit. Follow your gut feeling. Remember, a simple habit is easily broken, but a need does not go away easily. Your baby may truly need to nurse at night a little while longer. It will be easier to increase your own acceptance level than to change your baby's behavior. Try to get a nap during the day.

Finally, remember that it's okay for a baby to nurse once or twice a night quite a while longer. Night nursing won't last forever. The time spent in your arms, at your breasts, and in your bed is a short blip in the total life of your child, but the memories of love and trust will last a lifetime.

WAKES UP TO PLAY

My eighteen-month-old wakes up wanting to nurse and then play in the middle of the night, but I want to sleep. How can I teach her that nighttime is for sleeping?

Try playing possum. Baby wakes up and expects you to wake up, too. Instead, you and your partner pretend to stay asleep (well, *you* pretend to be asleep). Maybe you open one eye and say, "It's nighttime; sleep now," but you don't start a discussion on the subject. You might even tell a child who wants to nurse that mommy's breasts are resting and they'll be awake again when the sun comes up. (It's a good idea to talk about this with your child during the day and again at bedtime if you're taking this approach.) If baby is upset about not being able to breastfeed, then enter dad as night "nurser" (see the father comforting tips in chapter 10). If she's happy to just play in the dark, let her, as long as you know she's safe. Eventually she'll go back to sleep because it's just not very interesting being awake in the dark alone.

CHANGING SHIFTS

Sometimes we approached nighttime parenting as shift work, especially with our seventh child, Stephen, who has Down syndrome. Stephen tired easily if he nursed for long periods, so he tended to nurse frequently around the clock, and Martha had trouble getting enough rest. So here's what we did. One night, Martha would stay up late and breastfeed Stephen to sleep. When Stephen woke during the night, Bill would father nurse him so that Martha could sleep—at least for a while. The next night Bill would wear Stephen down in the baby sling and Martha would go to bed early in preparation for taking the late shift. As Stephen grew older and stronger and able to breastfeed more during the day, he did not wake as often at night, and when he did, he was more willing to accept father nursing as an alternative to the breast.

If you have a toddler who persists in protesting this approach by crying or screaming, realize that it is okay to say no to her at this age—after all, she is not crying alone in a dark room down the hall. You will be teaching her by example that nighttime is not for playing. Her protests may be hard for you to ignore (you've responded so lovingly in the past), but she's old enough now to handle this frustration and she'll handle it better if she senses that you are not anxious about her.

FREQUENT EAR INFECTIONS

My baby gets frequent ear infections, and my doctor believes that night nursing is contributing to this problem. Is this possible?

Yes. When your baby lies flat, milk can enter the middle ear via the eustachian tube, the passage that connects the ear with the mouth. Milk in the middle ear can lead to a middle-ear infection. This happens often in bottle-fed babies, which is why doctors always encourage mothers to bottle-feed with baby in an upright position. There are three reasons why this is less of a problem for breastfed babies. Because of the different swallowing action in breastfed babies, milk is less likely to enter the eustachian tube. If it does, breast milk, being a human substance, is less irritating to the middle-ear tissues. Finally, breast milk itself contains a lot of natural infection-fighting cells and antibodies. Since your baby is prone to ear infections, it would be wise to prop her up to at least a thirty-degree angle during night feedings. It is also wise to eliminate dairy products from your diet (and your baby's diet), since cow's-milk protein in breast milk is a common allergen that can cause fluid to build up in the middle ear and become infected.

NAP-TIME CUDDLING

My two-month-old has no problem sleeping alone in her bassinet next to our bed at night, but the only way she'll nap during the day is in my arms, at my breast, or on my lap. Am I setting up a bad habit by allowing this? Will she grow out of it?

You are not setting up a bad habit by letting your baby sleep in your arms, on your lap, or at your breast. In fact, you are creating a good habit. Many kids ago we learned that babies have an inborn ability to communicate their needs to their caregivers. It's up to parents to learn how to listen. It is often difficult for parents to discern whether babies are communicating a need or merely a preference, but after many years, and after parenting eight children, we've learned that it's best to consider any cue a baby gives during the first few months as a *need* and respond accordingly. If your baby will nap only in your arms or at your breast or on your lap during the day and sleeps well alone at night, let it be. If you try to change a baby's daytime sleeping habits, you may wind up with a night waker. Most parents can handle any kind of napping habits during the day as long as baby sleeps well at night. Don't worry that you may be spoiling your infant or that she is manipulating you. This type of thinking will only create a distance between you and your baby and lessen your natural ability to read and respond to her cues. Besides, most mothers of two-month-olds need daytime naps themselves. Lie down with your baby and nap nurse together. This way your baby's need is translated into a restful habit for you—a pleasure you would not have indulged in if baby had not needed it.

It's easy for mothers to let themselves fall into the trap of focusing on "getting something done" while baby sleeps. Instead, we urge you to enjoy these special cuddle times while they last. Eventually your baby will outgrow her naptime cuddling need and you may long for the restful days when all she wanted was for you to hold and nurse her. Have you ever heard of a parent who looked back and wished she had held her baby less? We haven't! Most of us wish we had held our children more.

"NURSING" BABY TO SLEEP AT DAY CARE

My fifteen-month-old daughter will be entering day care part-time and I'm concerned about naps. At home she either nurses herself to sleep or I take her for a drive. How can I teach her another way of going to sleep?

The first thing to do is talk to your child-care provider about how she can create an environment for your daughter that mimics her home environment as closely as possible. It will also be less confusing for your baby if the child-care provider uses a parenting style that's similar to yours. Even if the caregiver can't breastfeed your infant, she can still lull her to sleep in her arms. Nursing is as much about comforting as it is about breastfeeding, especially at this age. Anyone can "nurse" a baby to sleep in this sense. Explain to the child-care provider that your infant is used to being nursed to sleep and you want her to put your child to sleep at nap time in her arms, either by rocking, singing, or lying next to her. (If your caregiver is unwilling to do this, consider looking for another caregiver.)

Finally, instead of taking your baby for a drive at nap time, show your caregiver our wearing-down technique (see page 194). Then if your baby doesn't fall asleep taking her bottle, the caregiver will have another tool.

10

The Father's Role in Breastfeeding

IT MAY NOT BE OBVIOUS, but fathers have an extremely important role to play in mothers' breastfeeding success. Sadly, most fathers go to every prenatal class except the one about breastfeeding. Many fathers feel left out of the inner circle of breastfeeding. They watch their wives developing a close symbiotic relationship with their newborns and wonder if there's any room left for dad.

When we talk with mothers in our medical practice about what has made it possible for them to breastfeed successfully, one factor stands out: a sensitive and supportive mate. As a father who took a while to find his way, Bill must admit that at first he did not see himself as crucial to Martha's role as a breastfeeding mother. When she decided to breastfeed our first child back in the late 1960s, when only about 25 percent of women chose to breastfeed, Bill was sort of lukewarm about breastfeeding. Even though he was a pediatrics intern and had heard a little bit about the benefits of breastfeeding, he offered only passive encouragement, and Martha coped on her own. Now, many years and seven babies later, after seeing the benefits of breastfeeding in thousands of breastfed children in our practice and having watched Martha log eighteen years of breastfeeding experience with our eight children,

Bill is absolutely convinced that breastfeeding makes a crucial difference. If we sound passionate about breastfeeding, it's because we are. Bill also learned in those years that his support made a difference to Martha's ability to nurture our babies at the breast, especially those children who were more challenging to nurse.

Sure, there will be times when you'll wonder if you'll ever get your wife back. But when you come to appreciate the physical, emotional, and intellectual advantages of breastfeeding to your wife, your children, and your family (which includes you), you will want to bend over backward not only to encourage your wife to breastfeed but also to do what you can to make breastfeeding a happy and memorable experience for all of you.

NORMAL FATHER FEELINGS

Fathers of breastfeeding infants will often share these kinds of feelings about their wives: "She's too attached to that baby," "All she does is nurse," "I feel left out," and "We need to get away — alone." These are real feelings from real fathers who sincerely love their children but feel displaced in their wives' affections by the breastfeeding baby. If you are a father feeling pushed aside, let us reassure you that your feelings and your wife's attachment to your baby are both very normal. How you handle these feelings and the effect they have on your wife is what's important. Perhaps an understanding of the biology behind mother-infant attachment and the changes your wife undergoes after birth will help you appreciate her intense focus on your baby.

While it's neither accurate nor fair to blame everything men don't understand about women on hormones, lactation hormones do explain why breastfeeding mothers behave the way they do. Before pregnancy, at least the first one, you are the center of your wife's attention, and romance abounds. Her hormones are geared up for reproduction, and her interest in you, her mate, is high. During pregnancy you have nine months to get used to a shift in that focus. And once birth happens, the mothering hormones definitely overpower the mating hormones for a while. Not only is she directing all her care and concern toward your baby, but her body also knows that it would not be wise (or even possible) to get pregnant at this time. This shift in hormones is part of nature's design to ensure that the young of a species get the care they need to survive and thrive. A new mother is programmed to be attached to her baby physically, emotionally, and chemically. This does not mean that the father is being displaced by his baby but rather that much of the energy previously directed toward him is now being directed toward his infant. In time, this energy will come back to him. We have learned from our practice and in our own family that when a husband is caring, involved, and supportive during this early attachment period, a wife's interest will return at a much higher level. One day Bill explained this hormonal tale to a "left-out" new dad, who commented, "This seems to be part of the 'for better or for worse' clause in the marriage vows: better for baby, worse for daddy." That may be the short-range viewpoint.

We call this early attachment period a season of the marriage—a season for nurturing your baby and your wife. If the marriage is tended carefully during this season of growth, the harvest will be a good one.

My husband did okay with our first two children, but with number 3 he really caught on. He was tender and nurturing, looked out for all my needs, took care of me and his daughter, and didn't make demands himself—on top of caring for two preschoolers! My libido returned in weeks rather than months, and I fell in love with him in a new way.

WHAT DADS CAN DO

Fathers have two roles when there's a new baby in the house. One is to care for the mother; the other is to share baby care (and child care if there are other children). Both jobs are important, and your wife will appreciate your taking them on without a lot of fanfare and complaining. For many men fatherhood marks the first time in their lives that they have had to center their attentions on someone other than themselves. What could matter more than nurturing the two (or more) most important people in your life?

Care for Her

As the breastfeeding mother takes on new roles, so does the "nursing" father. You now become servant, waiter, cook, housekeeper, chauffeur, and whatever else your wife and baby need. (Perhaps the late stages of pregnancy brought a glimpse of this.) Why should you be expected to take on these jobs? Traditional non-Western cultures have long recognized that a new mother needs time after birth to concentrate on her baby. During this time, special helpers and postpartum traditions and rituals relieve mothers of any outside

WHAT'S IN IT FOR DAD

Dads, did you know the following facts?

- Breastfed infants are smarter.
- Breastfed babies are healthier.
- Breastfeeding mothers are healthier.
- Breastfeeding costs less than formula feeding.
- Breastfeeding mothers miss fewer days of work.
- Breastfed babies have less smelly diapers.

Put the right milk into your baby now and you'll reap the rewards later. Breastfeeding is indeed a valuable long-term investment.

responsibilities that could drain energy away from the baby. Mothers are taken care of by others, are served special foods, and perhaps even live with their babies in a place set apart from others. This period of time usually lasts thirty to forty days, or in some cultures one moon cycle. These cultures believe (and they seem to have more wisdom about baby care than we do) that it's important for mother and baby to have this nesting-in period to build their attachment without a lot of distractions from everyday life.

Western cultures, on the other hand, make few provisions for the postpartum woman. She typically stays from one to three days in a hospital and then goes home, often with no special help in place or for a short time only. Mother gets the message (if she didn't already expect it) that it's back to business as usual; she will quickly take on all the household tasks again—in addition to caring for herself and her baby (and the other children, too). Mother quickly becomes overburdened. The demands on her exceed her ability to give, and soon she is headed for burnout.

Burnout is a condition in which the mother feels overwhelmed by her circumstances with little or no reserve energy available to cope with the demands on her time, her emotions, her whole being—physical, mental, emotional, and spiritual. Unrecognized and untreated, mother burnout can progress to mother meltdown and postpartum depression.

Dads have a major role to play in preventing burnout and in addressing it when it does occur. Recognize warning signs. Don't expect your wife to suddenly put her arms around you and beg for help. She won't, and she shouldn't have to. Mothers are usually unable or unwilling to ask for help for fear of shattering their own carefully built "supermom" image. And husbands may assume that unless they hear otherwise, all is well. A stressed-out mother of a high-need baby once confided to us, "I'd have to hit my husband over the head before he'd realize I'm giving out," but there are plenty of more subtle signs to watch for. One is when a woman seems unable to find joy in her mothering and in her marriage. If you and your wife begin to view your baby as a chore rather than a child, that's a red flag. Other signs include diminishing attention to grooming, no sense of humor, acting or looking depressed, angry outbursts, making mountains out of molehills, feeling overbooked and overbusy, loss of appetite, and loss of interest in intimacy.

Dads, keep in mind that a burned-out mother is a burned-out wife. Preventing burnout is not only in your child's best interest, it will also benefit you. You may believe that because your wife is such a "good mother" and has all those relaxing breastfeeding hormones working for her, she's above burnout. Wrong! It's the best and most dedicated of moms who are prone to burnout.

Here's what you can do to prevent burnout in your wife, or turn it around if it does occur.

Protect Her

Yes, you will both want to share the joys of a new baby with friends and relatives, and it's good for new mothers to be on the receiving end of praise and fuss over the baby and the birth story. But it's up to dad to stand guard against well-meaning but annoying visitors who use up time and energy that would be better spent on the developing mother-baby relationship. There will be times when you need to turn your phones off and put a DO NOT DISTURB sign on your front door. Be especially vigilant when it comes to defending your wife against critics (even your own mother)—well-meaning friends and relatives who insist that she do things their way and who imply that she is not a good mother if she doesn't.

Having a new baby opens your life up to a whole parade of advisers, some helpful, some harmful. Their comments can undermine the confidence of a vulnerable new mother, especially in the early weeks after birth. People who know little about breastfeeding offer unhelpful and counterproductive advice, such as, "Are you sure you have enough milk?" or "I couldn't breastfeed, either," or "You're spoiling that baby by holding him so much," or the comment that we hear so often aimed at mothers of fussy babies, "It must be your milk."

Don't expect your wife to waste energy defending herself against critics; that's your job. You can disarm critics by framing your baby's behavior in a positive light. When someone says, "He sure is demanding!" with a disapproving scowl, you come back with, "Yes, he sure is determined" or "Our son sure knows what he needs!" When another critic offers the classic comment "That baby is manipulating you—you have to show her who's boss," you reply, "Well, sure, she's smart enough to want first-class care." Lay an affirming hand on her shoulder and stand by the mother of your child. Keep in mind that the postpartum period is a time when women are particularly sensitive to the way they believe others perceive them. (Imagine yourself trying to master a new job, one with unpredictable demands, while everyone from your boss to your mother-in-law watches your every move.) Affirming out loud your belief that your wife is a good mother, saying it to her in person and to friends and family in her presence, is an effective way to combat the intrusions of unhelpful criticism.

Serve Her

Stan, a professional tennis player, once asked us how he could help in the care of his newborn. Bill responded in the language of Stan's trade: "Improve your serve." Be sure your wife gets plenty of nutritious food to eat. Offer her refreshments during the day. Restock her nursing station with fresh water and nutritious snacks. Ask what particular foods she needs and wants. (For a crash course in nutrition for a breastfeeding mother, see chapter 4.) And remember, breastfeeding mothers need to nibble on nutritious snacks throughout the day. In the early weeks, be sure there is something healthful and ready to grab in the fridge, especially for breakfast if you leave for work before she and baby are up. On your days off work, encourage her to go back to sleep or indulge in a tub soak while you take baby for a walk.

Obtain Help for Her

In many cultures after a birth, a mother enjoys the help of a doula (from the Greek word for "one who ministers" or "bond servant"), a woman who specializes in mothering the mother, *not the baby*, and relieving her of chores that drain her energy away from the task of learning to mother her baby. Anybody can be a doula: hired help, relatives, friends, and especially dads. When someone asks, "What do you need?" be ready with a reply: "Bring over dinner" or "Take Emma to play group tomorrow." If you're lucky enough to have offers of help, set up a schedule, marshal the troops, be in charge of who does what when. Doula services are springing up throughout North America, so if you can afford it or if someone wants to give your wife a rather expensive baby gift, hire a doula to help her in those first weeks postpartum.

Clean for Her

Some new mothers carry their late-pregnancy nesting instincts into the postpartum period. They feel calmer when the house is clean, neat, and organized. Dads, keep in mind that an upset nest often means an upset mom, which leads to an upset family. If you have trouble making housework a priority, hire help. Bill noticed that during the first months postpartum, a single dirty dish in the sink could get on Martha's nerves, though usually she can ignore a whole sink full. An acronym that Bill used to remind himself to keep our nest tidy was just that—TIDY: Take Inventory Daily Yourself. Walk around the house and try to notice the little things. (Men, she'll love you for noticing little things. Women don't expect it!) When you walk past the bed, make it. Pick up the nightgown on the floor and drape it over the chair, and pick up your dirty socks. Load last night's dinner dishes in the dishwasher before you leave for work, and make a mental note to bring home a supply of paper plates. If the older kids have trashed the house, get on their case to clean it up—and help them. (In fact, this is a good time for you to hold a family council and let older, school-age children know that for the next few months, they get to do more giving and less taking.) If Bill saw one of our children about to do something that he knew would upset Martha, he would quickly intervene with "That's disturbing Mom's peace." This was a phrase they could understand. Give kids a title and a job, such as "waiter," "cook," "bed maker," "drink server"—

whatever needs to get done that kids can do. Even a three-year-old can fetch a water bottle from the kitchen while mommy is nursing the baby. Fathers, model this behavior for your children and teach them how they are to treat their mom. And remember, you may be bringing up someone's future husband. One day a burned-out mother confided to us during her newborn's visit, "I'm tired of teaching my husband how to help around the house. That's a job his father should have done."

Drive Her

Many new moms have such zeal for taking good care of their babies that they forget to take care of themselves. And if burnout is setting in, inertia is not far behind. At that point mother not only loses interest in caring for herself but also no longer knows how. You need to remind her. Not by offering platitudes such as "Honey, just relax and take it easy" but by being proactive. Make her an offer she can't refuse: "I've made an appointment at the spa for you today, which I've already paid for. After you nurse Clara, I'll drive you there, wait for you, and Clara and I will have a little daddy-daughter time together. We'll pick up something for dinner on the way home." You're giving her permission to focus on herself, even if it's only for an hour. New mothers often find it difficult to admit they need help with their babies, let alone accept it. Veteran mothers usually know they should glom on to any help they can get.

Counsel Her

Sometimes it's up to dad to bring some perspective and balance to the mother-baby relationship. One day when Martha was overwhelmed with our high-need baby, Hayden, during one of those marathon nursing sessions,

Bill noticed that she was getting frazzled. He suggested she relax and take a shower. Martha snapped back, "I don't have time to take a shower because this baby needs me so much." Whereupon Bill put up a sign on our bathroom mirror that read EACH DAY REMIND YOURSELF THAT WHAT OUR BABY NEEDS MOST IS A HAPPY, RESTED MOTHER. And then Bill took Hayden for a walk.

FILL IN FOR HER WITH YOUR TODDLER OR PRESCHOOLER

If your new baby has an older sibling, the postpartum demands on your wife's energy will be enormous. This older child needs reassurance and lots of attention as she copes with the new baby usurping her privileged place in the family. It's up to dad to spend time with her by participating in fun activities, telling stories, playing on the floor—whatever it takes to help the child feel that she is still an important person in the family. You want her to decide that being herself instead of a baby has definite advantages. Be proactive about spending time with your two- or three-year-old. Don't wait until she is tired and whining for mom to offer an alternative. Plan ahead for things you can do together, even if it's just a trip to the store for milk and bread.

"NURSING" FOR FATHERS

While only mothers can breastfeed, both mother and father can nurse, if you understand the term *nursing* to mean comforting and caring for baby. Dads, don't settle for the downgrade to babysitter, feeling like you're pinch-hitting until mom returns. Fathers have their own unique way of caring for babies. It's different from moms', and babies thrive on this difference.

Men don't get a hormonal boost at the beginning of their parenting careers the way women do. The more time you spend caring for your baby, responding to his signals (even if you don't always interpret them correctly), or just watching him and looking at the world through his eyes, the better you will feel about yourself as a father. Here are some tips to get you started:

The neck nestle. One day Martha left our apparently settled and well-fed six-month-old Matthew with Bill while she went shopping. All was well until a half hour later, when Matthew went into an unexplained crying jag, probably because he was missing mommy. All Bill's usual rocking and walking measures didn't work. Just as he remembered that Matthew always settled for Martha when she offered him her breast, it dawned on Bill that he had something Martha didn't—a deep voice and a hairy chest. So he put those uniquely male characteristics to work and came up with the neck nestle. Nestle your baby's head against the front of your neck, his head cradled under your chin, chest-to-chest, skin-to-skin. Sing a droning song, such as "Ol' Man River," or make up your own:

> Go to sleep, go to sleep,
> Go to sleep, my little baby.
> Go to sleep, go to sleep, go to sleep, my little boy.

A tiny baby hears with the vibration of his skull bones in addition to his eardrums, and the male larynx (Adam's apple) protrudes more than the female's. When you place baby's head against your larynx in the front of your neck and hum or sing to your baby, the slower, more easily felt vibrations of the lower-pitched male voice will often lull baby right to sleep. An added attraction of the neck nestle is the warm air baby feels from your breath on his scalp. Experienced mothers have long known that sometimes just breathing onto their babies' faces or heads will calm them. They call this magic breath. Also, you can sway

baby's tense abdomen. We also call this position the colic carry. Dad's larger hands and firmer grasp have an edge over mother's softer touch and worn-out arms.

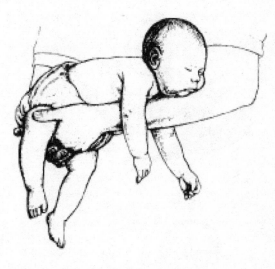

Colic football hold

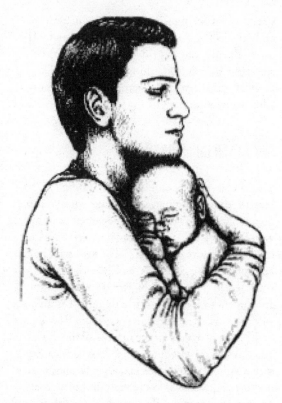

Neck nestle

back and forth, dance, or rock baby in the neck-nestle position. Our babies have enjoyed this holding pattern better than any other position.

The warm fuzzy. This comforting measure offers another opportunity for you to shine. Drape baby skin-to-skin over your chest with her ear over your heartbeat. The rhythm of your heartbeat plus the rise and fall of your chest as you breathe will usually lull baby right to sleep.

The colic football hold. Tuck your baby against your body as if she were a football, draping baby's stomach down over your forearm, head in the crook of your elbow, and legs straddling your hand. Grasp the diaper area firmly, with your forearm and the palm of your hand pressing on

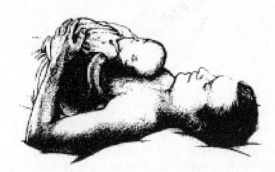

Warm fuzzy

Baby bends. Flex your baby's body to untense him. This is the position that stimulates the relaxation pathways in the brain. Extension of the body, with the back arching and limbs flailing, creates tension. This is why mothers bend their babies around them while breastfeeding. Hold baby with either his back or his legs flexed against your chest. If baby has a tense abdomen from lots of gas, try the tummy tuck: support baby's bottom with one hand, his back against your chest, and place the palm of your other hand over baby's navel. Lean baby forward against your big, warm hand.

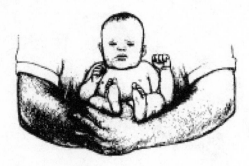

Baby bend

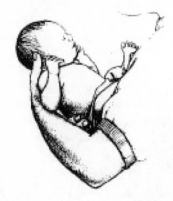

Baby bend (side view)

Wear your baby. Become a participant in the family art of babywearing. Put your baby in a sling-type carrier and wear her as much as possible so that she gets used to the rhythms of your walk, your voice, and your dance. Go for the triple play and use all three of these methods together. Put baby in a sling, let her head rest against your bare, fuzzy chest and her ear over your heartbeat, and nestle her into your neck. (This is guaranteed to impress mom. Nothing turns a woman on like watching her man sensitively tend to "her" baby.)

Freeway fathering. Place your baby in a car seat and take a long nonstop drive. Babies usually fall asleep during long car rides. Meanwhile, insist that your wife do something just for herself at home. Or do the drive together to share some adult conversation.

SEX AFTER CHILDBIRTH

Yes, there is sex after childbirth and during breastfeeding, but it may not be quite what you are used to. Left-out fathers often share their feelings with Bill: they say, "All she does is nurse"; "We haven't made love for weeks"; "The heck with mom hormones—I've got needs, too!" We want to reassure you that your feelings and your wife's strong attachment to your baby are both normal. Your wife's shift of attention from you to your baby is part of the normal design for the survival of the species. You can survive without sex, but your baby cannot thrive without an attached and attentive mother. It's not that your wife has lost interest in you; it's that her interest is temporarily refocused onto baby.

Besides these biological causes, another reason for your wife's lack of interest in sex is that she's just too tired. Mothers often feel so drained by the incessant demands of the baby—and the household—that at bedtime all they want to do is sleep. Mothers have described this end-of-the-day feeling as being "all touched out" or "all used up."

Note for husbands: Put enough pressure on your wife to have sex, and that's how she'll feel about it—pressured.

For the first few months after birth, and sometimes longer, most women do not have the energy to sustain a high level of interest in being both a mother and a sexual partner. Rather than pouting and pressuring, consider this season of your marriage a time to delay your gratification a bit and give love and support to your wife in a way that will woo her back toward intimacy. Here's how.

Be Sensitive

Your wife needs you to be sensitive during these times when her energy is low. Even though sexual intercourse may be the last thing your wife wants, emotional intercourse is high on her need list. For most men, sex equals a physical connection. Not so for women, especially during the postpartum period. Women have to be emotionally ready before they are physically ready. Her body is not ready for sex until her mind is.

PROVE YOURSELF

Dads, let us share with you some secrets we've learned about new mothers. When a mother develops a strong, healthy attachment to her baby, she experiences an incredibly strong biological and hormonal bond. So she is naturally reluctant to share the care of her baby with anyone else. You will notice this when your baby cries. Suppose you hear that your baby is awake from his nap and needs comforting. You calmly start for the bedroom only to be shoved aside by your wife sprinting in from the backyard to scoop up her baby. You may feel a bit insulted. You know you could have handled this. Doesn't your wife trust you?

Mothers are made that way. When a baby cries, the blood flow to a mother's breasts surges, and she has a hormonal need to pick up and comfort her baby. Even the most sensitive father doesn't experience the same hormonal change when his baby cries. When you do win the race to the crying baby, be prepared for your wife to hover around you, waiting to rescue baby with the unintended but definite put-down, "I'll comfort her, dear." Because baby seems to settle down more quickly in your wife's arms or at her breasts, you back off from becoming a baby comforter, and your wife readily lets you off the hook.

Two unhealthy situations occur as a result. You never get a chance to develop your own nurturing skills, and your wife falls into the exhausting trap of believing that she is the only one who understands baby's needs. As a result, she doesn't allow herself the luxury of a soak in the tub, coffee with a friend, or even a much-needed shower because "there's no one else who can comfort my baby." This situation is a red flag for approaching mother burnout, mate burnout, and family burnout. You can keep your wife from falling into this trap by sharing in the comforting of your baby early. Right from the start, show her that baby sometimes accepts comfort from you, too, so that she can feel comfortable releasing "her" baby into your care and can take a break now and then.

Fathers, don't make the mistake Bill made with our first two children. He thought Martha was such a good breastfeeding mother that our babies really didn't need him to comfort them. He decided he would wait to get involved with them until they were old enough to throw a football. Big mistake! This was a lose-lose-lose situation. Bill lost the opportunity to hone his skills as a baby comforter and to connect with our children at a sensitive period in their lives. Our babies lost a chance to get used to their father's unique way of providing comfort. And Martha lost a much-needed support person.

By becoming an early expert in father nursing, you can teach your baby that the breast is not the only source of comfort in the world. This will make baby more able to accept alternatives during night wakings, colicky periods, and days when the breasts, and the woman they are attached to, are giving out.

Go Slowly

Pressuring your wife to give too much too soon is bound to fail. Besides, as all men know, sex given out of love and desire is so much better than sex given out of obligation. Even though the obstetrician may say it's okay to have sex again, the doctor is not the one who had the baby. Nor is he or she the one who is breastfeeding. Court your wife all over again. While you may not be able to compete with the hormones in her bloodstream, you can work your magic on her heart and mind. Look for things you can do during the day to help her conserve energy, anticipating a warm-up period in which the two of you gradually reestablish your sexual relationship. Don't pounce on her on that doctor-okayed "due date." Help her, hold her, caress her, love her, and share the baby care. Spend time just cuddling, not as foreplay for that night but perhaps as foreplay for the next week.

Go Carefully

Be gentle and sensitive to the physical changes in your wife's body as she recovers from giving birth. Some fathers have described sexual reunion with their wives as "getting to know her body all over again." On the plus side, the bulge is gone, and you'll be able to snuggle close again. But her perineum could still be tender and her breasts extremely sensitive.

Sexual responsiveness after birth and during lactation varies greatly among women. Some women actually experience a heightened enjoyment of sex during lactation. Others experience highs and lows—one week feeling very sexually responsive and the next week feeling very uninterested. Some women find that breastfeeding helps them become more comfortable with their breasts, and therefore their bodies, and this carries over into lovemaking.

During lovemaking, expect a few biological reminders that you are a new father:

- The same hormone that is released during sex (oxytocin) also stimulates the milk-ejection reflex, so it's not unusual for a woman's breasts to spray milk, especially during orgasm.

- Leaking milk during lovemaking is a natural side effect of breastfeeding, which is easy to handle with understanding and humor. Don't give your wife messages that leaking bothers you. Instead interpret leaking as a sign that your wife's body is being aroused by your lovemaking—and keep a towel handy.

- You don't have to assume that the breasts are off-limits to you just because they are being used to nurture a baby. If nipple stimulation has been a mutually enjoyable part of your previous lovemaking, there's no physical or biological reason that this can't continue. You don't have to be concerned about germs or about stealing milk that belongs to the baby. Some women, however, find that their responsiveness to breast stimulation during sex changes while they are breastfeeding. This may be related to changes in nipple sensitivity, engorgement and tenderness, or the feeling that the breasts belong to the baby. These changes are temporary, but you need to respect them.

- Vaginal dryness is common after childbirth and during lactation because of low estrogen levels. If intercourse is painful because of dryness, irritation, or a still-tender perineum, use a water-soluble lubricant.

- Schedule time for lovemaking. One thing that is common to all postpartum parents, whether breastfeeding or not, is that sex becomes less spontaneous. You have to plan ahead for your intimate time together.

- Remember that the master bedroom is not the only place where lovemaking can be enjoyed. If your baby has nursed to sleep peacefully on your bed, head for the living room or the guest room. You will learn to be more creative.

- Nursing the baby right before lovemaking may prevent untimely interruptions and will minimize leaking. However, it often seems that breastfed babies have a kind of radar that wakes them up just when things are getting interesting between mom and dad.

You may sometimes feel that you are making love to a split personality: your wife's body is in your arms, but her mind is on the baby. Avoid giving your wife the message that your baby is spoiling your sexual relationship with her. When baby cries just as you are getting amorous, don't let loose with an angry "foiled again" reaction. You can't compete with your baby's heart-wrenching, milk-stimulating cries. Turn this biological interruption into an opportunity by giving your wife the message that you can wait: "Relax — I'll get her and bring her to you for a feed." Leave out any expectations that you'll get back to having sex later. Mom will probably be asleep by then anyway. You will win lots of gratitude by encouraging your wife to tend to baby's needs before yours. A new mother is really turned off by sexual selfishness in a man. Although at some level you may feel deprived and consider baby an intruder, try to work through those feelings. A surly message from dad that "baby has had enough attention and now it's my turn" is a guaranteed turnoff.

Fathers who feel that they are suffering from an acute lack of sex in the first few months after birth but develop the maturity to accept delayed gratification of their needs usually find that their overall relationship with their mate improves. Understanding and respecting the natural design for parenting in the early months motivates a husband to seek ways of achieving intimacy with his wife outside of intercourse. In ancient times writers described sexual intercourse as "knowing" another person. And this is exactly what happens when you court your wife all over again after childbirth. Yes, there is sex after birth! It's a fuller, richer kind of sex that matures a man as a person, a husband, and a father.

Talk to Her

Tell your wife how you feel — openly, honestly, but gently. Confiding in her will help you feel heard and understood and will open up her soul to you, as you are opening yours to her. Airing feelings in a sensitive way can keep resentment and bitterness from building up. Maybe you can even have a good cry together. You don't want her to see you as pathetic and needy, but you do want her to understand you. And she will love you for it.

Love Her

A new father once asked Bill, "When will our life get back to normal?" Bill informed him that after you become a father, this new life *is* your normal life. Embrace the changes in your life and the changes that are going on in your wife. One of the greatest gifts a father can give his children is to love their mother. She can breastfeed better, be a better mother, and be a more attentive wife if she believes that you affirm and support her chosen style of mothering.

FOR MOTHERS ONLY

Moms, realize that even though your hormones change after birth and during breastfeeding, your mate's do not. As a result, fathers are not as driven to nurture their babies, and their sexual needs remain what they were before the birth. The two greatest concerns that new fathers have are the lack of intimacy with their wives and the baby's obvious preference for mother. They end up feeling inadequate both as a mate and as a father. Here's how you can help.

Have "The Talk"

Pour out your feelings to your husband. Explain to him the changes that are going on inside you to help him understand that you are feeling and acting the way you are because of your new role as mother, not because of anything he has done to turn you off. Be sure he knows that it's not his fault that sex is not the same as it used to be. Mothers, remember that for most men intimacy equals intercourse.

Show and Tell

Your husband may be feeling that you no longer want or need him because your baby is taking his place. It's easy for your husband to feel that there is no room for him in the relationship you have with your baby. It's time to let your husband know that you now need him even more. You need and want to be held and cherished. You need his support and his friendship.

Here's a story of how a mother in our practice handled her husband's sexual feelings. Susan worked hard at becoming both a giving mother and a giving wife. She and her husband were blessed with a baby who woke frequently at night. Dad felt he needed his sleep and moved out of the bedroom when baby was about one month old and spent most nights on the living room couch (not an unusual—or recommended—arrangement). Instead of adopting the attitude that many tired mothers have ("I need my sleep more than he needs sex"), Susan recognized that while baby's needs came first, the two of them needed each other. She would occasionally tiptoe into the living room and "surprise" her husband after baby had fallen asleep. These midnight surprises did wonders to help her husband accept her commitment to being sensitive to her baby's needs at night. And it was a happy day when the night waking lessened enough for all three to be able to share sleep as a family.

Watch for Red Flags

Is your husband enjoying work more and coming home less? If you find that you are drifting apart as a couple and your husband is drifting away from your child, it's time to refocus your family priorities. What your baby needs most is two happy parents. This could be a time for both of you to talk things over with a counselor. Obviously, you will want a counselor who is supportive of your breastfeeding and of your parenting priorities.

Set Dad Up to Succeed

It's understandable that you may want to handle nearly all the baby care during the first few months, both because you believe you can do it better than anyone else and because breastfeeding gives you two built-in surefire sources of most of what baby needs. As we mentioned earlier, this can become a lose-lose-lose situation. You lose the help of your mate, father doesn't get an opportunity to develop his baby-nurturing skills, and baby doesn't get a chance to connect with dad.

To get your husband to be more involved in baby care, you have to build his confidence. Avoid this scenario: baby is fussing and daddy picks her up, trying to comfort her. He's struggling, while you know exactly what baby wants. You hover around the pair and finally rescue fussy baby from fumbling daddy. Dad feels incompetent, and the next time baby cries he leaves the comforting to you, right from the beginning.

When dad is taking care of baby, mothers should back off a bit. Take a walk. Let daddy and baby work it out. You'll be surprised at what creative comforting measures your husband can come up with in a pinch. Be sure that your words and your actions convey the message that you trust him in the care of your baby. Show him and tell him about different comforting techniques that work, and then let him develop some of his own. When you leave baby with dad, pick a time when you know from experience that baby is usually in a good mood. Nurse him, fill his tummy, and then leave to go shopping. Give your husband the message that you respect his fathering abilities. Remember: only you can breastfeed, but both parents can nurse.

V

SPECIAL SITUATIONS

Now that more mothers understand that breastfeeding matters, they are finding ways to nurse their babies in a variety of challenging circumstances. Breastfeeding helps a mother of an infant with special needs take advantage of what we call the need-level concept. Some babies have a higher level of emotional, physical, and nutritional needs, and these needs must be satisfied in order for these babies to thrive. (*Thriving* means not just getting bigger but also growing to one's fullest physical, intellectual, and emotional potential.) To meet the higher need level, parents must respond with a higher level of giving. When the need level of the child and the giving level of the parent match, the family thrives.

Breastfeeding gives you an extra boost in challenging situations. Your milk is nature's built-in medicine for a variety of physical and developmental needs. And the very act of breastfeeding raises your level of intuition a notch, so that you're better able to meet the higher needs of your baby. Lactation hormones also make it easier to handle stress. If you have a sick or hospitalized baby, breastfeeding makes you an actual member of the medical team, because breast milk has valuable healing properties.

Not only are more mothers nursing babies with special needs, they are also nursing their infants longer. Breastfeeding a toddler brings benefits and unique challenges. Finally, all good things do come to a timely end, and every baby weans eventually. We'll show you how to do this at different ages and stages with minimal stress for both mom and baby.

There will be days when you're ready to quit breastfeeding but your baby isn't. You will wonder whether the frequent feedings and night nursings are really worth it. When you have those moments—and you probably will—remind yourself that the time in your arms, at your breast, and in your bed is a very short period in the total life of your child, but the memories of your love and availability during breastfeeding will last a lifetime.

11

Breastfeeding for Babies and Mothers with Special Needs

"BREAST IS BEST!" IS especially true for babies with health problems or special developmental needs. In fact, if there were a word that was better than *best,* we'd use it here. Breastfeeding offers an edge to babies who face special challenges. With all its nutritional, immunological, and developmental benefits, human milk helps babies with special needs concentrate their energies on growing and learning. The beauty of breastfeeding is that in nearly every case there is a special something in either the breast milk or the act of breastfeeding that helps fill these special needs.

This doesn't mean, however, that it's easy to breastfeed a baby with health or developmental problems. Mothers of these babies may have to work harder at breastfeeding, especially in the early days, the time when they are also learning to cope with their baby's difficulties. But for many mothers, breastfeeding helps them feel more "normal" and more connected to their children.

PREMATURE BABIES

When you and your baby are temporarily separated after birth because of illness or prematurity, it's easy to feel displaced by other caregivers. But breastfeeding makes you a valuable member of the medical team. You give your baby the "medicine" that no one else can make—your milk. Human milk offers exciting benefits to premature infants. Here's a partial list:

- Research has shown that premature babies who receive mother's milk have better visual development and a higher IQ later in childhood. Research at Brown University involving extremely premature babies found that for every teaspoon per pound (or 10 milliliters per kilogram) more breast milk they ate every day, their scores for mental development, psychomotor development, and behavior increased and their rates of hospitalization decreased. This visual and intellectual advantage is thought to be attributable to the special brain-building fats, especially DHA, in breast milk. Formulas made in the United States may contain DHA, but even so, DHA in formula has not been proved to function the same way as it does in human milk.

- The proteins in human milk are better suited to infant metabolism, and the fat, thanks to the presence of the enzyme lipase, is easier to digest. This makes more energy available for growth.

- Breastfeeding offers protection against necrotizing enterocolitis, a life-threatening bowel disease that affects premature babies.

WHY PERSIST

Breastfeeding a baby with special needs makes extra demands on a mother. Family, friends, and even health-care providers may wonder why she *persists* when pumping her breasts regularly and working with the baby at the breast takes lots of time and seems to create more stress. They may urge her to give up on breastfeeding. Formula feeding not only looks easier but may seem like the answer to mother's anxiety.

These advisers, though well intentioned, are missing the point. Breastfeeding may be the one variable in the whole situation that a mother feels she can control, or it may be the one thing she feels she can give her newborn that doctors and nurses can't. It reminds her that she *is* his mother and she is important to her child. Working through breastfeeding problems is a mother's way of giving her baby not only the best in nutrition but also the best of herself. She needs support to get through the tough times, not a way out.

Besides giving extra help to a special-needs infant, breastfeeding gives mothers that extra intuitive edge they will need to make on-the-spot decisions. Breastfeeding is an exercise in baby reading; the higher the baby's needs, the more cue-reading help a mother needs.

- Human milk offers protection from infection that is simply not available to formula-fed infants.

- Milk from mothers who give birth to preterm babies is specially "engineered" by nature to match the infant's unique nutritional needs. It contains higher levels of protein, fat, sodium, iron, chloride, and other nutrients that correspond to the needs of these small babies.

Even in the high-tech world of neonatal intensive care, old-fashioned mother's milk is the superior food.

Pumping for Your Preemie

When a preemie is too young or too sick to nurse directly at the breast, mother must express her milk. This signals her body to continue to produce milk, so that when baby is finally ready to nurse at the breast, there will still be lots of milk. Meanwhile, the milk mother pumps can be saved and given to her baby through a tube. Mothers of preemies may soon feel "bonded" to the pump. Emptying the breast frequently is important in the early weeks even if baby can't nurse. Here are some suggestions to help you pump enough milk for your preterm infant:

Follow a nursing schedule similar to a newborn's. At first mothers should follow a schedule similar to a newborn's nursing, which means pumping at least every three hours. Ideally mothers should try to get in eight pumping sessions in twenty-four hours. This may sound overwhelming, but it keeps you from being at higher risk for losing your milk supply in the long term. It's better to have frequent short pumping sessions than infrequent long pumping sessions. Rather than pumping every three hours around the clock, do it every four hours at night and do it every two or three hours during the day (for example, 7:00 a.m., 9:00 a.m., noon, 3:00 p.m., 5:00 p.m., 8:00 p.m., 11:00 p.m., 3:00 a.m.). Using a double-pump setup, pump for fifteen to twenty minutes per session. At least eight short and frequent pumpings per day is the key: ideally, pump every three hours during the day and four at night, with the first pumping of the day only two hours from the next one. If you miss a pumping, you can pump ten minutes every hour until you are back on schedule. Measure your supply in terms of total output for the day, not per pumping session, and don't get discouraged if more frequent pumping yields less per pumping. It's the total amount for the day that counts.

Pump often to build up your supply. Frequent pumping builds up a good milk supply, so that even if a mother's supply diminishes while she's pumping, she will have plenty of milk once her baby is nursing at the breast. Recent research into the physiology of lactation suggests that emptying the breast often in the early weeks sets a mother up for better milk production two and three months later. Infrequent emptying of the breasts allows milk-suppressing substances to accumulate that slow milk production. Try "power pumping": pump ten; rest; pump ten more. It takes at least three days of increased pumping frequency to measurably increase your supply, so be patient.

SEPARATING THE CREAM

Milk from later in a feeding is higher in fat, and it can be used to supplement babies who are not gaining weight well because of a weak suck or increased nutritional requirements. Here are three different ways to separate the cream from your expressed milk.

- Pump milk right after feeding your baby at the breast. The milk in the collection bottle will be richer than milk pumped before baby nursed.
- If your baby is not yet nursing at the breast, separate the hindmilk from the foremilk by switching collection bottles partway through your pumping session, after you have triggered the milk-ejection reflex.
- When you refrigerate expressed human milk, the cream rises to the top. Skim this off and give this to your baby first.

Hand-express or pump as soon as possible. Start expressing milk for your preemie as soon after the birth as you are able to. Those first drops of colostrum may not look like much, but they are the ideal first feeding for any baby—especially a preemie who is not quite ready for the big world. Save every drop (the nurse can take what you pump and dilute it as necessary with sterile water to make as much of this liquid gold as possible) and ask that your baby be given your colostrum as his very first tube (or oral) feeding, whether that's in a few days or a few weeks.

Nursing tip: Reduce the travel time from mom to baby. If you pump at the hospital when you visit your baby, the nurses may be able to give him your milk only minutes after it has left your breast. And you're likely to pump more milk after you've spent some time with your baby. Some mothers even arrange to pump at their babies' bedside.

Use a high-quality pump. Don't waste effort or get stressed out using a less-than-efficient pump. When you must pump to maintain a milk supply, you need to rent a hospital-grade breast pump to use at home. (See chapter 7.) These pumps have been shown to produce the highest prolactin levels in mothers, and mothers of preemies need all the hormonal help they can get. With signed orders from your baby's doctor, your health insurance may cover the cost. A lactation consultant or someone on the neonatal nursery staff can help you arrange a pump rental before you are discharged from the hospital.

Store your milk for later use. The hospital staff can tell you how to store and label your milk so that it can be given to your baby later. Ask that your baby be given fresh (rather than frozen) milk whenever possible, since some of the live infection-fighting white blood cells are destroyed by freezing. (For more tips on expressing and storing your milk, see chapters 7 and 8.)

SUPERMILK FOR TINY BABIES

Preterm infants need extra amounts of some nutrients in order to grow quickly. By a marvelous feat of nature, for about one month mothers who deliver a preterm baby also deliver milk that is higher in these nutrients. Preterm milk is notably higher in calories, protein, and fat. It's especially high in the brain-building fats LC-PUFAs (see chapter 1). The immature intestines of premature infants have difficulty absorbing fat, especially formula fat. Again, enter mother's milk, which is rich in the enzyme lipase, which helps the fat be more digestible. Preterm milk is also higher in growth-building and immune-boosting proteins. Preterm babies need extra nourishment and protection. With their mothers' milk, they get both.

Sometimes human milk given to preterm babies in the neonatal nursery is fortified with a commercial human milk fortifier. Don't interpret this as an indication that your milk is somehow not good enough for your baby. It's true that preterm milk contains extra amounts of many nutrients, but it may not be able to deliver all the nutrients a baby needs to grow as he would have grown in the womb. Still, the protective shield against germs and foreign proteins that comes with your milk can't be matched by any factory-made concoction. If the doctors are concerned about your baby's growth on human milk alone, consider pumping in a way that gives the baby nothing but "cream" (see box above). This is a way of getting your body's own technology to work for your baby in the high-tech nursery.

Keep the pump clean. Because these babies are more vulnerable to infection, mothers who are pumping for a preemie or a baby who is ill must take more care with cleaning and sterilizing milk containers and the parts of the pump that touch the milk. Besides following the hospital's instructions about cleaning and sterilizing equipment, you should thoroughly wash your hands (including under your nails) before pumping, and pump your milk directly into special sterile collecting bottles rather than risk contamination by transferring the collected milk into another container. There are special milk-collecting containers from which milk can be given directly to the infant. Ask the nurses if they can provide sterile containers for your milk.

MOTHERING YOUR PREEMIE

You may feel that there is little you can do for your baby during the time he is cared for in the neonatal nursery. But even now you are an important person in his life and an indispensable member of the medical team. If you feel you're being pushed aside, remind yourself: you are the baby's mother. Ultimately you and your partner are responsible for this tiny person's life.

Visit your baby in the hospital every day, and plan on spending several hours there. If you are a first-time mother without a toddler or preschooler at home, you might even spend most of the day with your baby. This will help you feel more like his mother, and he will get to know the sound of your voice and the comfort of your touch. Set up a meeting with the neonatal doctor and head nurse and tell them your desires about parenting your preemie. Tell them you want to begin kangaroo care (skin-to-skin contact) as soon as possible (see below).

If distance or the needs of other children make it difficult to be with your baby, get help. Friends and relatives can assist you with older children, household chores, and meals and can even drive you back and forth to the hospital and keep you company while you're there. Accept all offers of help and provide specific instructions about what you need. Focus your energies on the things only you can do, and let others take care of the rest.

RESOURCES FOR THE CARE AND BREASTFEEDING OF PREEMIES

The Premature Baby Book: Everything You Need to Know About Your Premature Baby from Birth to Age One by William Sears, M.D., Robert Sears, M.D., James Sears, M.D., and Martha Sears, R.N. (Little, Brown, 2004)
Breastfeeding Your Premature Baby by Gwen Gotsch (La Leche League International, 1999)
Kangaroo Care: The Best You Can Do to Help Your Preterm Infant by Susan Ludington-Hoe, Ph.D. (Bantam, 1993)
Online resources: GrahamsFoundation.org; MilkyWayFoundation.org; Prematurity.org

---

READING A PREEMIE'S SIGNALS

A premature infant is easy to overstimulate because she needs to conserve nearly all her energy for growth. First feedings at the breast will be short so that your baby doesn't get overtired. Go easy, and be gentle and encouraging but not aggressive. Don't jostle the baby to keep her sucking. If she becomes frustrated, stop the feeding. Calm her, let her sleep if she wants to, and try again later. (The same goes for you: if you're getting frustrated with a feeding, take a break. Relax with baby held upright, or have your helper comfort baby while you grab a few moments for yourself.)

Kangaroo Care, or Skin-to-Skin Contact

This parent-friendly innovation in the care of premature babies is more than just a feel-good gimmick. Babies and mothers benefit physically as well as psychologically.

In kangaroo care, mother holds her tiny baby skin-to-skin, upright on her chest between her breasts. A lightweight blanket or the mother's shirt or nightgown covers them both. Mother's body keeps baby warm, and the touch of her skin and her gentle breathing motions often soothe baby to sleep. Babies' heart rates and breathing become more regular during kangaroo care, and they achieve a level of peace that they don't often exhibit in incubators or cribs. Some even smile.

Babies in kangaroo care often seek the nipple. They may lick it or make a tentative effort to suck. Their efforts may even be rewarded with a few drops of milk that leak from the nipple as mother's body responds to the stimulation with the milk-ejection reflex. Mothers often pump more milk than usual following a kangaroo session with their babies.

Kangaroo care has been used more widely as the body of research behind it has grown and more nurses and doctors have become aware of the benefits. Kangaroo care can be used with infants in incubators as well as those ready for open-air cribs. Babies born at thirty-four to thirty-seven weeks' gestation can be placed skin-to-skin with mother right from birth. Studies have shown that babies who receive kangaroo care gain weight faster, have fewer episodes of apnea (times when they stop breathing for a moment or two), and have shorter hospital stays. They cry less in the hospital and at six months of age.

Kangaroo care is not just for mothers. Fathers, too, can enjoy the closeness with their babies. It's a wonderful way to help both parents get attached, despite the stressful circumstances of a preemie's birth. When these babies leave the hospital, their parents feel more confident about caring for them, and they know that they have the tools for soothing their little ones. Skin-to-skin kangaroo care should continue at home, with the added stimulation of gentle walking or rocking and the convenience of a baby sling.

TEACHING YOUR PREEMIE TO FEED AT THE BREAST

First Feedings: When?

Conventional wisdom in the neonatal unit used to be that babies had to demonstrate that they could bottle-feed well before they were allowed to breastfeed. So babies would have their first feeding experiences with an artificial nipple, and when it was time to try breastfeeding, mothers would have great difficulty getting them to latch on and suck efficiently. Often these babies ended up being formula fed despite their mothers' best efforts at pumping and breastfeeding. We know that nipple preference is a potential problem for full-term infants, so we certainly shouldn't expect a preterm baby to handle this challenge easily. It's better if a preemie's first nipple feedings are at the breast. Avoiding bottles entirely is best of all.

Published research shows that it's easier for a baby to coordinate sucking, swallowing, and breathing during breastfeeding than during bottle feeding. Studies show that preemies maintain higher and more stable breathing patterns and higher levels of blood oxygen during breastfeeding than when they are bottle feeding, and the more stable their oxygen and breathing are, the better they grow. Babies have more control over the milk flow and can establish a more regular suck-swallow rhythm at the breast. It takes less energy to breastfeed, and babies' heart rates are more regular than they are during feedings from artificial nipples. Experts on breastfeeding preemies have found that these babies can go to the breast at a younger age than they would if they were given bottles. Preemies should be allowed to learn to breastfeed before they are offered regular bottles.

AVOIDING BOTTLES IN THE PREEMIE NURSERY

You won't always be available to breastfeed your baby while she's in the neonatal nursery, and at first she may be able to nurse only once or twice each day. Meanwhile, she has to be fed. How do you avoid or minimize bottles?

• Talk to the staff and tell them that you want to do everything possible to avoid nipple confusion so that you will succeed at breastfeeding your baby. Let them know when you will be there to feed the baby and work out a feeding and visiting schedule that maximizes opportunities for breastfeeding.

• Ask if your baby can continue to receive tube feedings as an alternative to bottles while she is learning to nurse at the breast.

• Preemies can also be fed by medicine dropper, syringe, finger, nursing supplementer, or even with a cup. In fact, studies show that premature infants who are cup fed maintain higher blood-oxygen levels during feedings than bottle-fed preemies do. Researchers are currently studying these alternatives to artificial nipples in breastfed babies. A feeding technique we have used successfully with mothers of preemies is the

AVOIDING BOTTLES IN THE PREEMIE NURSERY(continued)

syringe-and-finger-feeding method. Breast milk is put in a sterile syringe or special container that is then connected to a feeding tube taped to the mother's or the nurse's clean finger. The finger is inserted into baby's mouth. Depending on baby's ability to suck, you can either squirt a few drops of milk to coordinate with baby's sucking or remove the plunger from the syringe and let baby's sucking action draw milk from the tubing. With this method, baby learns efficient sucking, since with each suck she is rewarded with milk.

- As your baby nears the day when she will go home, plan on staying at the hospital all day or even around the clock. Some neonatal units have

special rooms for parents where they can practice caring for their preemies for a day or two before they are released from the hospital. You can breastfeed your baby on cue during this time and figure out how you will give any necessary supplemental feedings. Neonatal intensive care unit schedules of three hourly feedings do not have to be followed once you are home. Baby is likely to want more frequent feedings, at least during the day.

If your baby gets some bottles, or even a lot of bottles, all is not lost. It may take more time and patience, but your baby can learn to nurse well at the breast.

MEASURING WHAT GOES IN

If you feed a baby a bottle you can measure how many milliliters or ounces end up in his tummy. Breasts, however, don't come with markings that show how much milk they contain before and after feedings.

There are times when caregivers need to know how much breast milk a premature baby or a baby with a health problem is taking from the breast. This information can be used to calculate how much supplementary milk the baby needs or to determine other things about the baby's medical care.

You can find out how much a baby has taken at the breast with a process called test weighing. You weigh the baby before the feeding and

weigh him again afterward, in exactly the same clothing and the same dry diaper. The difference in weight tells you how much milk he has taken.

Only a sensitive electronic scale for test weighing gives accurate results. The hospital nursery should have one of these. You can also rent one to use at home; to rent one, check with your lactation consultant, your local hospital, or a local breastfeeding boutique.

Don't think of the information obtained from test weighing as a "grade" or a measure of breastfeeding success. It's just another piece of data that tells you how your baby is progressing and helps you and others make decisions about his care.

First Feedings: How?

Nursing a very tiny baby in the hospital requires some special techniques. Most babies do better in the football hold (see chapter 2) or reversed cradle hold because of the extra support and control of baby's head. Since a soft areola is easier to latch on to, start with an "empty" breast for practice so baby isn't overwhelmed by having to deal with a full breast. You can simply have a pumping session beforehand, leaving enough milk in your breast both for baby to drink and for your MER to be triggered so baby gets milk without having to work at it the first few times. If baby seems hungry enough, the feeding can be supplemented at the breast with a syringe or feeding tube using the milk you pumped. With this practice, you'll know when baby is ready to manage all his feeding directly from the breast.

The R-A-M technique described in chapter 2 will probably not work well with a tiny preemie, especially one who has to be cajoled into taking the breast. Instead, use your hand to make a nipple sandwich, flattening the breast tissue between your thumb on top and fingers underneath (see page 34). Pull back slightly to make the nipple and areola stand out, or push forward with the fingers well off the areola, to the compress the areola into a smaller oval. Both methods make a more manageable mouthful.

Encourage your baby to open her mouth by brushing downward on her bottom lip with your nipple. Then ease the breast into baby's mouth. It may take several sessions to teach your baby to latch on consistently. Keep trying, and you'll develop your own technique for getting as much of your breast as possible into baby's mouth.

An extra pair of hands is very helpful at these first breastfeedings. An experienced lactation consultant or neonatal nurse can help you teach your baby to latch on and suck. She can help support the baby at the breast, or use a finger on baby's chin to keep his mouth open wide. She can also help you interpret your baby's signals during these early feedings.

When first learning to breastfeed, a premature baby may latch on and suck briefly and then fall asleep. This is a good time just to hold your baby skin-to-skin and be at peace. When he wakes, you can try getting him to nurse again. Here is where the nipple sandwich can help—the breast compression can help push milk down to baby and trigger swallowing, which in turn will trigger sucking.

TAKING CARE OF YOURSELF IN THE HOSPITAL

When your baby is hospitalized, all your worry, all your concern, is for her. You stay with her, you hold her, you nurse her, you comfort her, you worry. You forget to eat, you forget to drink, you don't sleep well, maybe you don't pump your breasts when you should—not a good situation. Your baby needs a healthy mother now more than ever. Here are some suggestions:

- Carry a water bottle and healthful snacks with you at all times.
- Wear comfortable, lightweight clothes that make it easy to nurse or pump.
- Sleep when your baby sleeps. To minimize unnecessary interruptions, hang a PLEASE DO NOT DISTURB BABY OR MOTHER sign on baby's crib when you are napping.
- Arrange to have an electric breast pump at your baby's bedside.
- Talk to the nurses about getting food trays for yourself at mealtimes. Since you are baby's food source, the hospital should feed your baby by feeding you. Hospital staff can also tell you where to get juice and snacks between meals.

The time when a baby is learning to latch on and suck efficiently is probably the hardest part of nursing a preemie. It takes patience and time and confidence, but you can do it! Seek the support of people who believe in what you're doing: a lactation consultant, a supportive hospital staff member, or an experienced breastfeeding mother.

Continue to pump during the time that your baby is learning to nurse so that your breasts receive plenty of stimulation. If your milk supply has dwindled during long weeks of expressing milk, now is the time to pump more frequently, so that you will have more milk for your baby. His sucking alone may not be enough to build up your milk supply. Having a bit of an oversupply is a good thing at this point. You'll experience a stronger letdown that actually pumps milk into your baby's mouth.

Nursing tip: *Relax your milk in.* In one study, mothers whose premature infants were in the intensive care unit increased their milk delivery by more than 60 percent after listening to a twenty-minute tape on relaxation and visual imagery.

Homecoming

When it's finally time to take your little one home, you're likely to feel both relief and apprehension. You're glad to be through with the hospital routine but worried about being your baby's only caretaker. Plan on spending the first weeks at home just nesting and nursing. Your baby will tire easily and take frequent naps. Encourage him to nurse often but respect his cues about when it is time to rest. Carry him in a baby sling to keep him close to you, even when he is napping. Skin-to-skin contact and the gentle stimulation of your movement will help him sleep peacefully. Once home, nurse baby at least every two hours. Baby will gain weight faster.

Until your baby masters efficient breastfeeding, you may still need to offer supplements of expressed milk or formula. You'll also need to continue to pump to ensure a good milk supply. Offer the breast first, then the supplement. If your doctor or lactation consultant advises you to, consider using a nursing supplementer or a feeding tube; both can deliver supplemental milk to the baby who is nursing at the breast. See "If You Must Supplement: Alternatives to Bottles" in chapter 7. And ask for help with feeding chores such as cleaning the pump parts and cup feeding or finger feeding baby. This is a good way for dad to become involved in the care of his baby. For a while you may feel like all you do is feed your baby and pump your breasts. But you will see your baby thriving on your milk, and usually within a week or two of your due date, your amazing baby will have mastered the art of nursing.

Babies who are born a few weeks early but are otherwise healthy will often go home with their mothers when they are only a few days old. These infants may not need high-tech care, but they may be more of a challenge to breastfeed than full-term infants. With time and patience, they will nurse just as well as other babies, but you may have to pay special attention to how they are latching on and sucking. Lots of skin-to-skin contact, as well as rocking, walking, and carrying in a baby sling, will help these babies in their early transition to the outside world.

TWINS, TRIPLETS, AND . . .

No doubt you've heard it said that twins are a double blessing—and a double challenge. Your body will make enough milk for two babies, even for three. You can breastfeed multiples, and it's well worth the effort. Breastfeeding ensures that you spend time with each of your babies rather than with the laundry, the cleaning, and the preparation of bottles of formula. In the first months, you will spend almost all your time, day and night, feeding and caring for your babies.

Everything that this book has to say about resting and setting priorities, getting help with household tasks, and putting aside nonessentials goes double or triple for the mother of multiples. Household help that's considered a luxury with one baby is an absolute necessity for multiples. Use the latter weeks of pregnancy to line up the help that you are going to need, remembering that twins tend to come early.

NIGHT NURSING TWINS

Mothers of twins need the extra rest they can get if they sleep and nurse at the same time. This means bringing the babies into your bed (invest in a king-size bed) and working out a sleeping arrangement in which mom, dad, and babies all sleep well (see chapter 9).

One experienced mother who nursed and slept with *two* sets of twins found that nursing at night was much less complicated if she just slept topless. She could roll to one side or the other to nurse her babies without getting tangled or fumbling to find the openings in her nightgown.

A Double-Good Beginning

At first, nurse your babies one at a time, so that you can give close attention to latch-on. Since multiples are often born a bit early, one or both babies may be sleepy or may not suck well at first. Get skilled help from a lactation consultant while you are still in the hospital, especially if you are experiencing any latch-on difficulties. Room-in with your babies in the hospital, so that you can feed them on cue and get to know their different personalities. If you are tired from the birth or had a cesarean and can't move around easily, have your husband, the babies' grandma, or a friend stay with you much of the day to lend a hand. With twins, there's always an extra baby to hold!

RESOURCES FOR BREASTFEEDING TWINS

Mothering Multiples: Breastfeeding and Caring for Twins or More by Karen Kerkhoff Gromada (La Leche League International, 3rd ed., 2007)
The Womanly Art of Breastfeeding by Diane Wiessinger, Diana West, and Teresa Pitman (La Leche League International, 8th ed., 2010)
Multiples of America: MultiplesOf America.org

Your babies will have distinct feeding personalities. One is probably bigger than the other, and one may want to nurse more often than the other. As the babies become more adept at latching on, it will be easier to nurse them at the same time, at least for some feedings. (Feeding on both breasts at the same time will really boost your prolactin levels.) At times, you may want to encourage the less demanding baby, or the one who is not very hungry yet, to nurse at the same time as his sibling, especially at night so that you can get some rest. There will be other times when you want to give each baby individual attention at the breast. You may want to develop a system for switching babies from one breast to the other. If one baby is a more efficient breastfeeder than the other, this will ensure that both of your breasts receive plenty of stimulation.

Breastfeeding Two at Once

Mothers of twins need lots of pillows for everyone to be comfortable. A special nursing pillow that fits around your lap is a big help when there are two babies and you have only two hands (see chapter 7). If you don't have nursing pillow you can try rolling up and taping a large towel and tucking it in around you. A nursing footstool, or something else under your feet, will help raise your lap to better contain the babies. Another tool is a baby sling; latch the first baby on and secure him with the sling so that he is more likely to stay in place when you latch the second. Try these positions:

Double football hold. Position the babies on pillows along each side or on a nursing cushion on your lap. Their heads go at the breast, and their bodies extend along your sides, under your arms. Hold each baby in close to you with pressure against the nape of the neck from your hands. This helps them stay latched on. Use pillows behind your back and be sure to bring the babies up to the breast rather than hunching your shoulders forward.

Double cradle hold. Each baby lies in the crook of an elbow on their sides so they are facing toward the breast. Their bodies crisscross in your lap. Use pillows under your elbows for support.

Cradle-and-football hold. Nurse one baby in cradle hold and the other in football hold. The head of the baby in football hold lines up with the bottom or legs of the baby in cradle hold.

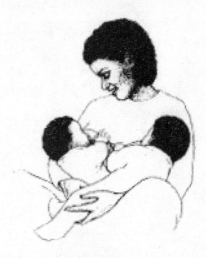

Double cradle hold

Lying down. Lie on your back with two pillows under your head and shoulders. Cradle a baby in each arm, with their bodies on top of yours, their knees meeting in the center. You will need pillows at your sides to support your arms.

Mothers of twins soon figure out a favorite position and a favorite place for simultaneous

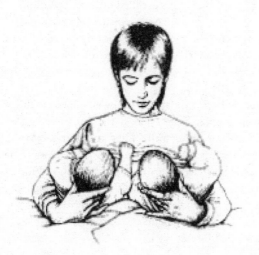

Double football hold

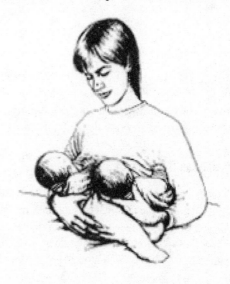

Cradle-and-football hold

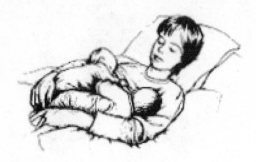

Lying down

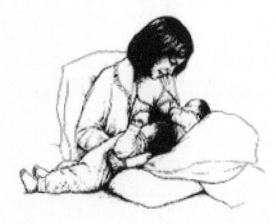

Nursing twins who are older

feedings. This might be a big easy chair or a big recliner with wide armrests, or it might be a corner of the couch where an older sibling can sit by mom and read a story while the babies nurse.

Surviving and Thriving with Twins

Dad really has to pitch in and help when there are multiple babies in the family. He can't breastfeed, but he can do everything else, including diapering one baby or walking one to sleep while mom feeds the other(s) in a kind of baby-care assembly line. If there are other children in the family, dad can really shine. What they may be losing in attention from mom they can gain in increased time with dad.

While the typical cue-feeding (or demand-feeding) approach could be too tiring for mothers of twins, the babies may not thrive on a rigid schedule. Somewhere in between is a feeding routine that will work for your family, one that meets the needs of the babies and lets the parents get enough rest.

When there's more than one baby in the house, expect that little else will get done. Say no to all outside commitments, at least for now. Get help with housework, with meals, with errands. When friends offer assistance, be ready with specific suggestions. Accept that you won't get through this challenging time all by yourself.

THE ADOPTED BABY

Where there's a will, there's a way. Yes, you can breastfeed a baby who is not biologically yours. Nipple stimulation will bring in a milk supply, even in women who have never been pregnant, and mother and baby can enjoy the closeness of breastfeeding. This is called induced lactation.

Martha breastfed our adopted daughter, Lauren, for ten months. Here's what we learned about adoptive nursing from our own experience and that of other mothers.

Set realistic goals. Mothers who choose to nurse their adopted babies believe that breastfeeding is more than giving milk. They put their babies to the breast because they want the unique bond that comes with breastfeeding. The benefits of human milk are an added bonus. While some women do manage to produce enough milk for their babies, most must continue to offer supplements along with their breast milk.

MEDICATIONS TO HELP MAKE MILK

Medications that boost levels of milk-making hormones such as prolactin can boost a mother's milk supply in situations such as relactation, adoptive nursing, or when a mother has been trying to maintain a milk supply by pumping for a baby who can't feed at the breast.

The medication with the best record for being safe and effective is metoclopramide (Reglan). This medication is generally used to treat reflux in adults and even premature infants, so it is safe for baby. It works to increase milk supply because it also happens to increase prolactin levels. However, it has not been approved for milk production, so this is an "off-label" use. Despite being off-label, it is quite effective and works about 75 percent of the time. Like every medication, it can have side effects and risks, but most mothers who take it experience no side effects aside from tiredness. Mothers who have a history of seizures or are depressed, however, should not take it. Mothers should stop the medicine if they experience mood changes or uncontrolled muscle movements of the head or neck (note that these side effects are extremely rare). Other occasional side effects are diarrhea, headache, and restlessness. Side effects can be minimized by lowering the dosage. Various lengths of treatment are needed to help mothers attain a full milk supply. Some mothers will need to take the medicine for only ten to fourteen days, and others may need to continue for the duration of nursing. The starting dose is ten milligrams three times a day. Mothers who wish to halt medication should always taper off so that if the supply starts to drop they can immediately taper back up.

A similar medication called domperidone is available by prescription at compounding pharmacies in the United States and over the counter in many other countries. This medication is also very effective and does not pose fatigue, depression, or seizure concerns. It can, however, have a very rare side effect on the heart, which prompted the FDA to issue a warning. As a precaution, mothers who use this medication should have their hearts checked with an electrocardiogram prior to starting it and again after they have been on it for a week or so. The starting dose is twenty milligrams four times a day. Again, some mothers will need to take it for only ten to fourteen days, and others will need it for the duration of nursing.

Oxytocin nasal spray, which stimulates the milk-ejection reflex, is no longer widely used, but it is available by prescription at a compounding pharmacy. If you have a special situation that seems to warrant the use of medication to increase your milk supply, consult your doctor.

These medications should be used in combination with other techniques for building up your milk supply, especially increasing the frequency of nursing or pumping. They can also be used with most herbal treatments. (See "Herbs to Increase Breast Milk," pages 111–113.)

Get some support. Breastfeeding an adopted baby makes a lot of sense to some people but seems totally crazy to others. A breastfeeding support group leader is a good source of encouragement, and she may be able to put you in contact with another mother who has breastfed an adopted baby.

Seek professional help. Find a lactation consultant in your community who has experience with adoptive mothers. Choose a pediatrician who is knowledgeable about lactation and willing to support your efforts.

Preparing for Baby's Arrival

If you know when your baby will be born or when the baby will join your family, you can begin to stimulate your milk supply ahead of time. Breastfeeding is an exercise not only of the body but also of the mind. In addition to professional help, pumps, and supplementers, you mainly need high doses of *commitment*. Here's what to do:

• Start pumping as early as six weeks before baby is due. If baby is arriving sooner, then just start pumping as soon as you know. Rent a hospital-grade electric breast pump, which mimics the action of the baby at the breast and will eventually stimulate your body to produce milk. Start by pumping each breast for five to seven minutes. Then spend a few minutes massaging your breasts. Next, move the milk toward the nipple by lightly stroking from the base to the nipple, then lean over and jiggle your breasts, using gravity to move the milk forward. Finally, pump another five to seven minutes. Pump both breasts at the same time, and pump as often as a newborn would nurse—every three hours and at least once during the night. You may see "milk" within a few days, but typically it takes at least a few weeks. The first milk to appear will be drops of colostrum, a thick yellow liquid. Mature milk will follow.

• Talk to your doctor about using medication to prepare and stimulate your body to produce milk. Not much research has been done on the best ways to help moms start lactation. However, in one study, the majority of adoptive mothers who had never breastfed were able to adequately lactate with the following medical regimen: one injection of 100 milligrams of Depo-Provera (synthetic progesterone) one week before beginning to induce lactation, followed one week later by ten milligrams of metoclopramide four times a day, taken orally until the breasts make enough milk. But there other methods frequently used as well. The most well known are the Lenore Goldfarb protocols, which can be accessed at AskLenore. info. Medications used for stimulating milk supply include birth control pills in combination with metoclopramide or domperidone prior to pumping, then either metoclopramide or domperidone alone for as long as needed. Many lactation consultants also recommend herbal supplements or foods that increase supply, such as fenugreek, oatmeal, and brewer's yeast (see pages 111–113).

• Purchase a nursing supplementer, a container-and-tubing device that delivers the supplemental formula to a baby who is sucking on the breast. Mothers breastfeeding adopted babies can use the supplementer for many months, so that baby can do all his sucking at the breast while getting the extra milk he needs.

• If possible, arrange to be at the hospital for the birth. Offer the breast as soon as you can. If you are present at the birth, there is no need to have the supplementer in place for that initial bonding time. Ask the hospital nurses to avoid giving your baby artificial nipples. Babies can be fed with a cup, a syringe, or with a nursing supplementer hooked up for finger feeding. Be there yourself for as many feedings as possible.

- Depending on your relationship with the birth mother, consider asking her if she would be willing to express colostrum, which can be given to your baby by cup, spoon, or syringe. (She may even be willing to supply mature milk for a while to augment your milk supply.) This amount of pumping should not make much difference in the way her milk comes in because even a mother who does not breastfeed has to cope with her breasts filling up with colostrum and then milk.

When Baby Arrives

Some adopted babies take to the breast immediately. Others must be coaxed. It depends on how old the baby is, whether he was ever breastfed by his biological mother, his sucking needs, and his personality. In general, babies who come to live with their adoptive mothers when they're only a few days old will take to the breast much more readily than babies who have been bottle fed for several weeks or months. Once your baby is finally in your arms, plan on doing little else besides getting to know him and working on breastfeeding. Here are some ways to teach him to seek comfort and nourishment from the breast:

- Offer your breast frequently throughout the day and night. Encourage the baby to suck for comfort as well as nourishment.

- Baby may be more willing to take the breast when he is not desperately hungry or sleepy. Try offering the breast in a darkened room, while walking, while rocking, when baby is awake, or when he is asleep. You'll soon figure out what works best for you and your little one.

- Give baby lots of skin-to-skin contact. Sleep with your baby and carry him in a sling

during the day. Take baths with your baby and offer the breast as baby is surrounded by warm water, totally relaxed and secure in your arms.

- Use the nursing supplementer to give baby formula, expressed milk, or banked milk (banked milk is expensive and is available only by doctor's order) while he sucks at your breast. Ask your lactation consultant to show you how to use the supplementer and help you develop a plan for feeding baby supplements at the breast.

- Don't give your baby bottles or pacifiers while he is learning to nurse at the breast. You can give supplements using a cup, medicine dropper, or feeding syringe or at the breast with a nursing supplementer. Encourage baby to do all his comfort sucking at the breast.

- If you are giving bottles while your baby makes the transition to breastfeeding, give them while baby is cuddled against your bare breast. Switch him to the breast for comfort sucking after his tummy is full.

- If your baby is nursing well at the breast, there is no need to continue to pump your breasts. A baby who latches on and sucks frequently and efficiently can build up a milk supply more effectively than a breast pump can.

- Keep a close watch on your baby's urine and stool output to be sure he is getting enough to eat. As your milk increases, his stools will become softer and yellower.

- As your body begins to make milk, you may notice other changes related to the presence of lactation hormones. Your menstrual periods may be lighter or irregular. Your milk supply may be less during your period and increase again once the flow is over. Some adoptive mothers experience mood swings as their bodies begin to produce milk.

- Be patient. Don't get into a struggle with your baby over feeding. If a feeding session is not going well, stop and try again later.

- Remember that your main goal is to enjoy this special time with your new baby. Focus on breastfeeding as a mothering tool rather than on how much milk you are making. In reality, a few mothers produce very little milk, a few others produce a full supply, and the rest produce varying amounts in between.

Like biological mothers, adoptive mothers get something back as a result of giving their babies the breast. The hormones of lactation will enable you to relax and enjoy your baby more, and the whole process of getting started with breastfeeding will help you know your baby and grow in confidence as a mother.

BABIES WITH DOWN SYNDROME

We have a special place in our hearts for babies with Down syndrome and the parents who care for them. Our seventh child, Stephen, has Down syndrome, and while we knew when he was born that breastfeeding would benefit him greatly, we also discovered that getting him started at the breast was an uphill struggle. We have since talked to many other mothers who have nursed babies with Down syndrome, and they have had similar experiences. But these mothers persisted, and those lucky babies have been fully breastfed—as was Stephen.

The Benefits of Breastfeeding

The benefits of breastfeeding are magnified in babies with Down syndrome. Here are some examples:

- These infants often have trouble with respiratory infections and the ear infections that

follow, but studies show that breastfed babies have fewer and less severe colds.
- Breastfeeding provides oral stimulation and helps with the development of muscles in the mouth and jaw. This will be important for speech later on.
- Breast milk contains nutrients needed for optimal development of the brain and nervous system.
- Constipation is often a problem in babies with Down syndrome, but breastfed babies are rarely constipated.
- Infants with Down syndrome may grow slowly, especially if they also have a heart defect (a problem in 40 percent of infants with Down syndrome). Nursing at the breast requires less energy than bottle feeding.
- Children with Down syndrome often have vision problems. Breastfeeding improves visual development.

Problems You May Encounter

Some of the problems common in babies with Down syndrome can make breastfeeding challenging in the early weeks. Here's what mothers may encounter, along with some suggestions:

- Babies with Down syndrome have low muscle tone. They need extra support to stay at the breast. Try nursing in the football or reversed cradle hold (see chapter 2). Use gentle pressure behind baby's neck and continue to hold your breast throughout the feeding to help him stay on the breast.

- Newborns with Down syndrome are often very sleepy in their first weeks of life. (Stephen rarely opened his eyes until he was two weeks old.) Try to wake your baby to nurse every two hours throughout the day and at least twice at night. Undress him, hold him skin-to-skin, talk to him until he becomes more alert and is ready to feed.

- If he tends to fall asleep or lapse into flutter sucking or comfort sucking after only a few minutes at the breast, take him off, wake him up again, and nurse on the other side. Repeat this switching back and forth until you have observed at least ten to fifteen minutes of sucking *and* swallowing. Then you can let him nurse off to sleep.

- Low muscle tone in the mouth and tongue means that babies with Down syndrome often have a weak suck and latch-on difficulties. They may have trouble cupping their tongues and using them to milk the breast. Try some suck training with your finger to teach the baby to keep his tongue down while latching on. Insert a clean finger into the baby's mouth, pad side up against the palate. As the baby sucks, slowly turn your finger over and press down gently on the tongue, working your way to the tip and out of the baby's mouth. Repeat this exercise several times before putting baby to the breast. Gentle massage around the baby's lips will help improve muscle tone. Make little circles along the upper and lower lip, or stroke the lips from the center outward. Stroke the baby's cheeks down toward the mouth as well.

- During the time that a baby with Down syndrome is learning to breastfeed, he may need supplements. Your own pumped milk is the best, and pumping your milk will also help bring in a better milk supply. Rent a hospital-grade electric pump and pump after every feeding. You can give your baby the extra milk using a syringe, cup, nursing supplementer, or medicine dropper (see chapter 7).

- To stimulate your milk-ejection reflex, pump briefly before offering the breast to your baby. Or tuck the breast-pump collection bottle between your arm and your breast and pump one side while the baby nurses the other. This will bring down more milk for him with less effort on his part.

- A lactation consultant can help you make a feeding plan for your baby, set you up with a pump, and show you how to teach him to breastfeed better.

- Stay positive: every week, these infants get more proficient, feedings get easier, and most of these special babies become efficient breastfeeders around three or four months of age.

The birth of a baby with Down syndrome is a scary and emotional time for parents. There is much to learn. You need to tell family and friends about your baby and talk to experts about her care. You need to grieve, but at the same time, you need to get attached to this baby. Working on breastfeeding problems is one way to get to know your baby and love her. Be sure that you are also spending time holding your baby (even while she's sleeping), talking to her, and enjoying her. Babies with Down syndrome are wonderfully cuddly, and you'll find that as she grows, there are many things you will enjoy about your child and many things to take pride in.

Martha breastfed Stephen for three and a half years. In light of new research correlating the length of breastfeeding with improved visual and intellectual development, it's comforting to know we gave our child a good head start.

BABIES WITH CLEFT LIP OR CLEFT PALATE

Cleft lip and cleft palate are common birth defects, and they can be corrected with surgery early in life. The opening (cleft) in the upper lip or the palate appears when the two sides of the lip or the roof of the mouth fail to fuse together while the baby is developing in the womb. Babies with cleft lip or palate are prone to speech problems and ear infections. Breastfeeding helps lessen both these potential problems.

Cleft Lip

A cleft lip is usually repaired when the baby is quite young—only weeks old. The opening in the upper lip can make it harder for the baby to form a good seal on the breast and maintain suction during feedings. However, he can still milk the breast with his tongue and gums and with a little help will be able to nurse efficiently. The mother's soft breast tissue will fill in at least part of the cleft, and she can also use her thumb to close off the opening. Lots of practice in the first hours and days after birth will help this baby learn to nurse correctly before the mother's milk "comes in" and her breasts become more firm.

RESOURCES FOR BABIES WITH CLEFT LIP OR CLEFT PALATE

"Breastfeeding with a Cleft Lip or Cleft Palate" by La Leche League International (available online at: https://www.lllc.ca/thursdays-tip-breastfeeding-baby-cleft-lip-or-palate)

Smiles craniofacial support group: Cleft.org

ACPA Family Services: Call 919-933-9044 or visit their website at CleftLine.org

---

Some surgeons prefer that babies not nurse while the repair of a cleft lip is healing. Others find that sucking at the breast does not present problems after cleft lip repair and that babies who breastfeed recover quickly. Work with your medical team to create a feeding plan for your baby. If breastfeeding will be restricted for a time after surgery, you will need to rent a pump to keep up your milk supply. Your milk can be given to your baby by another feeding method, and it will help speed healing and his return to the breast.

Cleft Palate

A cleft palate presents greater problems for breastfeeding, depending on the location and size of the opening in the palate. The opening in the palate makes it impossible for the baby to use suction to keep the breast in her mouth. It is also difficult for the baby to compress the areola against the palate to milk the breast. Milk may go up into the nose and also flow more easily into the eustachian tubes and the middle ear. However, breast milk will be less likely to cause ear infections and less irritating than formula to the tender mucous tissues inside the nose. Babies with cleft palates do benefit from receiving breast milk, even if they cannot obtain it directly from the breast.

A baby with a small cleft in the soft palate at the back of the mouth may be able to breastfeed with little difficulty. A baby with an extensive cleft will probably have to be fed breast milk with a special feeding device and may not be able to nurse at all until the cleft is repaired. Babies whose problems fall between these extremes may be able to obtain milk from the breast with some special individualized techniques. A mother learning to breastfeed a baby with a cleft palate needs to work with a lactation consultant who is experienced with cleft-palate babies.

Here are some techniques to experiment with:

- Feed baby in an upright version of the football hold, with his head a little higher than the nipple. This makes it easier for him to swallow and cope with the milk flow.
- Aim the nipple at the part of the palate that is intact. If you change the angle at which baby takes the breast, he may be able to compress the areola.
- Use the Dancer hand position (palm supporting the breast underneath, thumb and forefinger in a U shape supporting baby's cheeks and chin) to keep the breast in baby's mouth. During your

consultation with a lactation specialist, this will be demonstrated.

- Some cleft palate specialists suggest the use of a dental appliance to cover the opening in the palate. This can make feeding — including breastfeeding — easier.
- Encourage baby to comfort suck, even if he isn't getting much milk.
- If baby is unable to take milk from your breasts, pump your milk and give it to him via a special bottle called a SpecialNeeds Feeder (a.k.a. Haberman Feeder [see page 141]) or via a special soft cup. These feeders are available from Medela and from certain online retailers.

A cleft palate may not be repaired until a baby is nine months or older. This is a long time to persist with special feeding techniques or expressing milk for a baby who can't nurse at the breast. We suggest you look for a provider who will repair the cleft at three months. Feeding a baby with a cleft palate is time consuming, no matter how you are getting the milk into baby. Providing your milk adds another step, but the benefits derived from breast milk last a lifetime.

BABIES WITH HEART DEFECTS

Babies with congenital heart defects benefit from receiving mother's milk. Human milk's lower sodium level is easier on the heart, and its immune-building properties help protect babies from illness and keep them healthy before surgery.

Babies with heart defects tire easily, and their hearts use more energy, leaving fewer calories for growth. Though these babies may gain weight slowly, research has shown that breastfed babies with heart problems grow just as well as those who are formula fed. In fact, babies conserve more energy during breastfeeding than during bottle feeding. They need small, frequent feedings, a lot

of encouragement, and patience. If supplements are needed, the mother's own high-fat hindmilk can be given at the breast with a nursing supplementer or a cup or syringe.

WHEN MOTHER OR BABY IS ILL

Breastfeeding is the best medicine. You can go right on breastfeeding if you or your baby has a cold, the flu, diarrhea, and many other illnesses. Your milk will help your baby fight the germs. If you are sick, baby may get only a mild case of what you have or not get sick at all, thanks to the immune-building properties in your milk.

If you are feeling under the weather, just plan on taking your baby to bed with you. Or camp out on the couch with a water bottle, clean diapers, tissues, and a few snacks. Plan on doing the same thing if your baby is ill. She'll probably want to nurse very often, so get a good book, a stack of videos, and the remote control and take it easy for a day or two.

Vomiting and Diarrhea

It's okay to keep breastfeeding when baby has a tummy upset that is causing her to vomit or have frequent loose stools. When babies suffer an intestinal infection (gastroenteritis), the germs injure the intestinal lining and damage the glands that secrete the milk-digesting enzyme lactase. As a result, infants with gastroenteritis often can't absorb the fat and lactose in cow's milk or formula. The leftover lactose ferments and causes discomfort and diarrhea. Not so with mother's milk, which contains biological helpers to facilitate absorption of lactose and fat. Because breast milk is so intestines-friendly, infants with intestinal infections who are breastfed are less likely to need hospitalization for treatment of dehydration. Small, frequent meals will keep baby from getting dehydrated. Babies with diarrhea usually recover faster and lose less weight if they continue to breastfeed. They also recover faster because human milk contains antiviral and antibacterial factors that help combat the infection.

If your vomiting baby wants to suck for comfort, it might be wise to express much of your milk before nursing her. She'll get only a small amount of milk as she nurses, not enough to irritate her stomach into sending it all back up again. If she does spit the milk back up, remind yourself that at least some of what she got at the breast was absorbed and is fighting the infection.

BABIES IN THE HOSPITAL

When a baby must be hospitalized, we encourage parents to stay with their children as much as possible and to participate in their babies' care. Babies need the familiar presence of a parent when they are sick and in a strange place. Parents are valuable members of the medical team. They help babies feel better sooner and often provide valuable insight into their children's behavior that can help medical personnel treat the illness more effectively.

When babies are ill, they usually want to nurse more often. Even babies who are eating solid foods and drinking other liquids may, for a time, depend completely on mother's milk for their nutrition. This is no time to wean—even if your "baby" is two and a half years old and nurses are looking at you like you're a real weirdo. Just say, "Yeah, I know he's old to be nursing, but I certainly don't want to wean him *now,* when he's so sick and upset. And I know my milk is good for him."

Feeding Restrictions Before Surgery

Food and liquid intake are restricted before a person has general anesthesia because of the risk

of vomiting and the risk that the vomitus can get into the lungs. In adults, "nothing by mouth" orders often mean no food or drink after midnight on the night before surgery. However, an eight-hour (or longer) fast can be very stressful for infants and small children, and eight hours without nursing is unimaginable for most breastfeeding pairs.

Hospitals and anesthesiologists are beginning to recognize that children and babies require different fasting guidelines. A recent survey of pediatric anesthesiologists found that practices differed from one hospital to the next but that the majority of hospitals followed the 2-4-6-8 rule for intake of food and liquids before surgery:

- Up to two hours before surgery: clear fluids (for example, water, apple juice, clear Jell-O)
- Up to four hours before surgery: human milk*
- Up to six hours before surgery: infant formula
- Up to eight hours before surgery: solid foods

Keeping a breastfed baby happy and comfortable during the three or four hours before surgery when he is not allowed to nurse can be a challenge. This might be a time for dad to take over the baby comforting. Or use your baby sling and walk the halls with baby held in an upright position. Sitting down may frustrate both of you, since baby may interpret this as a sign that you're going to nurse him.

Once baby goes into surgery (and in some hospitals, you may be able to stay with him until he is asleep), you will need to pump your breasts. Continue to pump every two or three hours if baby is not nursing well in the hours and days after surgery. Ask the nurses if there is a hospital-grade pump and a special room for pumping somewhere in the hospital (probably near the

---

* Because it is so rapidly digested, some anesthesiologists classify human milk as a clear fluid and therefore allow babies to breastfeed two to three hours before surgery.

neonatal unit). Ideally you should have your own pump at baby's bedside, so that you don't have to choose between being there when your little one wakes up and being away from him so you can pump your breasts.

BABIES WITH OTHER MEDICAL PROBLEMS

Babies with cystic fibrosis and phenylketonuria (very rare) can continue to breastfeed. Breastfeeding makes management of these serious diseases easier for both mother and the medical team.

Cystic Fibrosis (CF)

This congenital disease can affect a baby's breathing and digestion. Sometimes babies with CF need additional enzymes to help them digest their food so that they can gain weight adequately and grow. Breastfeeding offers these babies protection against the respiratory infections that may plague them. Breast milk is also easier to digest, so that enzyme supplements may not be needed until baby is older or weaned.

BABIES WITH JAUNDICE

Jaundice (also known as hyperbilirubinemia) is the cause of the yellow tinge that colors the skin and eyeballs of newborn infants in the first week or two. Jaundice happens because babies are born with more red blood cells than they need. When the liver breaks down these excess cells, it produces a yellow pigment called bilirubin. Because the newborn's immature liver can't dispose of bilirubin quickly, the excess yellow pigment is deposited in the eyeballs and skin of the newborn. This kind of jaundice is called physiological jaundice because it is part of a normal body process. Once the newborn's bilirubin disposal system matures and the excess

red blood cells diminish, the jaundice subsides (usually within a week or two) and causes baby no harm. Jaundice is more common in premature infants, who are less able to cope with excess bilirubin.

In some situations, such as ABO incompatibility or Rh incompatibility, jaundice may be the result of problems that go beyond the normal breakdown of excess red blood cells. In rare instances, the bilirubin levels can rise high enough to damage baby's brain. For this reason, if the health-care provider suspects that something more than normal physiological jaundice is the cause of baby's yellow color, bilirubin levels will be monitored more closely using heel-stick blood samples. If the bilirubin level gets too high, your doctor may try to lower the bilirubin level using phototherapy, which dissolves the extra bilirubin in the skin, allowing it to be excreted in the urine.

Because of a biochemical quirk that is not yet completely understood, jaundice tends to be more common in breastfed babies, in whom bilirubin levels average two to three milligrams higher than they do in formula-fed infants. The difference is thought to be the result of an as yet unidentified factor in breast milk that promotes increased intestinal absorption of bilirubin into the bloodstream rather than movement of it into the liver. Higher rates of jaundice in breastfed infants may also be related to lower milk intake in the first days after birth because of infrequent or inefficient feeding. It is normal for jaundice to last a bit longer in breastfeeding infants, sometimes until the third week after birth. This small difference in bilirubin levels between breastfed and formula-fed infants is insignificant, but jaundice phobia on the part of parents and health-care providers can lead to unnecessary disruption in the beginning breastfeeding relationship. Watch out for what we call the yellow flags that signal an overreaction to jaundice in the breastfeeding baby. Shake off any suggestion that something about your milk is bad for your baby. Instead, try these suggestions for lowering the bilirubin level in your baby and your own worry level:

- Follow the suggestions for getting started in chapter 2 — namely, early, frequent, and unrestricted breastfeeding with efficient latch-on techniques. The more breast milk baby gets, the faster the bilirubin is eliminated from baby's intestines. Bilirubin exits the body in the infant's stools, and because breast milk has a laxative effect, frequent breastfeeders tend to have lots of soiled diapers and thus lower bilirubin levels.

- Don't worry; make milk. If your baby is jaundiced, be sure you understand what type of jaundice your baby has. If it's normal physiological jaundice, you have absolutely nothing to worry about. If it's jaundice caused by a medical condition such as a blood-group incompatibility, be sure you understand that this is easily treated and should not interfere with your breastfeeding. Worry may cause you to make less milk and doubt your ability to nourish your baby at the breast. This gets in the way of breastfeeding success.

- Bear in mind that jaundice sometimes makes babies sleepy, so they nurse less enthusiastically. The higher the levels of bilirubin, the sleepier the baby may be. Babies need to eat to get rid of the bilirubin, but they tend not to wake up often enough or to eat for a long enough period of time and may need help.

- If phototherapy treatment is necessary because of a high bilirubin level, be sure your health-care provider works with you so the treatment of the jaundice does not interfere with breastfeeding. Bringing the baby out from under the lights to breastfeed will not take long enough to interfere with the light treatment, so

you can keep breastfeeding unless baby is too sleepy or is unable to effectively breastfeed. In that case you will need to pump your milk and feed it to your baby.

- If you are advised to give your baby supplements in order to provide him with more calories and decrease his intestinal absorption of bilirubin, use your own pumped breast milk or banked human donor milk if you can't express enough. (New insights reveal that banked human milk is preferable to formula if you want to preserve your newborn's growing microbiome; see page 123.) Only on rare occasions, such as when your baby is very ill, will formula need to be used when breast milk is available. Also, it's best to work with a lactation consultant who can help you administer this supplement via a supplemental nursing system, a syringe, or the finger-feeding method (see chapter 7).

- Giving breastfed babies bottles of sugar water in hopes of reducing bilirubin levels has been shown to be ineffective. Studies show that it may even aggravate the jaundice, because babies whose tummies are full of glucose solution may nurse less often, reducing their milk intake and the opportunities for bilirubin to be excreted in stools. Water doesn't push stools through; food (milk) does.

In some breastfed babies, bilirubin levels may exceed twenty milligrams, and jaundice may last well into the third week of life or longer. It was once thought that this was caused by a distinct type of jaundice called breast milk jaundice, which was found in a small group of mothers whose milk contained a substance believed to interfere with bilirubin absorption. Treatment for this type of jaundice involved taking baby off the breast for twenty-four to forty-eight hours. Doing this brought bilirubin levels down but sabotaged the course of breastfeeding. More recent research suggests that high bilirubin levels and prolonged jaundice in otherwise healthy breastfed babies are just normal variants of ordinary physiological newborn jaundice. There may well be a substance in the milk of some mothers that inhibits the absorption of bilirubin by the intestines, but whether a baby has a little jaundice or a lot is largely attributable to individual differences between mothers and babies. Nevertheless, some health-care providers may suggest a period of temporary weaning (twenty-four to forty-eight hours) to bring down bilirubin levels. Work with your doctor to determine if there are other alternatives, such as phototherapy, that would allow breastfeeding to continue without restrictions.

Above all, it's important for parents and health-care providers not to develop a jaundice phobia. It's vital that both the bilirubin level of the baby and the worry level of the parents be appropriately managed, since the usual physiological jaundice of newborns is harmless. For more information on managing jaundice in a breastfeeding newborn, see the website of the Academy of Breastfeeding Medicine (BFMed.org/jaundice).

BABIES WITH HYPOGLYCEMIA

If the doctor or nurse says that your baby may have or is at risk of developing hypoglycemia, or low blood sugar, there are ways you can help the situation. Low blood sugar occurs when the body's demand for glucose is greater than its supply. While an occasional dip in blood sugar is harmless, prolonged periods of low blood sugar can damage the central nervous system. Because of this, health-care providers are especially careful to ensure that a newborn's blood sugar remains adequate. Babies at risk for developing hypoglycemia are preterm or postterm babies, infants of diabetic mothers, babies of mothers

who were given a large dose of glucose solution intravenously during labor, small- or large-for-gestational-age infants, infants who experience respiratory distress or breathing difficulties, and infants who are the product of a complicated delivery.

Here's how a breastfeeding mother can help keep her newborn's blood sugar stable:

- Take good medical and nutritional care of yourself during pregnancy.

- If you have diabetes, try to maintain stable control during pregnancy. Also, we suggest asking your health-care provider if you can do a little pumping before birth so you can supplement with your breast milk afterward.

- Unless medically necessary, avoid high doses of intravenous glucose solution during labor. High maternal blood sugar triggers insulin production in the baby, which can cause baby's blood sugar to plunge soon after birth.

- Newborn stress can also deplete baby's glucose stores. See page 30 for a list of good reasons to delay bathing baby, one of which is avoiding hypoglycemia.

- Begin frequent breastfeedings right after birth. Feed your baby as frequently and as long as baby is willing and mother is able. Basically, this frequent early nursing is the standard treatment for hypoglycemia: small, frequent, high-protein, high-calorie meals. Protein and calories are exactly what colostrum provides. It is two to three times higher in nutrients and calories than what's in the sugar-water bottles that may be offered to newborns.

- If medically indicated, use formula supplements or banked milk rather than glucose and water, which can cause baby's blood sugar to go up too fast and then suddenly drop. Recent studies indicate that if newborns do need supplements to treat hypoglycemia, as they do when they have jaundice, they should be given formula rather than glucose and water. Since this happens on the first day only, using your own milk is not an option unless you have some banked.

- A newborn of an insulin-dependent diabetic mother, especially a premature infant, will often need a day or so of intravenous glucose solution and/or bottles of formula until mother is able to produce sufficient milk. If possible, these supplements should be given in addition to, not instead of, frequent breastfeeding. If baby is not breastfeeding yet, mother can pump colostrum, dilute it as necessary with sterile water, and feed it to baby in a syringe. The nurse should help with this.

Remember, one of the ways of keeping a newborn's blood sugar stable is to keep baby from wasting energy. Breastfeeding has an energy-sparing effect. Babies use less energy breastfeeding than they do bottle feeding. So if your baby's health-care providers are concerned about hypoglycemia, realize that you have the cure. Again, the breastfeeding mother is an important member of the medical team.

MOTHERS WITH SPECIAL PROBLEMS

There are surprisingly few situations in which a mother's health problems or disabilities keep her from breastfeeding her baby. Mothers who are determined and who get the support and information they need not only breastfeed successfully but also have a keen appreciation of the ease and naturalness of breastfeeding.

WHEN MOTHER IS HOSPITALIZED

Most hospitals do pretty well when it comes to accommodating the needs of a sick baby who is nursing. But when it's the nursing mother who lands in the hospital, it becomes more difficult to keep mother and baby together. Of course, the most important thing is that your baby has a healthy mother for many years to come, but medical problems don't have to lead to weaning. Some of these suggestions may help minimize the separation time that your baby experiences and help maximize breastfeeding during your treatment.

- Find out if your baby can be brought to you in the hospital for breastfeedings or if she can stay in your room with you as long as you provide a helper to care for her.

- Investigate whether outpatient care is an option for you. Can you go home sooner if there is someone at home who will care for you and for your baby?

- If your baby cannot be brought to the hospital for breastfeeding, you will need to express your milk every two to three hours using a hospital-grade electric breast pump. This is important for keeping up your milk supply and avoiding a breast infection, which could complicate your illness. If you are too sick to express your milk yourself, hospital staff or another helper should assist you. Have your doctor write this into the order for your care.

- Your baby should be cared for at home by someone who is responsive to her needs and who can offer support and comfort during the time she is separated from her familiar source of security. See chapter 7 for suggestions on getting baby to accept nourishment from sources other than the breast.

Herpes

Herpes infections can be fatal to newborn infants. That is why mothers with active vaginal herpes infections must give birth by cesarean—so that their babies can avoid contact with the sores. A mother with an active herpes sore on her breast must cover the sore so that the baby does not come in contact with it. If the sore is on the nipple or the areola or anywhere near it, she must express her milk from that breast and discard it. She should nurse the baby only on the unaffected breast until the sore has healed. She should also consider taking medication to prevent future outbreaks for the duration of breastfeeding.

Diabetes

The key to successful lactation for diabetic mothers is good control. Breastfeeding can actually help a mother manage her diabetes following pregnancy. Lactation provides a more gradual return to the prepregnant state, making it easier to balance out diet and insulin needs. (Insulin taken by a breastfeeding mother will not affect her baby.) Every woman will react differently, but many diabetic mothers find they need less insulin during breastfeeding. Insulin and dietary requirements may fluctuate in the first week after birth, but once a woman's body settles into the process of lactation, she will learn to manage her condition better. Growth spurts, when the baby nurses more, may require some adjustments in diet or insulin, as will weaning. It's important for a diabetic mother to wean gradually, so that her body can make the adjustment.

The biggest problems faced by the diabetic mother may occur in the early days of her baby's life, while she is still in the hospital. Infants of diabetic mothers may be kept in a special-care nursery for observation following birth, and the separation between mother and baby makes frequent nursing difficult in the early days. Ask if you can keep your baby with you so that you can nurse frequently and avoid supplements. If your baby is given glucose water or other supplements, ask that she be fed with a syringe, medicine dropper, or cup rather than with an artificial nipple. Get prompt help from a lactation consultant if you are having difficulties with latch-on.

Diabetic breastfeeding mothers are more prone to mastitis and yeast infections. Frequent feedings and prompt attention to any plugged ducts will minimize problems with mastitis. If you have persistently sore nipples, especially after the early postpartum period, yeast or incorrect latch-on is probably to blame. (A yeast infection of the baby's mouth is called thrush.) Seek treatment promptly.

Remember, as we mentioned in chapter 1, breastfeeding can lower the chances of your infant getting diabetes.

Other Chronic Illnesses

Whether it's epilepsy, rheumatoid arthritis, lupus, multiple sclerosis, or something else, there's probably someone somewhere who has breastfed her children despite having the disease. Breastfeeding makes life easier for a mother who must keep her stress level down to stay healthy. The hormones of lactation may actually help alleviate symptoms of some chronic conditions. Breastfeeding will ease the transition from the pregnant to the nonpregnant state, and this can be important for mothers with autoimmune diseases.

If there are any concerns about a mother with a chronic disease breastfeeding, they usually center on medications. However, there are very few drugs that are not compatible with breastfeeding, and there may be alternatives to those few drugs that should not be taken while a mother is nursing a baby. Talk to your doctor about breastfeeding before your baby is born so that you have ample time to work out any medication problems. Specialists who do not often have nursing mothers as patients may need to do some checking around beyond the *Physicians' Desk Reference* to find out more about the effects of a drug on a breastfeeding baby. Two resources are readily available. The first is a government website called LactMed, at Toxnet.NLM.NIH.gov/NewToxnet/LactMed.htm, and the second is the Infant Risk Center, part of Texas Tech University's Health Sciences Center, at InfantRisk.com. You can check these sites, and you can ask your doctor to do this for you if he or she has concerns about the medication's effect on your baby. This may mean talking with the baby's doctor, with a pharmacologist who has some knowledge of lactation, or with an expert on drugs in human milk. (For more on medications while breastfeeding, see chapter 5.)

POSTPARTUM DEPRESSION

Most mothers go through the "baby blues" sometime in the first week or two after birth. They'll feel weepy, discouraged, and anxious about their ability to care for their new babies. Hormones may be partly to blame, along with lack of sleep. Your body is worn out from pregnancy and birth, and it may feel as though your life is in complete upheaval. The big birth event is over, and it may not have turned out as planned. Or you come face-to-face with the letdown that follows any event that you've looked forward to for a long time. At some point in these first postpartum days, many a mother has wanted to grab the next flight to the Bahamas—alone.

For most women, these feelings pass, and they soon feel like their usual selves, only changed by the wonders and demands of motherhood. For a smaller group of women, the baby blues come to stay. These women don't (and can't) snap out of it.

How do you know if what you're feeling is within the range of normal or is something that needs special attention? Here are some signs (in increasing order of severity) that normal baby blues are drifting into full-blown postpartum depression or even postpartum psychosis:

- Persistent feelings of sadness and helplessness
- Anxiety that makes it difficult to care for baby
- Sleep disturbances—either sleeping too much or not enough
- Crying jags
- Appetite changes
- Lack of interest in your surroundings, in how you look, in your partner
- Inertia—lack of energy to do simple chores or even have fun but also the inability to relax
- Mental confusion
- Thoughts or fears about hurting the baby
- Distorted perception of reality
- Suicidal thoughts

It's estimated that 10 to 20 percent of women develop some degree of postpartum depression. Recent studies show that the greatest risk factor is a history of depression rather than "demand" feeding or even breastfeeding in general. This isn't a sign of weakness of character or ambivalence about the mothering role. It's simply your body and mind telling you that the changes and demands of your life are, at the moment, exceeding your ability to cope.

Mild postpartum depression will often respond to various self-help measures. Try some of the following suggestions if you are struggling with symptoms of postpartum depression. Some of these are ways to cut back on the demands in your life. Others will help to fill your emotional tank so that you are better able to cope with stress.

Respect your need to nest and nurse. In many traditional societies women are waited on hand and foot for weeks after the birth of a baby. They are not asked to worry about meals or cleaning or entertaining visitors. They concentrate on their babies and themselves. Take your cue from these wise ways. Relax, nurse your baby, and make sure that anything else you try to do is something that nourishes your spirit. Ask for help from your family and friends.

Set priorities. You are doing the most important job in the world: mothering a new human being. Nothing matters more than this. Talk to your spouse, and use this time to establish priorities in the new alignment of your family. Newborns can't wait. Adults can. It will be easier to accept this situation if you remind yourself that this all-consuming baby-care stage doesn't last forever.

Get some exercise. "Yeah, right," you say. "All I can manage to do is sit on the couch and nurse the baby all day. And I'm so tired." Exercise doesn't use up energy, it creates it. It burns off anxiety and worry and releases endorphins—the body's own feel-good substances. Naps are good, but sometimes physical activity is even better. The best exercise for new mothers is brisk walking, which you can do with baby in the sling or stroller. (The more anxious you feel, the longer you walk—even as much as one or two hours in the morning and then again in the afternoon.) Getting outside every day, even if the weather isn't exactly beautiful, will do you good. You may have to make a daily appointment with yourself to get this accomplished. Be flexible and schedule your daily walks around your baby. As baby grows, your exercise plan can become more ambitious. Some mothers exercise at home with a treadmill or an exercise video while baby naps (plan on being interrupted when baby wakes up). Others head for a workout at the health club or pool when dad gets home from work.

Eat well. Good nutrition, like exercise, will help you cope with the stress of your new life. This doesn't mean complicated meals, just good, healthful food. (See chapter 4.)

Look nice. Mothers with new babies usually can't spend forty-five minutes every morning on hair, makeup, and getting dressed. You can, however, make an effort to comb your hair, to dress neatly, to grab a shower. Get an easy-care haircut (bring someone along to hold the baby). Buy some new clothes that fit your postpartum figure. You deserve it—and you'll feel better.

Talk to other new mothers. Hearing that other mothers have problems similar to yours can give you a whole new perspective. Find some outlet where you can share your mothering worries and joys with others. Try getting together with new mothers from your childbirth class, or look in your neighborhood or local church for friends with small children. Breastfeeding support group meetings provide the support that many women say keeps them breastfeeding, even when family and friends are less than supportive, and these meetings may be the one place you can complain about breastfeeding without having someone tell you that you should give your baby bottles of formula.

Treat yourself. Whether it's a massage, a stroll through the park or mall, a phone call to a good friend, a long soak in the tub, or an hour's escape with a good book, do something every day just for yourself. Choose something that does not require separation from your baby.

Consider counseling. Becoming a parent (even for the second or third time) is a major life transition, and many women find that professional counseling helps them understand and cope with the changes in their lives and in themselves. Look for a counselor who specializes in postpartum depression. Your doctor may be able to recommend someone. In many areas, you can also find support groups specifically for postpartum depression.

Breastfeeding and Postpartum Depression

Lactation hormones make it easier to cope with the demands of a new baby, but ongoing problems with breastfeeding can make it hard for you to feel good about yourself and your baby. Weaning to formula would end the breastfeeding problems, but it might not leave you feeling any better (and it may bring a whole new batch of problems). If sore nipples, engorgement, and frequent feedings are leaving you wondering if breastfeeding is right for you, *get some support.* See a lactation consultant for assistance. Attend a breastfeeding support group meeting.

Make a plan for solving your problem. Write it down and chart your progress daily. Talk to other breastfeeding mothers with babies a little older than yours so that you can adjust your expectations and learn how to get out of the house with your breastfeeding baby. Set a goal for yourself, such as to try breastfeeding for at least three weeks.

As we have said before, breastfeeding is not just a feeding method, it's a lifestyle, one that is sometimes at odds with our culture. We're not always comfortable with the utter dependence of a breastfed baby on mother. American culture thinks everyone should be independent. But this is not good for babies or mothers. It's not really good for anyone. As you build your relationship with your baby, think of the two of you as *interdependent.* Each needs the other, and each has something to give the other. This is a wonderful way of looking at family life and a way to raise children to be adults who can form intimate, interdependent relationships with others.

Medication for Postpartum Depression

Antidepressant medication is an increasingly popular way of treating depression and related mental-health problems. The safety of these drugs for breastfeeding mothers and babies, however, is not well established. Your provider can consult the LactMed database for the most up-to-date information on specific drugs for breastfeeding mothers. Previously, the American Academy of Pediatrics stated that the effect of psychoactive drugs on the breastfeeding infant was "unknown, but may be of concern." These drugs do appear in human milk in varying amounts, and there is concern about whether they may affect the developing nervous system of a nursing baby. However, pediatrician Jack Newman, director of the breastfeeding clinic at Toronto's Hospital for Sick Children, has pointed out that while we don't know the long-term effects of antidepressants on breastfeeding infants, "We also do not know all the long-term effects of not breastfeeding. We do know they include negative effects on the central nervous system, the very concern cited by physicians who are reluctant to counsel continued breastfeeding." Bottom line: the risks of weaning far outweigh the risks of taking most antidepressants.

If you are a breastfeeding mother caught in the middle of the antidepressant dilemma, consider these alternatives:

- Counseling is an effective alternative to medication in many situations.

- The self-help measures described above can help you overcome depression. They require self-discipline, but your desire to continue breastfeeding will be a powerful motivation.

- Healthful omega-3 fats, in both wild salmon and in supplement form, can help alleviate postpartum depression (see page 86). For more information, read *The Omega-3 Effect,* which Bill wrote with our son Jim.

- Abrupt weaning can make depression worse. Women who must wean quickly may feel devastated and may grieve for the end of the breastfeeding relationship with their babies. This feeling is more intense when weaning was not the mother's choice.

BREAST LUMPS

Lactating breasts are often lumpy (especially the breast tissue under the arm). Painful lumps are usually associated with plugged ducts or infection. A lump that doesn't go away after a week of being treated as a plugged duct should be evaluated by a physician.

Don't work yourself into a frenzy worrying about a breast lump. Most are benign—nothing to worry about—but it's important to have your doctor check it out. Even though mothers are often told they must wean, it is unnecessary to do so before having a mammogram, an ultrasound of the breast, or a biopsy. Be sure that doctors and technicians know that you are breastfeeding. Lactating breasts are more dense, and this can make it more difficult to read a mammogram. If there is any uncertainty about the results, consider having an ultrasound.

COSMETIC BREAST SURGERY

Breast Reduction

It's hard to predict exactly how breast-reduction surgery will affect breastfeeding years later. Much depends on how the surgery was done, how many milk ducts were severed, how many milk ducts remain intact, and whether nerves were cut. During some breast-reduction surgeries, the entire areola is cut from the breast and then replaced after the surgeon has removed the excess breast tissue. While there are reports of milk ducts regrowing or reconnecting themselves after surgery, a woman who has had breast-reduction surgery may not be able to nourish her baby

completely at the breast. The breast will make milk in the first days postpartum, but there may be no way for that milk to reach the nipple and the baby. If it has been at least five years since the surgery, many of the ducts will have regrown, the milk will flow, and these mothers will have the best chances of succeeding. That is not to say you won't succeed if it has been less than five years, however.

What to do? Give breastfeeding a try, but work with a lactation specialist and have your doctor monitor your baby's weight gain closely. You should pay special attention to the number of wet and soiled diapers your baby has in the first weeks postpartum. If your baby is not getting enough to eat at the breast, you can continue to breastfeed while giving supplements, either at the breast with a supplemental nursing device or other alternatives or with a bottle.

Breast Augmentation

Silicone breast implants have received lots of media attention, and many women who have implants have become concerned about long-term effects on their health. Studies have shown that no increased concentration of silicone was found in the milk of mothers who had implants compared with the milk of mothers who didn't. Media-generated worries have not been borne out by dispassionate scientific study, especially when it comes to the effects on breastfed children. Even if a mother's silicone implants were leaking, it is highly unlikely that the silicone could appear in her milk.

Whether a mother who has had breast-augmentation surgery can nourish her baby completely at the breast depends again on how the surgery was done. If incisions were made in the fold under the breasts or near the armpit, the milk ducts will not be affected and therefore the surgery should not affect your ability to breastfeed. So give it a try. Do everything you can to get off to a good start. In most cases you can breastfeed even though you have implants. If there were incisions around the areola, milk ducts and nerves may have been severed, and this could lessen your milk production or delivery, even though the severed ducts and nerves may eventually regenerate. So keep a careful eye on baby's diaper output and weight gain so that you can start supplements.

12

Funny (and Not So Funny) Things That Happen on the Way to the Breast

BREASTFEEDING IS MORE than just a way of getting nutrients into a baby. It's baby's first social relationship. Babies reveal much about their personalities when they breastfeed, and mother and baby both use this special time to bask in each other's presence and enjoy the trust and affection they share. Babies love to nurse. You can see this in the eagerness with which a one-month-old attacks the breast or in the smile that a four-month-old flashes as he stops nursing long enough to look up at mother. And then there's the satisfied grin on the face of a nursing toddler, whose demands to nurse have pulled mother away from the dirty dishes and gotten her to sit in the rocking chair and concentrate on just him. A baby's behavior at the breast changes as he or she matures. Each new stage of the breastfeeding relationship presents joys and challenges. Here's an overview of what you can expect as your baby grows.

BREASTFEEDING PERSONALITIES

Some babies gulp down their milk in five or ten minutes, and that's it—see you in three hours, Mom! Others breastfeed in leisurely fashion, savor

every mouthful, and it seems would nurse forever if only mother would sit still that long. Maybe your baby's breastfeeding style is something in between these two extremes, or maybe baby nurses one way in the morning but takes a different attitude in the late afternoon.

Your baby's nursing style will give you a clue to his or her temperament. We enjoy giving these different breastfeeding personalities names:

The Gourmet. He relishes everything about breastfeeding—the taste of the milk, the feel of mother's skin, every suck, every swallow. He licks, fondles, nestles, and goes to great lengths to prolong the experience. Just when you think he's done, he latches on for yet another after-dinner drink.

The Efficiency Expert. She gets right down to business. She can drain a breast in five minutes and finish the other side just as quickly. She has places to go and people to see—even if her vantage point is looking out of the baby sling. She doesn't miss much.

The Nip 'n' Napper. He alternates between eating and sleeping—sucking awhile, sleeping in mother's arms, rousing to nurse again, and then sleeping some more. Newborns often exhibit this sort of personality. If baby is gaining enough weight, there's no need to be concerned about this nursing style. Just put your feet up and enjoy the enforced leisure. If your doctor is concerned about your baby's weight gain (or if you just can't sit on the couch all day), you can encourage your baby to nurse actively for a longer stretch of time. Take him off the breast when he begins to drift off, sit him up, and burp him. When he's alert again, latch him on to the other side. Repeat the waking-up routine at least twice more so that baby sucks actively for fifteen or twenty minutes before you finally let him fall asleep.

Mr. Suck-a-Little, Look-a-Little. He is easily distracted. This on-and-off-the-breast behavior is typical of two- to four-month-olds, who can at this point see across the room. Newborns are nearsighted. Their eyes focus on mother's face while nursing, and the world beyond is a blur. But once babies can see well, they want to look at everything. When someone walks by, or even if they hear a voice or noise, they have to turn their heads and look. Sometimes they do this while still attached to the breast. (You'll be amazed at how far your nipple can stretch.) To get a good feeding into this baby, you may have to practice sheltered nursing, in which you take him into a darkened quiet room to breastfeed. When this isn't possible, nurse him in a baby sling, with the fabric pulled up over his head. This is an especially good strategy when you're nursing in public, since every time Mr. Suck-a-Little, Look-a-Little cranes his neck around, he leaves you exposed.

The Luxuriator. She loves to breastfeed so much that she often settles into a comfortable nursing position, as you would in an easy chair. She plays with your nipple, your hair, and

whatever else is within patting distance. While luxuriating, she may pause and gaze adoringly at your face and reward you with an appreciative smile, as if saying, "Thanks, Mom. I like being here."

NURSING NUISANCES

Not everything a baby does at the breast is interesting and delightful. In fact, some breastfeeding behaviors are downright annoying, and some hurt. Just as you shouldn't put up with sore nipples but should take action and fix what's causing them, you don't have to endure things about nursing that irritate you. Shaping your baby's behavior is part of your job as a parent. If he's doing something that bothers you, find a gentle way to change what's going on.

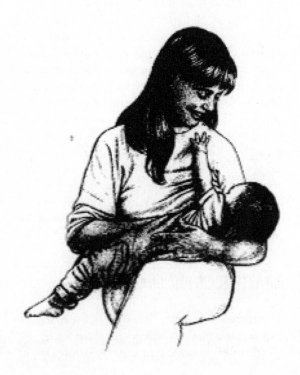

PLEASURABLE FEELINGS WHILE BREASTFEEDING

Breastfeeding is supposed to be pleasurable. That's how nature makes sure that babies will get fed. The oxytocin and prolactin released during breastfeeding make a woman feel relaxed, happy, and loving. These same hormones are released during sex, another activity needed for the human race to survive. Oxytocin is the orgasm hormone, and it is responsible for female erections of the clitoris and nipple. This hormone accounts for the increased skin temperature or "hot flash" some mothers experience while breastfeeding. It also contributes to the increased thirst.

Sometimes the physical sensations associated with breastfeeding can make a mother feel sexually aroused. This is more likely to happen as baby grows older, and it may worry some mothers. These feelings are perfectly normal. Their sudden appearance doesn't mean that something in your breastfeeding relationship has suddenly gone wrong. Your body is responding naturally to your baby's sucking.

Most of the time, the physical sensations of breastfeeding are translated by the mind into an overall sense of well-being or as great tenderness toward the baby. Mild sexual arousal is just another part of the spectrum of loving feelings supported by the hormones of breastfeeding. If this is part of your experience of breastfeeding, you might as well relax and enjoy it. If you feel irritated or restless, it's okay to end the feeding and nurse again later.

Biting, Teething, and Chomping

Many mothers nurse comfortably right through a whole set of teeth, but some babies do "bite the breast that feeds them." Talk of babies biting makes breastfeeding mothers wince, even mothers whose breastfeeding years are long in the past. But don't let the prospect of being bitten frighten you into weaning as soon as you see those pearly whites emerge from baby's gums. When baby is nursing correctly, even a full set of incisors, top and bottom, won't get in the way of comfortable breastfeeding for mom.

That doesn't mean you won't get bitten. Usually this happens by accident as baby is experimenting with these new tools in her mouth. Or maybe she chomps down because she is trying to make her gums feel better while teething. (As a prevention, firmly massage her gums with your finger before a feeding.) Some babies bite down as the breast slips out of their mouths when they fall asleep. Whatever the reason, mother's startled reaction is often enough to persuade baby not to try again.

When biting catches you unawares — as it does the first time it happens — you may have no control over your reaction. "Ouch!" you holler, and then you pry baby's jaws apart with your finger to get that tender piece of flesh back to safety. What you do once you've rescued your nipple depends on your baby's personality.

Some very sensitive babies will burst into tears at the sound of mother's shriek or at the look on her face. Mother's reaction is enough to persuade this little one never to bite again. Calm baby down, then offer the breast again to get her back into her usual "nursing is calming" groove. Reassurance is important for sensitive babies; we've heard of babies refusing to nurse again because they've been so startled.

Some babies will be puzzled by your reaction. In this case, you may want to end the feeding so that baby can learn that biting has consequences. Offer to nurse again in twenty or thirty minutes.

Instead of the yell-and-yank response to biting, as soon as you sense baby's teeth coming down, draw her in very close to your breast so she will automatically let go in order to open her mouth and uncover her nose to breathe. Or try another approach. If baby is in a biting phase, keep a finger in the corner of her mouth, ready to break the suction if you sense clamping. Another option is to place your finger on the cheek in the groove between the jaws and press inward when necessary. It should take her about a week to learn not to clamp down. For the older baby, try the "pull off and put down" technique. If baby bites, immediately disengage her from the breast and put her down, not in a punitive way but with enough firmness for her to make the connection between biting and being put down.

If your MER is delayed, baby may bite to express her impatience. She also may bite if you try to rush her to breastfeed when she's not ready, such as before you leave home. Biting happens often toward the end of a feeding, when baby is no longer actively sucking and swallowing. You can frequently prevent baby from sinking his teeth into your breast if you pay attention to his behavior during comfort sucking. A certain glint in the eye, a certain movement of his mouth will signal what's about to happen. You can intervene and end the feeding before someone—you!—gets hurt. Be ready to offer your baby something acceptable to chew or bite, such as a frozen teething ring or a toy that he loves to gum. If you are firm and consistent with your reactions to biting, it will be a short-lived problem.

Cluster Feedings

Your baby may have periods called cluster feedings or bunching, usually in the evening or night, when she wants to nurse constantly. These periods are usually followed by a three-hour sleep period. This is normal. While some babies nurse predictably every few hours, others like to cluster their feedings and nurse five or six times in a three- or four-hour period during the day or night with a long sleep period later. They receive more high-fat milk this way. Smart babies soon realize what nursing pattern to follow in order to thrive—and this pattern may change at different stages of development. Babies also learn the best time of the day to nurse the most (which may not always coincide with mom's favorite time). At night you're available, not distracted, and your milk-making hormones are going strong. Baby settles in to enjoy these environmental and biological perks.

Nursing Strike

Some babies abruptly refuse to take the breast. It's as if they're carrying a sign that says I'M ON STRIKE. They're not very happy about the situation, but nevertheless they refuse to nurse.

Imagine how mother feels: rejected, puzzled, and worried about how to get food into her baby. Nursing strikes can be very frustrating for the whole family. They can last two or three days, sometimes longer.

What do you do? Try to figure out why the baby is rejecting the breast. Is he in pain in any way, especially when lying in the nursing position? Does he have a cold? Is something hurting his mouth? Has baby been upset by a long separation from mother? Has something changed about the way you breastfeed? Has something changed about you (for example, your perfume, your deodorant, your clothing)? Has your family moved, had houseguests, or just gotten too busy? Has baby gotten too many bottles? Has your supply dropped? Are your menstrual cycles resuming? Did he get scared when you reacted to his biting you while he was nursing?

If you have some suspicion about what caused the nursing strike, you'll have some ideas about what needs fixing. But many times, mothers are unable to find the reason for the nursing strike. They manage to entice their babies back to the breast but never discover what the problem was.

Negotiating with a Striker

Your negotiating position in this "labor action" is that baby's loss of interest in breastfeeding is only temporary and you are willing to work with him so that he can be happy back on the job. A nursing strike is different from weaning. Weaning happens gradually, over many weeks or months, and a baby who is weaning himself from the breast is content with his situation. When baby's on strike, it's as if he has suddenly walked off the job with little warning, and he is not happy about being "out on the street."

So you put your best contract offer on the table. You woo baby back to the breast. Put aside other obligations for a few days and concentrate on your baby. Give him lots of skin-to-skin contact. Take baths together. Lie down and nap together, with baby's cheek cradled against your bare breast. A striking baby may be willing to accept the breast when sleepy, either when falling asleep or waking up. Wear your infant in a baby carrier much of the day and sleep with him at night. Re-create the atmosphere around breastfeeding that baby loves. Most babies, after a few days of comforting and reassurance, resume breastfeeding.

You should pump to relieve engorgement and maintain your milk supply during this trying time. Your milk can be given to your baby in a cup, with a spoon, a syringe, or a medicine dropper. Don't use bottles when you're trying to entice your baby to the breast, and don't use pacifiers, either. You want to encourage your baby to satisfy his sucking need at the breast, not with substitutes.

Nursing strikes are tough on mothers (tough on babies, too). It may feel as if your baby is rejecting you, but his apparent misery should make it clear to you that he wants to nurse but just can't for some unknown reason. This is a good time to call a breastfeeding support group leader or a friend who breastfeeds. You need someone to talk to who can help you puzzle out the cause of the nursing strike and support you while you're trying to get baby back to the breast.

If all your best efforts do not succeed in getting your striking baby back to the breast, it may be that baby has just plain decided to wean. (This rarely happens before nine months, so if your baby is younger, don't give up prematurely.) This may leave you feeling sad if you had hoped to nurse longer. Recognize your need to grieve a bit for the end of this stage in your life, but realize, too, that you are still your baby's mother and his world revolves around you. Many more exciting adventures are ahead for the two of you.

One-Sided Breastfeeding

Many babies have a favorite breast. It might be something about the shape of the nipple, or the milk may let down faster or slower on that side. There's no need to worry about this. Your breasts will adjust, even if baby decides he wants one side exclusively. Babies soon learn which breast works best, and they prefer that breast first. The breast that baby prefers will make more milk, and the other side will make less. This may leave you lopsided for a while, but you can live with this. Here are some suggestions to get baby to nurse more at the less preferred side:

- Begin each feeding and nurse frequently on the less favorite and often smaller breast. You may need to pump a few drops at first to entice the one-sided nursing baby onto the less preferred breast.

- If your milk-ejection reflex is very forceful on one side, less nursing at that breast may eventually reduce the supply, which will make the milk flow less overwhelming.

- If the milk doesn't flow as quickly at the less preferred breast, try stimulating your milk-ejection reflex with a pump before latching baby on. Or start the feeding on the preferred side and switch to the other side after you notice your milk-ejection reflex. Be sure baby empties the favored breast. This may be the one that stores the most milk and could be more prone to plugged ducts and infection.

- Sometimes ear infections, tight neck muscles, or other problems are more bothersome to a baby when he's lying on one side as opposed to the other. Try nursing in the cradle hold at the preferred breast, then sliding baby over to the other breast and nursing in the football hold (see chapter 2).

If baby still would rather hold out than switch to the less efficient breast, don't worry as long as baby is thriving on getting most of the needed milk from one breast. Just go with the flow, literally. Eventually, at least when you are finished nursing, your breasts will return to a more even size.

"No Bottles for Me! Nope, Not Me!"

Some breastfed babies refuse bottles. They know where milk is supposed to come from, and they refuse to settle for anything else. Some babies have even gone as long as twelve hours without eating. But you will both get through this, and it will become a nonissue at around nine months.

This presents challenges when mom goes back to work or needs to get away for more than the two or three hours her baby can go without a feeding. We've heard of grandmothers who just plain refuse to babysit for breastfed grandchildren for anything longer than ninety minutes.

Yes, we know—we told you to avoid giving your baby bottles and artificial nipples during the early weeks of breastfeeding. And yes, we know— other advisers said, "Get that baby used to bottles right from the start." We understand that you are probably blaming us and other breastfeeding "fanatics" for your dilemma, and you are promising yourself that you will do things differently the next time.

But remind yourself that if you'd given those early bottles, you might not even be breastfeeding at this point. The danger of early bottles is that you could end up with a nipple-confused, breast-refusing baby. This can be a very difficult problem to solve and can easily lead to weaning before a baby is even two weeks old. Not giving your baby bottles in the early weeks may make it more challenging to introduce the bottle later on, but this is a problem you can solve. Besides, your baby can also get milk from a cup or a spoon when you're gone, and once he has started solid foods, grandma can feed bananas and other goodies when she's in charge of filling baby's tummy.

For suggestions on getting a breastfed baby to take a bottle, see chapter 8.

The Gymnast

As babies learn to crawl and get around on their own, they stay in motion even while nursing. They wiggle, they twist, they kick. They nurse with their bottoms in the air. They surprise you by crawling over your shoulder to nurse at the breast hanging upside down.

This is cute—and irritating. Nipples were not meant to undergo 180-degree twists, nor were mothers meant to double as trampolines. As for nursing in public this way, forget it!

Here's how to control the gymnast and give baby a lesson in mealtime manners:

- *Try the toddler tuck.* With baby in the cradle hold, use your arm to wrap baby's legs around your body and keep them there.

- *Use the hook.* With baby in the cradle hold, put your free arm between his legs and grab him by the diaper. The squirmer's upper leg hooks over your arm. He'll feel more secure.

- *Nurse in a place that makes acrobatics more difficult.* The couch and your bed invite bouncing around. It's harder to climb and wriggle when mother is sitting in a narrow rocker.

- *Use reminders.* Use simple words in conjunction with these other strategies to remind your baby to lie still while nursing.

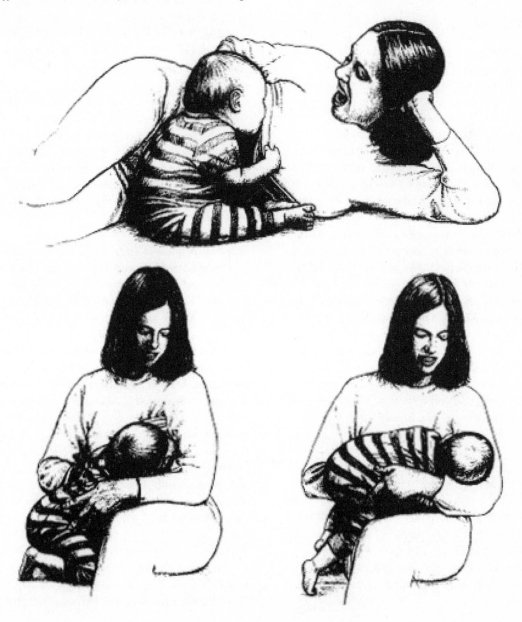

The Twiddler

Babies have at least one hand free while nursing. They'll find lots to do with it. They explore mom's face, mom's clothes, mom's skin under her clothes, and her hair. Sooner or later those little fingers find her other nipple and they begin to twiddle. This is more nipple stimulation than most mothers can handle. They grit their teeth, they take deep breaths, they end the feeding. Pulling on your lip or exploring the mole on your breast or midriff may be other ways your baby makes breastfeeding less than pleasurable for you.

The best solution for this problem is prevention. In the words of one veteran breastfeeding mother, "Hold that little hand when it starts to fumble around." Kiss it, stroke it, adore it, just don't let it go off on its own. Ending twiddling behavior once it takes hold is a matter of being firm, gentle, and consistent. You don't want breastfeeding to become a battleground, but you do want the twiddling to stop. Try holding baby's hand. If that doesn't work, offer a toy or something else for baby to explore with his fingers while he nurses. One mom put a Band-Aid over the nipple not being used. (Keeping the bra flap closed doesn't work, as you'll find out.) You may have to simply end the nursing session a few times (as you would with biting) until your baby understands that you will not tolerate a behavior that is annoying to you. Firmly and calmly let him know what your limits are.

LAUGHTER IS THE BEST BREASTFEEDING MEDICINE

One evening during a parenting seminar, we were asked what one needs in order to be a happy parent. We offered, "A sense of humor." Here are excerpts from our collection of breastfeeding stories:

During lovemaking, my nipples went off like sprinklers and got my husband right in the eye.

I was nursing while visiting friends in a college dorm room. There were a number of women sitting around talking. A male friend came to the doorway and joined in the conversation. Several minutes later, he suddenly realized what I was doing. He sputtered, "Uh, er, I'm, uh, sorry . . . I, uh, didn't mean, uh, to . . . I'll leave so I don't, er, embarrass you!" I wasn't the one who was embarrassed!

One night while nursing three-year-old Jason for what seemed like forever, I said, "Jason, when I count to five you will have to stop nursing." He immediately let go and said something I did not understand and latched on again like there was no tomorrow. I said, "What did you say?" He very quickly let go and said in a clear voice, "I said, count to twenty-one!"

When my two-and-a-half-year-old is about to nurse and sees my breasts, he exclaims, "Ho, ho!" He gets really excited. He often smacks his lips while nursing and says, "Yum, yum!" and then offers some to Ginger Cat. (No, she's not interested.)

My daughter Julie had always been a no-nonsense nurser: she got what she needed and then was off! I was envious of the other mothers as they talked about how their babies gazed at them with love as they nursed. Would that ever happen to me, I wondered? One evening, when Julie was almost two, I looked down, and there it was—that look! She was staring into my eyes, almost transfixed. Ah, this breastfeeding really pays off, I thought. With this, she pulled off and exclaimed, "Mommy, I can see the TV show in your glasses!"

When Bethany was about fifteen months old she was very verbal, and because of a lack of forethought on my part we didn't have a cute name for nursing. When she was tired or hungry she would just look at me and say, "Mamma, sit and nurse." We were visiting my father-in-law in the hospital, and Bethany became very tired, increasingly restless, and really needed to take a nap. We were saying our good-byes when a nurse came in to check my father-in-law's blood pressure and temperature. Bethany, who was becoming more insistent by the minute, grabbed my shirt and said, "Nurse, Mommy, nurse!" The nurse looked around and said, "Isn't that sweet! She knows I'm a nurse!" We just smiled and excused ourselves.

We were at a farm where kids (and parents) get to hold and play with many farm animals. When my daughter saw the great big mommy pig nursing a gazillion piglets at one time, she almost crawled right in to join them. She said quite loudly, "But Mommy, I've had your milk, cow's milk, goat's milk, and rice milk, but I've never tried pig's milk before!"

My husband and I own a dairy farm. Our first child weaned shortly before our second was born, and he was very verbal at that time. He also loved to spend time in the barn with Dad and the cows. So when I was nursing his little sister, he'd tell people that he drank Daddy's milk while Katie drank Mommy's milk!

"Mommy's moo: no sugar, no caffeine," quipped one of our little patients when we asked her why she liked nursing so much.

More wonderful than anything is how my daughter pets and strokes me during our feeding time together, as if to say, "I love you, thank you, and everything will be okay."

When my toddler was twenty months old, I had a very dear friend come stay with me along with her three-month-old. She sat down to nurse her very sweet and calm infant, and my little guy decided that he would like to nurse as well. My friend was curious. She had never seen a toddler nursing before. When he saw my exposed nipple, he dove in like he was in a pie-eating contest, and she gasped. Once well attached, he continued to climb on my lap until he was standing on my legs and bent over at the waist. She said, "Surely he's not still nursing," and just then he thrust both arms out airplane style — while still nursing, of course! We all had a good laugh, including my guy, who stopped nursing just long enough to participate in the fun!

In the 1980s, when the US government decided to promote breastfeeding, a Senate subcommittee asked a California lactation consultant to advise them on why breastfeeding was so important. The chairman opened the meeting by saying, "Please tell us why breastfeeding is so important. After all, I was bottle fed, and I'm a senator." The lactation consultant replied, "Senator, if you had been breastfed, you might be president."

13

Toddler Nursing and Natural Weaning

MAYBE YOU PLANNED to nurse for six months. Maybe you planned to nurse for as long as a year. And here you are, nursing a child of ten months, twelve months, fourteen months who shows no sign of losing interest in the breast. You can't imagine weaning him—how will you get him to sleep at night?—but you and your husband are starting to wonder, How long is this child going to breastfeed?

THE BIG PICTURE, OR WHY EXTENDED BREASTFEEDING IS BECOMING MORE COMMON

In 2012, the American Academy of Pediatrics released a statement that recommended breastfeeding "until at least twelve months of age, and continuation of breastfeeding for as long as mutually desired by mother and baby." This statement not only affirms the importance of breastfeeding for a baby's entire first year but also reminds parents and pediatricians alike that breastfeeding can continue for much longer and that baby and mother both play a part in the weaning process.

However, extended nursing is relatively rare in the United States, Canada, and other Western nations. One of the challenges of nursing a toddler is that you become aware that your attitude about breastfeeding and weaning is a little bit different from other families'. Unless you're hanging out with like-minded moms, you may not know anyone who is nursing a child as old as yours. Meanwhile, there are people in your life who think you're a little strange (or worse) and don't hesitate to tell you so.

While mothers who nurse children of one and two and three may be out of step with the prevailing parenting culture, it's really the culture that is out of step with the needs of growing humans. A look beyond Western culture reveals that in many human societies, children are nursed until they are three years old or more. The World Health Organization recommends at least two years of breastfeeding for babies around the world.

Children in the second and third year of life are still very dependent, and modern psychological research confirms the importance of filling these dependency needs rather than pushing a child to become more independent. Babies and toddlers with a secure attachment to their mothers actually grow to be more independent, separate more easily from their mothers when they are older, have better relationships with teachers and peers, and are easier to discipline.

Extended breastfeeding seems to be nature's way of assuring that baby's needs for emotional closeness and dependency on other human beings get met. Humans thrive when they get along with one another, and this requires trust and mutual sensitivity, skills in human relations that can be learned even at the age of one or two while breastfeeding. Yes, your child may seem clingy or very mom centered at the moment, but your acceptance of this behavior in a toddler or a preschooler will produce a trusting relationship with your child that will make family life easier for many years to come.

THE BREASTFEEDING YEARS

We have a sign in our office that says EARLY WEANING NOT RECOMMENDED FOR BABIES. While there may certainly be circumstances beyond a mother's control that may lead to weaning before a baby's first birthday, we urge mothers to think in terms of years, not months, when they are contemplating how long to nurse.

The occasional baby will be ready to wean before a year, but this is unusual. If a baby who has been exclusively or almost exclusively breastfed suddenly indicates a lack of interest in the breast, this is more likely a nursing strike than true self-weaning (see chapter 12). When you breastfeed frequently in response to your baby's cues, and your baby nurses regularly for comfort as well as for nutrition, you may well find yourself nursing a child who walks—and even talks. In our parenting career, we have enjoyed this wonderful continuum immensely. Extended breastfeeding has shaped us as parents and our children as "little nursing persons" in ways we could measure as each birthday slipped by.

In our pediatrics practice, we are now enjoying the privilege of seeing teens who as infants were not weaned before their time. One quality stands out—sensitivity. These are kids who care. Attachment-parented young men and women are able to get behind the eyes of others (they practice empathy) and think through what they're about to do (they are more considerate and less impulsive).

WHY TODDLERS BREASTFEED

If you are currently breastfeeding a baby who is turning into a crawling-walking-climbing toddler, you probably understand very well why he continues to nurse. His eagerness as he settles in to nurse and his contentment when he's done say it all: breastfeeding makes him feel good. But if you are reading this when your baby is still quite young, or if you are having doubts about the wisdom of continued nursing, consider these advantages of breastfeeding for toddlers:

A balanced diet. Even for babies past their first birthday, human milk provides significant nutrition. While nursing toddlers eat other foods, human milk rounds out their diet, providing protein, fat, energy, and lots of vitamins and minerals. You worry less about what your toddler is eating or not eating when you know that he is still receiving your milk.

Immunities. Levels of immune-boosting ingredients in mother's milk actually increase during the second year of breastfeeding. So even if baby is taking less of your milk than he did as a six-month-old who was totally dependent on the breast, he is still getting lots of the good things that protect him from tummy upsets, ear infections, and other medical problems big and small.

Illness. When a breastfed toddler does get sick, mothers find that they really appreciate being able to comfort the child at the breast. A child who is under the weather may nurse much more frequently than usual while refusing other foods and liquids. As long as he is nursing, he will not get dehydrated.

Comfort. Sucking continues to be an important way for baby to settle himself when stress, fears, or

THE NATURAL AGE FOR WEANING

What anthropologists call culture has a huge influence in determining how human babies are cared for and how long they are breastfed. But if you could remove the cultural influences, how long would babies breastfeed?

Dr. Katherine Dettwyler, an anthropologist and a nursing mother, has explored this subject extensively. By looking at breastfeeding behavior in primates—humans' closest relatives in the animal world—she has brought an interesting perspective to discussions of a natural weaning age for humans:

- Large mammals, including primates, typically wean when the offspring has quadrupled its birth weight. In humans, this would be around the age of two and a half.

- Other studies suggest that large mammals wean when offspring attain one-third of their adult weight. In humans, this would place weaning between the ages of four and seven years.

- In some animals, the period of lactation is approximately equal to the length of gestation (pregnancy), but Dettwyler reports that in gorillas and chimpanzees, the period of lactation is six times the length of gestation. Apply that formula to humans and you get a weaning age of four and a half.

- Many primates wean when the young get their first permanent molars. In humans, this happens between the age of five and a half and six.

Of course, we're not animals, and we have many resources available for feeding, nurturing, and protecting our young that are not available to gorillas. But the same complex society that provides medical care and a steady food supply sometimes makes it more difficult to understand basic human needs.

There's no single "right" weaning age. You need to do what works for your child and in your family, but you can use Dr. Dettwyler's perspectives on weaning for guidance beyond what everyone else does or even what your doctor suggests.

tiredness threaten to overwhelm his emotional resources. Lots of one-year-olds in the United States walk around with pacifiers in their mouths. How lucky your baby is to do his comfort sucking at the breast, which has a comforting person attached to it.

Security. Toddlers are beginning to explore their world, and the pattern of exploration is this: they venture out, they try new things, and then they return to their secure home base, mother, to affirm their discoveries and to renew their courage. And when they return to mother, what

better way than nursing to feel secure in her presence?

The baby inside. Others may see your child turning into a regular kid with a will of his own and his own daily agenda. A breastfeeding mother still sees the baby inside, the little person behind the child who can cope with independence some of the time, but not all of the time. A toddler is a little person with big needs, and you have to nurture those needs if he is to grow into a big person with manageable needs.

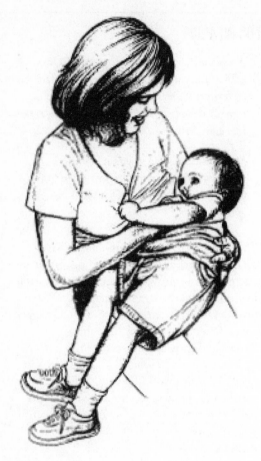

Toddler nursing

WHY MOTHERS CONTINUE TO BREASTFEED

Hasn't mother put in enough nursing time by the time her child arrives at his first birthday? Actually, there are advantages for mothers who nurse toddlers. Whereas once you thought of breastfeeding as primarily a form of nutrition, you now use it as an indispensable mothering tool. Here are the uses to which you'll put extended breastfeeding:

Comforting tool. Toddlers are known for their sometimes tempestuous tempers. Life has its ups

and downs and its bumps when you're learning to get around on your own. A few minutes of nursing can patch up many of the hurts and setbacks a toddler encounters daily. Since one-year-olds don't have much in the way of language skills (nor do two-year-olds when they're upset), mothers appreciate nonverbal means of dealing with difficulties. Breastfeeding is a quick and easy way to fix bumps and scrapes and soothe frustrations.

A chance to relax. Mothers of toddlers are on their feet much of the day, chasing children, getting to the teetering lamp before it hits the floor, keeping eighteen-month-old humans away from the dog's food bowl. If you can catch that child and nurse him, you get to sit down for a while, maybe even doze off, knowing that your intrepid little explorer is also headed for dreamland.

Bedtime enforcer. Think of your breasts as the ultimate secret weapon when it comes to getting your child to sleep at night or at nap time. The toddler who is wound up and "too tired to sleep" will usually consent to nurse. When he lets his guard down at the breast, sleep sneaks up and overtakes him. Mom's breasts win again!

A peacekeeping strategy. If you find yourself constantly saying no to your toddler, or if your two-year-old is constantly saying no to you, you'll appreciate nursing as a "demilitarized zone," a place to put conflicts aside and reconnect.

Health booster. The degree to which breastfeeding protects a woman against breast cancer and other diseases depends on how long she nurses. One study showed that women who had breastfed for twenty-five months or more in their lifetimes were one-third less likely to develop breast cancer than women who had given birth but never breastfed. Most women can also enjoy longer periods of infertility when they plan to nurse past a year. (See "Breastfeeding and Fertility," page 72.)

A special time. Life moves at a faster pace as children grow. Breastfeeding ensures that you still take time to give your little one your full attention several times a day. This one-on-one time is especially important when your little one must compete with older siblings for your attention. Any fears that you may be shortchanging the child at the end of the family parade can be alleviated by the special time you share while nursing.

THE CHALLENGES OF NURSING A TODDLER

From the time a baby achieves mobility — whether crawling, cruising, or walking — until age two and a half is the single most exhausting stage of parenthood. Your baby grows and changes so much during this time that it's hard to keep up, literally and figuratively. Breastfeeding behavior changes as your baby grows. The child who is nursing many times a day at the end of his first year will not be nursing nearly as often (if at all) at age two. Some mothers have told us, however, that around the age of two their babies increased the amount of nursing time for a few months, then dropped back to less than before, as though the stress of being two threw them into a temporary high-need period. We had this experience with two of our toddlers. Try not to compare one child's needs with another's. As with other developing behaviors, your job is to steer your child along the path that leads to maturity while allowing him to move at the pace most comfortable for him.

> ## TODDLER TALK
>
> As your nursing baby nears her first birthday, pay some attention to the words you and your partner use to refer to breastfeeding. Make sure that what she hears is something you can live with when she begins talking. "Booby, booby!" might be cute at home but embarrassing at the grocery store. If you don't want others to know that your two-year-old chatterbox is still breastfeeding, encourage her to use a code word. Often parents pick up the baby's own babbling term for nursing: *ma* or *nummies* or even *side* (as in *other side*).

Nursing tip: *Wean gradually.* In one sense, extended breastfeeding is really a very long period of weaning. Weaning begins when your baby starts to get nourishment from sources other than breast milk. Weaning is completed when the child no longer nurses at all. So when someone asks, "When are you going to wean that baby?" you can truthfully answer, "Oh, we've started weaning," even if that means your baby has had only a few bites of banana.

Dependency

During the toddler and preschooler years, children gradually learn to be more independent, but they do this at their own pace. They can't be hurried. Sometimes it seems that continuing to nurse keeps a child dependent on mother. "Wean her," say the critics, "so she won't be so clingy. You're spoiling her."

These advisers have things backward. Sensitive attention is not what "spoils" children. Spoiling is what happens to fruit that is left in the back of the refrigerator neglected. The same holds for children. If you fill the need, it will eventually go away. Neglecting the need will produce a mess — if not now, then later in the child's life. *Spoiling* is also the word we have for giving a child too much of what she wants but doesn't need. Giving a child too many things instead of giving of ourselves and even giving too much help instead of teaching her how she can manage some of her own needs are other ways to spoil a child.

So how can you tell if your child still needs to be nursing?

Generally, her desire to continue nursing is a sign that a child has needs that are still being met at the breast. It is usually that simple. At some point, however, you will find out (and so will she) that something else can also meet that need.

Just a Habit?

Breastfeeding toddlers and preschoolers often have regular times when they nurse—bedtime, nap time, when they awaken—or they may "pounce" whenever mother happens to sit down for a few minutes. Do they really need to nurse at these times, or is this a habit they have gotten into? Sometimes older toddlers will nurse out of boredom or because this is the one way they know they can get mother's attention.

How do you know if nursing has become a habit for your child, at least at certain times or in certain settings? Try distracting him from nursing at these times. Offer alternatives: a story, a back rub at bedtime, a trip to the park. If he stays happy with the alternative activity, you know that he was ready to give up that nursing time. If he becomes fussy or clingy, his need to nurse may be stronger than you thought. Wait a month or six weeks before trying again to offer alternatives.

Your Feelings

There are two people involved in extended nursing. Your feelings count, too. An important lesson children learn at the breast as they grow older is that mothers have feelings, too, and they sometimes have to change their behavior to accommodate mom. If you're not happy with something about breastfeeding, change it. If your toddler wants to climb all over the couch while attached to your nipple, you can tell her that this hurts you and remind her that "we lie still when we nurse." Or you can help a two-year-old learn the difference between private and public, if you're no longer comfortable nursing her at the mall.

Mothers of toddlers often feel drained at the end of the day, physically and emotionally. Sometimes all the closeness that goes along with breastfeeding becomes too much to handle. At this point, you may begin to resent nursing—and even your child. It's time to take some action and gain a sense of control over the situation. This might mean developing creative alternatives to nursing, at least part of the time. It might mean setting some limits on your child's nursing ("You can nurse for as long as it takes to sing the ABC song"), but be sure the child is able to understand and accept, at least somewhat, the limits you set. You need to have some time to yourself every day; perhaps dad can take over for a while when he gets home from work and you can go out for a walk or take a long soak in the bathtub.

If you're feeling resentful of nursing, look at your alternatives. This may be a good time for you to take the lead in weaning and step up your effort to provide loving activities that will substitute for breastfeeding. On the other hand, as you think about it, you may decide that although nursing isn't easy, you prefer continued breastfeeding to launching an all-out effort to wean. Just making a decision to do one or the other may leave you feeling more in control of the situation than letting the nurse-or-wean debate continue to rage in your brain.

Mothering Your Nursing Toddler by Norma Jane Bumgarner is a wise and insightful guide for anyone who is interested in extended breastfeeding. Another title is *Breastfeeding Older Children* by Ann Sinnott. There are also books written for the nursing toddlers. Many breastfeeding support groups sponsor meetings just for mothers of nursing toddlers. Talking with other mothers about breastfeeding growing children is often the best way to deal with doubts and resentments.

WEANING AT MOTHER'S PACE

While we advocate natural weaning, in which a mother follows her child's cues about his readiness to wean, we know that is not always possible and that some mothers will choose to breastfeed for a shorter period of time. Here, then, are some guidelines for weaning on mother's schedule.

What to substitute. If you are weaning a baby who is less than a year old, you will need to give bottles to replace breastfeedings because your baby still has a strong need to suck. Check with your doctor for a recommendation on what to put in the bottles. If your baby is older than six months, you can replace some breastfeedings with solid food. If you are weaning a toddler, you'll be substituting other kinds of "nursing" for breastfeedings — that is, other ways of spending nurturing time with your child.

Wean gradually. Stopping breastfeeding cold turkey is not good for baby or mother. Mother is likely to experience engorgement, plugged ducts, and a possible breast infection. Baby is likely to become very distressed. Instead, start with the least favored feeding and offer a substitute at that time. After a few days or a week, offer a substitute for another feeding. Gradually, you will cut out the breastfeeding and replace it with bottle feedings, solid-food feedings, or nurturing activities. Favorite feedings, such as those that take place at bedtime, nap time, or early morning, will be the last ones to go. Don't be in a rush to give up these treasured times.

Watch your baby. Fussiness, clinginess, anger, sadness, and tantrums are signs that weaning is going too quickly. Slow the process down, and be sure your child is getting lots of attention from you at the times when you are not offering the breast. If your child comes down with a cold or a tummy upset, he may want to nurse more often until he feels better. Be prepared for regressions, taking two steps forward and then one step back. Remember that you are helping your child into a new stage, not forcing him to do what you want.

Don't wean by desertion. Many a well-meaning grandma has suggested that dad and mom get away together for the weekend or for an entire week, leave the baby with her, and voilà! — he'll be weaned. Being deprived of mother at the same time he's deprived of breastfeeding is too much for a little one to handle. Weaning by desertion is traumatic.

Abrupt weaning. Sometimes in emergencies babies must be weaned quickly. Figure out how much time you have to wean, and space out the substituting of bottles for the breast over that time. You may need assistance from an experienced bottle feeder, since breastfed babies often refuse to take bottles from their mothers. When your breasts feel full, express some milk. Generally only pump enough to relieve the pressure. But for the first few days, pump until you're empty at bedtime so you can sleep comfortably and lessen the chance of contracting a breast infection. Offer baby lots of emotional support. If mother or father can't be with the baby during this time, choose a substitute caregiver who is patient, calm, and sympathetic to baby's distress.

THE JOURNEY TO WEANING

When your baby is nursing six or seven times a day at his first birthday, it may be hard to envision the day when he won't nurse. But gradually other activities and other kinds of closeness will take the place of nursing. You set the stage for weaning as you help your child try new experiences. Reading stories together, playing cuddling and tickling games, singing songs, enjoying outings, and building with blocks are all ways that your child can enjoy being with you. As the need for sucking wanes and the need for other kinds of stimulation increases, children really do move on to other interests. You can't push your child into new activities, but you can be ready and watchful and provide them when they are needed. And weaning does mean more work for you—it's harder to offer that alternative ("Let's walk to the park" or "Let's get out the puzzles") than it is just to sit down and nurse. If you are always tired, it's tempting to opt for what's easy, so be sure you are getting enough rest. And it helps to have a plan and some options.

Don't Offer, Don't Refuse

This time-honored method of weaning works well for many mothers. When a child asks to nurse, you agree, but you don't go out of your way to remind her to nurse. You might even avoid giving her cues that suggest it's time to nurse. You avoid sitting in the rocking chair unless it's bedtime or nap time. You get out of bed before your toddler wakes up and wants to nurse in the morning. When you are on the phone, keep it short and don't sit down.

"Don't offer, don't refuse" isn't a hard-and-fast rule. There will be times when your child is stressed or not feeling well, and offering to nurse her may seem like the best remedy. And there may be times when you refuse or ask her to wait until you're done with the dishes or until you get home from grandma's, for example.

When Weaning Is a Struggle

If you and your toddler or preschooler are locked in conflict over nursing (you want her to nurse less, she wants to nurse more), back off for a while. Sometimes trying to get a child to nurse less makes her want to nurse more to reassure herself that mommy is still available to help her with her feelings and needs. If you let up on the pressure to wean, you may well find that after a few weeks she will cut back on her nursing. You'll both be a lot happier.

My baby used to use his free hand while nursing to play with my bra strap. To help him wean, I cut the bra straps off and sewed them onto his favorite teddy bear.

Going to Sleep Without Nursing

You may wonder if your child is ever going to be able to go to sleep without nursing. Because the breast works so well, parents depend on this as the final "knock-out punch." You have to teach your child to associate other pleasant activities with going to sleep. You can begin to do this even when he is a baby. Mom nurses baby and then hands him off to dad for some final walking and patting and cuddling before he falls asleep. As your child approaches his first birthday, develop a bedtime routine that includes more than nursing to sleep: quiet play on the rug, a bath, a snack, toothbrushing, a story, a back rub, and then nursing. If he's truly tired at bedtime, he'll become drowsy and relaxed before he gets a chance to nurse.

NURSING DURING PREGNANCY

You're pregnant again and you're still nursing. Does this mean you must wean? No, not usually. You can nurse an older baby or toddler while pregnant and even go on to nurse two children ("tandem nursing") after the birth. However, nursing while pregnant does present challenges, and some mothers decide to help their older children wean before a sibling is born.

The medical question. Many obstetricians caution mothers about breastfeeding during pregnancy. Breastfeeding stimulates the secretion of oxytocin into your bloodstream, and this hormone also creates contractions in your uterus. New insights, however, show that oxytocin receptors in the uterus are not activated until the twenty-fourth week of pregnancy. With careful medical monitoring, most mothers can safely breastfeed during the first half of their pregnancies. At that point, if you are at risk for preterm labor, your doctor may advise that there be no nipple stimulation whatsoever (no uterine contractions caused by sexual excitement, either). If you have a history of previous late miscarriages (after twenty weeks) or are noticing strong contractions during breastfeeding, it is wise to stop nursing at this point. If you don't have any particular reason to believe that you are at risk for preterm labor, you can continue to breastfeed throughout your pregnancy with no worries about the safety of the new baby. The wisest course is to check with your doctor about whether it is safe for you to breastfeed.

What's happening in your body. The hormones of pregnancy overrule your lactation hormones sometime during the second trimester. The milk gradually changes to colostrum, and your milk supply decreases. Some toddlers report that the milk tastes different or that the milk is "all gone." This can be frustrating for a little one. Some wean as a result, while others keep nursing, never missing a beat and denying that anything about mother's breast has changed. If your nursing baby is still quite young when you become pregnant and is totally or heavily dependent on breast milk for nutrition, he may need extra nutrition when your milk supply decreases. You may have to encourage him to eat more solid food, or you may have to consider formula supplements.

Nipples become tender during pregnancy, which can make nursing sessions uncomfortable. It may be awkward to hold your toddler at the breast as your belly grows bigger, and you may find his squirming bothers you. Explain to your child that your nipples hurt, and tell him how you want him to nurse. Limiting nursing time may make feedings more bearable. Anticipate some tears as your child struggles to accept your limits. It will be easier for him if he sees that you are not anxious. Use relaxation breathing from your childbirth classes or try to think about something else if this makes nursing more comfortable for you. You can limit the time your toddler spends sucking and entice him into accepting nonbreastfeeding ways of being comforted. This might be reading stories, or it might be falling asleep with his cheek against your breast.

Some mothers feel very restless while nursing during pregnancy, or they begin to resent breastfeeding. It's as if their minds as well as their bodies are pushing one child aside to make room for the next. These are common feelings, and they strike even mothers who

NURSING DURING PREGNANCY (continued)

thought they were very committed to continuing to breastfeed during pregnancy. Heed these feelings and make some adjustments. It may be time to wean, time to put some limits on nursing, or time to rethink your own priorities.

Nursing siblings. If you still enjoy breastfeeding, one of the best ways to lessen sibling rivalry is to not wean the older child before her time. When breastfeeding during pregnancy, you have the needs of three people to consider: the baby soon to be born, the soon-to-be-older sibling, and yourself. Your toddler's emotional needs may be telling you to avoid weaning her before her time, while you may be struggling with continuing to satisfy her needs at the breast. This is quite normal. Some mothers persist despite these negative feelings, knowing how important nursing is to their children, although they may set some limits on the length of feedings or on night nursings. If you're beginning to feel increasingly drained (physically, emotionally, and perhaps nutritionally), then it's time to find other ways to meet your toddler's needs, with the help of dad. Some toddlers increase their frequency of nursing and overall demands on their pregnant mothers because they sense something is different. Others wean toward the end of the pregnancy because of the change in the milk. Our daughter Hayden, a high-need nursing four-year-old, exclaimed toward the end of

Martha's pregnancy with her sibling, "Mommy, I don't like your milk anymore. I'll wait until after the baby comes, when it's good again." (She waited, she tasted, and she went back to nursing, but very infrequently and not for long.)

Older nurslings are thrilled to discover that new babies also bring new milk. The bountiful milk supply combined with the presence of a tiny intruder at mom's breast often produces a child who suddenly wants to nurse a lot. Don't let this panic you. This stage will pass in a few days or weeks, and your older nursling will go back to something like his previous breastfeeding pattern. In the first few days, make sure the new baby has plenty of opportunities to get colostrum. Once your milk comes in, you will have enough for two.

When you're holding a tiny newborn in your arms, your older child will suddenly look much bigger to you. You may feel irritated by his need to nurse, especially if he's nursing more often, and you may feel quite protective of your little one. These are natural feelings, part of growing attached to your baby, but they may surprise you. Try to see the situation from the eyes of your older nursling, who may want to be a baby himself again. The arrival of a sibling brings complications, and you all need time to adjust. Remember, the word *nursing* implies not only breastfeeding but comforting, too. And here's one area where dad can take over a lot.

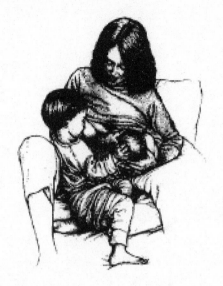

Tandem nursing

Night Weaning

The advice to never refuse a request to breastfeed is unrealistic, especially for an exhausted mother who wishes to night wean. Often, when we counsel exhausted parents on night weaning, we open our dialogue with, "Just say no." Initially, these breastfeeding-at-all-cost parents look as if they've heard a foreign language, and then we see a feeling of relief on their faces. A clue that you need to make some changes in night feedings is when you begin resenting going to bed because it's work rather than rest. It's okay to put limits on your toddler's night nursing, such as, "We only nurse when Mr. Sun goes down and when Mr. Sun comes up." You are not a bad mother if you say no to your baby.

Father's Role

Dad's role in baby's life gets more exciting during toddlerhood. As playing with dad becomes a bigger part of baby's life, nursing will become less important. Many fathers begin to take over bedtime routines as children grow. Mother may still provide the final nursing, but dad does the bath and the story. Eventually the child may fall asleep without needing to nurse, depending on how adept dad is at "father nursing," which could include watching a lulling video together or dad telling a long, unstimulating story.

WEANED AT LAST

Weaning is not a negative term, nor is it something you do *to* a child. Weaning is a passage, from one kind of relationship with mother to another. In Scripture, the Hebrew word for wean is *gamal,* meaning "to ripen." A child who is weaned before his time will neither be as ready for independence nor as well equipped to enter the next stage of development as a child who weans himself. A child who weans when he is ready will be at peace with his progress toward being more grown-up. The Old Testament's book of Psalms contains an evocative reference to weaning: "I have stilled my soul, hushed it like a weaned child. Like a weaned child on its mother's lap, so is my soul within me" (Ps. 131:2). There's a sense of peace and tranquillity in this description.

You might want to mark your child's weaning with a special family celebration: a party, an outing, a gift. Help your child truly appreciate what it means to be bigger and able to do lots more things on her own.

You may feel a tinge of sadness when your child finally weans. You can attribute some of this to shifting hormones, although with gradual weaning, the physical effect on mother is minimal. Most of what you're feeling is the passage of time; your baby is no longer a baby, and you are getting older. This is one of many such bittersweet passages you will experience with your child, and along with pride and happiness, you may feel a tear or two welling up in your eye and a lump in your throat. It's all part of being a mother.

Index

Page numbers of illustrations appear in italics.